"The generosity of knowledge, spirit and empathy is and has been deeply touching to me. As someone who has experienced postpartum depression and 'activity' after all three of my children's births. I can say from direct experience that Karen Kleiman walks her talk and offers profound space holding for the scary, overwhelming and terrifying parts of postpartum. As well as space holding for the possibilities available and the needs buried within the vulnerability of postpartum.

This empathy in the form of masterful space holding is the antidote to the abyss of pain and challenge that lies within the vulnerable postpartum time. The information in this book supports the healing of the strange and lonely and disorienting space of postpartum vulnerability.

Having experienced, three times, the perfect storm of hormonal, emotional, trauma triggering, cultural, circumstantial, social, physical challenge... I have had the privilege of being supported by Karen in the way that is described very eloquently and astutely in this book. To say Karen Kleiman helped me through a tough period post-birth is an understatement. I would go as far as to say she helped save my life.

And while Karen may quietly laugh at the passion of my appreciation for her, I am very clear: Karen's wisdom, knowledge, empathy, vision, insight, experience and humor helped me return to who I know myself to be during a time where all seemed lost and stuck in the tar and molasses of postpartum depression, anxiety and invasive/intrusive thoughts. One investigation at a time. With a kind of space holding that instantly heals and reconnects.

My gratitude for Karen Kleiman and her powerful work knows no bounds.

I wish for the emotional, somatic and holistic intelligence of Karen Kleiman to be available to every single birthing person who finds themself at a loss on every level during the postpartum period."

Alanis Morissette

The Art of Holding in Therapy

Written by a pioneer in the field, this second edition provides updated skill-building tools and a more developed, comprehensive understanding of how therapists can use the holding approach when treating perinatal distress.

First conceptualized by D.W. Winnicott, the "holding" approach refers to a therapist's capacity to respond to postpartum distress in a way that facilitates an immediate and successful therapeutic alliance. This model has continued to advance, and this newly updated edition will help readers learn how to contain high levels of agitation, fear, and panic in a way that cultivates trust and the early stages of connectedness. Filled with vignettes throughout, this book includes chapters on what holding is, how to prepare using this model, the emotions specific to postpartum mothers, the essential holding elements, and the practice of holding. This book uniquely addresses the needs of therapists who may find themselves confronting, struggling with, or recovering from their own reproductively related journeys, with chapters discussing the professional's identity, clinical challenges, and a new chapter on cultural humility.

This book is essential reading for all of those in the perinatal mental health community, such as therapists, social workers, and clinicians.

Karen Kleiman, MSW, LCSW, is a licensed clinical social worker and internationally recognized expert on maternal mental health. With over three decades of experience in the field, she is the author of several books on postpartum depression and anxiety and is the founder of The Postpartum Stress Center and The Karen Kleiman Training Center.

Hilary Waller, MS, LPC, is a psychotherapist in private practice and provides training to perinatal providers and women and their families.

The Art of Holding in Therapy

An Essential Intervention for
Postpartum Depression and Anxiety

Second Edition

Karen Kleiman
with Hilary Waller

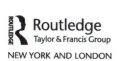
Routledge
Taylor & Francis Group

NEW YORK AND LONDON

Designed cover image: © Westend61 / Getty Images

Second edition published 2025
by Routledge
605 Third Avenue, New York, NY 10158

and by Routledge
4 Park Square, Milton Park, Abingdon, Oxon, OX14 4RN

Routledge is an imprint of the Taylor & Francis Group, an informa business

First edition published by Routledge 2017

ISBN: 978-1-032-51421-5 (hbk)
ISBN: 978-1-032-51420-8 (pbk)
ISBN: 978-1-003-40214-5 (ebk)

DOI: 10.4324/9781003402145

Typeset in Sabon
by SPi Technologies India Pvt Ltd (Straive)

Contents

Foreword

Maternal mental health disorders are known as the most prevalent significant complication of pregnancy and the postpartum period. Depression and anxiety are common manifestations, with prevalence rates up to almost 20% during pregnancy and the postpartum period. As research and public awareness gains momentum, more attention is being placed on medical protocols, interventions, and better access to treatment.

For many years now, Karen Kleiman has changed the face of maternal mental health for both clinicians and families. As a speaker reaching many through outlets such as The Oprah Winfrey Show and as an author, through her many books for families and clinicians, Karen is a pioneer in this field providing the mainstream community with an understanding of this devastating illness, validating the women who suffered and helping clinicians gain insight into the experience of postpartum depression.

Karen and I first spoke several years ago when I called her out of the blue to brainstorm solutions. I, as an advocate in maternal metal health policy and systems change was combing the landscape to learn *why* women weren't being screened, diagnosed, and treated routinely by their physicians. I knew that Karen had developed one of the only training programs for clinicians in the US at the time.

After speaking, Karen and I knew that more providers needed to be expertly trained so we could reach more women, augment recovery, and improve outcomes. Since then my organization, The Policy Center for Maternal Mental Health, along with Postpartum Support International has launched web-based training to easily reach clinicians all over the US and meet a growing demand to learn about this field. Though we have a long way to go, training is now available to more people than ever, and Karen's intensive postgraduate training program at The Postpartum Stress Center continues to produce expert clinicians and is recognized as a best-in-class training.

Recently the United States Preventive Services Task Force, the American College of Obstetrics and Gynecology, and the Council on Patient Safety in Women's Health Care joined in this mission and have highlighted the importance of screening and proper treatment of maternal depression. It is now more important than ever that we train providers.

Therapists in this highly specialized field often turn to Karen's books for guidance when working with the perinatal population. *The Art of Holding in Therapy: An Essential Intervention* introduces a novel strategy for treating women with postpartum depression and anxiety. At a time when we are finally paying attention to this widespread crisis in maternal mental health, this book provides a hands-on resource for therapists who are dedicated to making a difference in the lives of women seeking their help.

Clinicians, we need you now more than ever; moms and families are counting on you. Karen Kleiman, thank you for your extraordinary contributions to the field – without your work we would be several steps behind.

Joy Burkhard, MBA
Founder and Director
Policy Center for Maternal Mental Health

Preface

My clients have gotten so much younger.

Not so long ago we were all the same age. We were comrades in parallel worlds, raising our babies together, in a manner of speaking, navigating the ebbs and flows of new motherhood. I would observe through a therapeutic lens, and later reflect on the relevance to my own naive mothering experience. In the blink of an eye, my children turned into adults while my clients all seemed to stay the same age. One after the other, pregnant and postpartum women greeted me with tender tales of pain and loss. As years passed, young women continued to share stories of private anguish as I quietly aged in the background.

Today, clients tell me they worry that I will retire soon and abandon them. Or, not return from a vacation. Or, get sick and frail, or die. My clients never fail to remind me how old I am getting, how long I have been doing this work and the pièce de résistance – *how much older I am than their own mothers*. I take it all in stride, because, well, I am a resilient, thick-skinned professional.

Most of the time.

I am, at the very least, my best grown-up self when I sit with my clients.

Truth be told, I *have* been doing this a long time. I have reached the age where my peers and colleagues are retiring. Often a client mentions that her mother-in-law is way too old to help with the baby, though she is younger than I am. Or, she says her boss doesn't understand her because he's old so doesn't have any perspective. Turns out he is a decade younger than I.

The honored cliché is true, with age comes wisdom, and for many reasons, I feel more at ease with my work at this point in time than ever. I can sit with a postpartum woman in distress and know, for certain, that she will leave our session feeling better than she did when she came in. There is nothing mysterious about that. It comes with study, practice, the passage of time, and countless missteps.

The art of holding a postpartum woman in distress comes naturally to me. I suspect the same can be said by many therapists who specialize in the treatment of perinatal distress. As treatment for postpartum women has progressed, what originally felt like an instinctive and obvious response, holding has developed into something more substantial. Those who practice holding techniques understand this intervention as a fundamental therapeutic gesture, perhaps a prerequisite for optimal healing. The act of holding a client in distress does not merely represent our intuitive supportive response, as it might with a friend who is suffering. We know what it means to hold a friend who is hurting, both figuratively and literally. When we hold a postpartum woman, however, it is an intervention with a purpose and expected outcome.

Over the course of many years, our team at The Postpartum Stress Center has witnessed tired postpartum women meander from one inadequate therapy experience to another, only to reinforce their feelings of helplessness and perhaps their greatest fear – that they will feel like this forever. The development of the holding points was a natural and necessary product of this widespread pursuit of a reasonable and reliable response to the frantic cry for help. The holding approach tells the postpartum woman that we are listening. We are taking her seriously. We are skilled, determined, and able to help her find relief.

That has always been my number one professional priority and my greatest passion. Now, there is more.

As my clinical practice, interests, and ambitions evolve in predictable ways, I find my focus shifting. While The Postpartum Stress Center continues to provide services and support for treatment and professional training, I find my personal attention turning toward the succeeding generation of therapists. Passing on what I have learned simply feels like the next best thing to do. It feels indispensable and essential. Particularly in light of the recent surge of public awareness and positive momentum in the field of maternal mental health. Healthcare practitioners, mental health advocates, and consumers are desperately looking for excellent clinical resources. The outpouring of awareness points to the harsh reality that topnotch resources are scarce.

We must buckle down and make premium training a top priority. The community of perinatal therapists is a growing body of dedicated, exemplary clinicians. I have been honored to teach hundreds who present as a collective force of enthusiastic, warm, intelligent therapists with common goals and tons of heart. Training therapists who wish to focus their clinical practice in line with my decades of experience and commitment is infinitely gratifying and humbling. Offering guidance and inspiration to psychotherapists who seek clinical enrichment is nothing short of the peak of my career.

The transformation which has taken place is a parallel holding process, which will make more sense as you continue to read this book. While writing the first edition, it occurred to me that I am in the midst of a major professional pivot. As the development of holding practices and my desire to introduce this concept to other therapists gathered force, I realized that the tone of the book reflects my effort to hold *you*, the reader, the clinician determined to provide postpartum clients with the best possible options for relief and recovery. Working on this second edition was particularly meaningful to me. I have had the pleasure of working closely with Hilary Waller who has dedicated much of her practice to fine-tuning my work and turning it into her own. She has an impressive gift of being able to decipher my thoughts and my words and recite them back to me in ways that help me better understand my own thoughts. She is a brilliant thinker, and outstanding therapist and writer. I am honored to work beside her on this project. As with any project one devotes such extensive time and energy to, we found ourselves digging deep into the concept of holding – reworking, revising, relearning along the way. Ultimately our shared objective is to ensure that perinatal therapists understand that while holding may come naturally to many, our definition of holding within the context of perinatal women in distress is more than good instincts. It is an intentional intervention with specific guidelines designed to maximize a safe therapeutic environment within which the disclosure of her authentic suffering can take place.

In this second edition, in addition to overall updates and expanded revisions, we have added a chapter on the holding elements, broadening our perspective, as well as a chapter on cultural diversity (multiculturalism, implicit bias). Working on this book together has enlightened us further as we continue to refine our understanding of this delicate process and intervention.

We hold all the time. At work, at home, with loved ones, with people we meet for the first time. If you are a caring and sympathetic person, you probably hold someone or something much of the time and may wonder how holding a postpartum woman in distress is decidedly different. You may wonder what gives it more therapeutic value than simply being kind and attentive. You will learn that holding in the context of postpartum women is a supportive psychotherapy technique which, based on anecdotal and subjective observation, has shown to augment the therapeutic connection. This connection, subsequently, becomes the entry point to treatment options and recovery. You will learn that while your good instincts are paramount and instrumental to this process, your skills and aptitude for specific techniques bring credibility to your response. Caring about her is not enough. Assessing her symptoms and identifying her pain is not enough. Knowing what to say, why you are saying it, how to say it, and when not to say something can make the difference between her com-ing back and getting help or her leaving and surrendering to her suffering.

Holding is the gateway to healing.

Terminology within the postpartum community is a source of debate and some confusion. Among experts and the general public, maternal men-tal health terms are forever interchanged and overlapped with varying degrees of clarity. Those that are germane to this book will be defined in Chapter 1. The decision to use the phrase *postpartum women* did not come without significant consideration. My initial preference was to use a term more inclusive to the entirety of maternally related experiences. After all, women who are pregnant, or hope to get pregnant, or experience a pregnancy or infant loss, or adoption, infertility, and termination issues, also seek our help. The term *perinatal* was considered first because it is more all-encompassing. Ironically, it also felt too limiting. I realized that opening the discussion to the wide range of perinatal experiences distracted from the objective to underscore the needs that are unique to postpartum women, *when a baby is involved.* This is not to say the needs of pregnant women, or women who desire to get pregnant, or women who have lost a pregnancy are any less significant. It's just that they are different, thus, rerouting the content ever so slightly. It was decided that postpartum was most in sync with the message of this book, although its entirety is appli-cable to any perinatal woman.

Additionally, the word *depression*, like postpartum, doesn't come close to saying it all. The term postpartum depression, as an umbrella term which covers the spectrum of disorders, is understood to include anxiety disorders such as excessive worry, posttraumatic stress disorder, obsessive-compulsive disorder, and panic. We must also be careful not to exclude postpartum bipolar illness and postpartum psychosis, as they are serious concerns that are very much a part of the larger perinatal picture.

All holding principles in this book can and should be applied to any woman at any stage of any prenatal, postpartum, or reproductively related experience. Regardless of which diagnosis, symptom set, or psychological influences, if a woman in pain finds herself in a therapist's office, she should expect and deserves to be held in the precise manner described throughout these pages. For brevity, terms in this book were pared down to the use of postpartum depression and anxiety, sometimes postpartum depression, sometimes postpartum, and sometimes perinatal. Please do your best to generalize these references as applicable to the range of diagnoses or clas-sifications. Thank you for understanding that these references should not be construed as exclusive to other perinatal experiences.

Postpartum depression is increasingly being recognized as a serious and treatable condition. There is every reason to be optimistic about the recent government recommendations and pending legislation. The tide is definitely turning. Therapists wishing to specialize in the treatment of perinatal mood and anxiety disorders have never been in a better position to do so. Access to information along with the recent surge of public awareness makes this the perfect time for dedicated professionals to zero in on this passion. Holding is an intervention that bridges the passion you have for this work with treatment options that have been shown to reduce suffering and augment recovery. My hope is that you learn to use your inherent goodness and your strength as you guide each postpartum woman through the shadows that obscure her path.

Karen Kleiman

Chapter 1

Postpartum Women and Therapy

No matter how dark it is, I have you to care for. I may feel empty, but I make sure you know love. My arms feel heavy, but I put them around you. I am exhausted, but I pick you up. I kiss you despite my pain. You are my strength, my darling. I want the best for you. The best is a mother, no matter how broken she is. And that mother is me.

Elizabeth Broadbent, mother, writer (2015)[1]

Postpartum women do not want to go to therapy.

Every muscle hurts, and somewhat unexpectedly, full-body fatigue replaces the long-anticipated joy. Women who have recently given birth are tired, distracted, and weary from the overwhelming worry. When depression or anxiety is part of this picture, life with a new baby can feel, and be, unimaginably difficult.

Why are postpartum women not interested in therapy? They are bone-tired, exhausted from sleep deprivation, and inundated with tedious chores and fretfulness even on the best of days. They are both eager to fulfill the daily demands of their new and needy infant and overwhelmed by their baby's constant clinging to mommy for sustenance and shelter. The sheer pace leaves little room for lunch or a hot shower. For some women, without warning, things take a turn for the worse. Symptoms of depression and anxiety descend, crowding her frantic schedule with a thickening fog distracting them from the task at hand.

A new mother in the throes of depression quickly loses focus. She cannot think straight. She may wonder why she had this baby. She may think this was all a huge mistake. She longs to return to her life before the baby came. She feels resentful, lost, hopeless, agitated, and forever guilty. To make matters worse, she is told by friends, family, and her doctor that this is normal. If she feels bad enough, long enough, she is told she should talk to a therapist so she can find relief from her overwhelming emotions.

DOI: 10.4324/9781003402145-1

Are you kidding? I don't even have time to brush my teeth. And we don't have the money. And my partner will not understand. Besides, what good will it do to talk to a stranger about how I'm feeling? Can the therapist feed my baby at three in the morning?

Every postpartum woman is preoccupied, whether she is depressed or not. This may not be the best time to insert a therapeutic relationship and time-intensive healing process. But if her symptoms of depression and anxiety are acute enough, if she is sick enough, if her thoughts are distorted enough, she needs help.

And she needs help right away.

The taboo against mothers expressing negative feelings about their experiences or about their babies operates as reinforcement for their silence. Some try not to think about how terrible they feel, hoping it will all go away by itself. Others worry that this is a permanent state of being. Still others can't decide if seeking help will make things better or worse.

What if providers and policy makers take maternal mental health more seriously? What if we underscored the risk of untreated maternal depression and anxiety as the widespread healthcare crisis that it is? Even posing this question to healthcare providers makes many uneasy, and the public conversation subsides into a lull of good intentions. It is often claimed by various providers that mental health concerns fall outside the scope of their practice, but does it really? Can we afford to bypass the urgent needs of a postpartum woman in distress, whether they are physical, medical, or emotional? Furthermore, the provider barriers to diagnosis and treatment are only part of the conundrum. Even when providers care deeply, ask all the right questions, and have access to helpful resources, postpartum women in distress remain hesitant to reveal how much they are suffering.

While it is common for almost all new mothers to experience some moodiness during the first couple of weeks postpartum, approximately 13% of mothers experience more serious symptoms of postpartum depression (Gaynes et al., 2005; O'Hara & Swain, 1996). Remarkably, it has been shown that nearly half of new mothers with postpartum depression are neither identified nor treated (Beck, 2006), and we know that undetected depression and anxiety may have far-reaching consequences for the entire family system. Still, we understand the reluctance to follow through as a result of the overwhelming barriers. Mauthner (2002) found that many new mothers are afraid to disclose their symptoms of depression and anxiety because they are fearful that if they admit to having thoughts of harming their newborn or themselves, they will be hospitalized. Or have their baby taken away. They are also concerned about judgment from others, that they are different from all the other mothers, that they can't "cut it" as a mother, and that they will disappoint others, be viewed as less than, or further stigmatized by this illness. We are not surprised that women with postpartum depression and anxiety are often grateful to discover they have a diagnosable illness, instead of feeling that they are "crazy" or "bad mothers."

For these and other reasons, psychoeducation, along with collaborative and compassionate language, must be woven into each psychotherapy experience and each visit with a healthcare provider. Moreover, it behooves us, as professionals on the receiving end of the small percentage of women who find the courage to reach out for help, to arm ourselves with steadfast readiness. This readiness, armed with holding skills, can set the course for perinatal women in distress to feel heard and cared for, enabling a more transparent and reliable discussion of how they feel and what they need.

The first edition of this book noted the evolution of definitions and terminology used by researchers and healthcare providers. At that time the focus on postpartum depression was expanding to include issues related to anxiety and other disorders that onset both during pregnancy and the postpartum period. Since then, the field of reproductive mental health has continued to grow. Academic research, mainstream literature, advocacy efforts, and professional training focus on a gamut of reproductively related mood and anxiety disorders that present with a range of severity. It is widely recognized that depression (mood) and anxiety disorders can emerge throughout the period of pregnancy and the first year postpartum, a time frame defined as the *perinatal* period, in both gestational and non-gestational parents. The term *distress* is now used when anxiety and depression are manifesting concurrently, which is more prevalent than previously understood.

Because of the changing landscape of our field, some disclaimers need to be made at the outset of this book. You will notice that the language in the book will a) interchange postpartum depression and anxiety[2] with postpartum distress, and b) refer predominantly to the term *postpartum depression* at other times for simplicity's sake. This is not to exclude other diagnoses, such as bipolar illness, postpartum anxiety disorders, obsessive-compulsive disorder, or psychosis. c) This does not discount the profound experience of pregnancy, as there is evidence that prenatal depression is equally as common as postpartum depression (Milgrom et al., 2008), and as noted earlier, a significant number of postpartum depressions begin during pregnancy. Still, we use the terms *postpartum depression and anxiety (postpartum distress)* on behalf of succinctness as an inclusive reference and with sincere regard to all perinatal events. With this understanding, the postpartum time frame is the primary focus of this book to highlight the influences that are specific to the postpartum period, most notably the impact of the new baby, and how this directly shapes her world and your work. We will, however, continue to reference the perinatal period, which includes pregnancy, throughout the book.

Regardless of the reproductive life event, life cycle transition, or diagnosis, the holding practices referred to throughout each chapter apply to pregnant and postpartum women with depression, with anxiety, or with any related mood and anxiety disorder. They apply to women with the postpartum blues, women who are trying to or having difficulty getting pregnant, and women who have lost pregnancies or infants.[3] They apply to all birthing people, and to non-birthing parents, a group explored in greater depth in Chapter 13.

An Introduction to Holding

A postpartum woman who is concerned about the way she is feeling might find it difficult to reconcile the conflict of interest between having a baby and going to therapy. More specifically, did having a baby somehow *cause* her to need therapy? How could that be, when she has always wanted to be a mother? How can she now envy her childless friends who are feeling free and unencumbered? How could she not be enjoying what she has long desired? The mere recommendation of professional help only complicates things, and tensions rise. This hardly makes sense to her. When distress is high, it presents paradoxically as incompatible with psychotherapy.

Symptoms get in the way. Insight is limited. Depressed women may withdraw and isolate themselves. Intelligent, thoughtful women are grief stricken and humiliated by their own thoughts. Extremely anxious women may misperceive the advantages of therapy and tend to overfocus on their own counterproductive beliefs. Both of these scenarios interfere with the motivation for, and success of, traditional talk therapy relationships. The principal feature that defines therapy with postpartum women – obvious, yet often ignored – is that there is a baby involved. This is what distinguishes our work. Postpartum moms are hormonally compromised, sleep deprived, and besieged by demands placed upon them. When sitting in the room with them, the therapeutic energy feels especially urgent when we factor in the well-being of the infant.

Time is of the essence.

Despite the extent of her suffering, a postpartum woman might be appalled at the notion of needing/wanting/finding a therapist during a time in her life when she expects to feel joy and beam with anticipation. The contradiction feels nothing short of absurd. It is perceived as an embarrassing reversal of priorities. The dependence on another person (a stranger, no less) while wrestling with her infant's dependence on her own compromised self can be oppressive. Thus, her guilt deepens. Help-seeking behavior is not high on a postpartum woman's to-do list, particularly when she is grappling with the adjustment to motherhood through a dark, depressive lens.

Increasingly, therapists are choosing to specialize in this field of study and practice. Therapists who seek expert guidance on how to develop clinical skills tailored to this population admit they are attuned to the unique needs of postpartum women but may not yet understand the nuances that make this area of work different from other therapeutic liaisons. *The Art of Holding in Therapy* will look closely at this exceptional relationship between a perinatal woman with depression and anxiety and her therapist. Readers will learn that being an experienced therapist in other areas of therapy is not necessarily sufficient training to treat the complex influences intrinsic to the postpartum period. Intense symptoms can be disruptive or deceptively subtle. Learning how to discern that which is extremely uncomfortable from that which is clinically urgent, is crucial, and can be challenging for even the highly skilled, experienced perinatal therapist. Readers will also learn how this work can act as a trigger and ignite a host of countertransference issues that can either enhance or encumber the recovery process, depending on one's interpretation and response. Above all, this book examines the novel concept of what it means to therapeutically *hold* a perinatal woman in distress, highlighting the postpartum experience.

Holding is not a new concept within the psychotherapeutic arena. Conceptualized by pediatrician and psychoanalyst D.H. Winnicott, his description of the "holding environment" and the nurturing emotional environment of the "good-enough" mother (Winnicott, 1953) created a fitting parallel to the transitional space in psychotherapy. Winnicott and others extrapolated his foundational ideas into the wider world of psychotherapy and integrated the symbolic holding environment into the therapy session. With this analogy in mind, the holding approach becomes an understandable response to a woman in crisis.

Holding within the context of therapeutic work with postpartum women is defined as a loss-informed, strength-based approach that enables the therapist to contain high levels of distress and do so in a way that cultivates the early stages of connectedness. This attempt to contain her symptoms of agitation and despair is accomplished despite the innate pull she feels to repair this herself in order to preserve what she perceives as her dwindling sense of control. When it comes to postpartum women, holding must take place without delay and without the leeway of a longer-term therapeutic process. There is a great deal at stake. Often, you are faced with situations that cannot wait for the time it typically takes to develop a therapeutic relationship. Successfully holding a postpartum woman in distress can promote initial compliance and set the stage for healing. Symptoms of perinatal distress can abate with the right medication, and relief can come from even a mediocre therapist saying all of the right things. Meaningful and enduring recovery, however, is best achieved through the experience of empathy through holding within the therapeutic setting.

As you tease apart the strands of her resistance, her distractions, her predilections, and the essence of her wounded soul, you begin to learn who she is. Who she was before she had her baby and who you now see before you. Her symptoms do not define her, as she fears they do, but they are an important part of who she is at this moment in time.

The Development of The Art of Holding Perinatal Women in Distress™

Following years of studying perinatal depression and anxiety, Karen's work brought attention to a fundamental discrepancy that interfered with postpartum healing and the recovery process. If women aren't telling us how bad they feel, and providers are not asking the right questions, none of the evidence-based interventions, or the medications, or the tried and true therapies will truly bring about lasting change unless, and until, we gain access to the heart of a woman's suffering. And while we understand that perinatal mood and anxiety disorders are a very real medical condition, we also understand that they emerge within the context of the complicated developmental challenge of becoming a mother. This major life transition cannot be ignored while we seek to understand and treat the symptoms that scream for attention. Therefore, in our effort to address the enshrouded needs of a perinatal woman in distress, we must a) understand the larger context and how her transition to motherhood meets or fails to meet her expectations, b) understand what she desperately does not want us to confess, and c) simultaneously we must do our best to establish a trusting environment which unlocks her private suffering. In doing this, we must also pay close attention to how this process causes us to reflect on our own reproductive successes and failures, our own desires and expectations, which, to be sure, interface with hers in ways which may, at first, elude us. And while readers might acknowledge that their comprehensive psychological and therapeutic training has adequately prepared them to manage the presence of countertransference, I would argue that when it comes to our reproductive journeys, the process is more present, more precious, and more profound than any graduate teaching can prepare for or anticipate.

The Art of Holding Perinatal Women in Distress model of intervention was created to better understand the paradoxical presentation of perinatal distress distinguished by the contradiction between what a new mother feels and her disinclination to disclose it. This impressive incongruity, appearing as resistance or reluctance, is referred to as *authentic suffering*. Awareness and appreciation of authentic suffering (discussed in Chapter 7), and the skill to access it, is an essential key to her recovery. Holding provides a set of mindful, intentional skills which enable the therapist to simultaneously connect to their client's distress as well as their own response. Holding provides a framework with specific prompts for synchronized attunement to the client, the therapist, and the process. By applying the longstanding work of Winnicott to the precarious postpartum trajectory imposed upon by expected demands of and adaptations to this life stage, holding therapists learn how to sit with the suffering of a postpartum woman in distress and help her find her way back to her *self*.

The Common Experience

It may be helpful to begin by understanding the larger context of a new mother's anguish and how easily it is compromised by social, cultural, and personal expectations. One of your greatest challenges as first responders in any postpartum crisis is to decipher what *feels* like a crisis to any one woman from what may actually present as a crisis in more objective terms. If suffering is subjective, it is imperative that we determine the precise nature of this suffering and potential consequences. And while new mothers should not be expected to be able to know what they need to worry about and what is considered expected and normal for this time, providing a more universal set of expectations would be a good start to reducing their enduring uncertainty. After all, for generations, women have been told to expect that this will be the "best time of their life." In some ways, we've moved beyond this, but still, scary thoughts and strong negative emotions do not sit well with new mothers. At all times, we want to validate their experience, empower women to recognize the potential seriousness of the situation and guide them to appropriate resources. If postpartum women are not telling us the extent to which they are suffering, we need to understand this phenomenon better. Studies have shown that only a small percentage of women who are experiencing symptoms of perinatal distress seek help from a provider and of those who receive a referral for treatment a small percentage follow through (Goodman & Tyer-Viola, 2010).

Current research shows little change, and, in fact, some suggests that confusion about symptoms, stigma related to mental health disorders, and fear of judgment from providers continue to hinder help-seeking (Daehn et al., 2022). This is true despite thriving academic, clinical, and grass roots initiatives designed to increase mental health education among new parents. For this reason psychoeducation must be woven into each psychotherapy experience and each visit with a healthcare provider. While it may sound oversimplistic, talking about postpartum depression and anxiety is often avoided in the medical community. Straightforward, honest discussions are not the norm, partly because of time constraints, but more likely it's an attempt to pivot away from what might feel like a bottomless pit to providers who do not have the specific training or the resources on hand.

To this day, women report that their Ob-Gyn did not ask any questions about how they are feeling or did not mention the possibility of postpartum depression or anxiety. This gap in medical care further reinforces a woman's silence and uncertainty.

Open dialogues between providers and mothers are essential. We have learned that a mother's mental health cannot be separated from her physical and medical recuperation after having a baby. These discussions should be direct and include a) defining specific terms, b) possible symptoms that may overlap with what is normally expected during the postpartum period, c) a brief assessment of her current levels of distress, and d) a written list of reliable resources for support or treatment. In other words, it is incumbent upon providers to help every woman understand this fundamental concern which she often expresses:

How does she know if what she is experiencing is okay or not?

Postpartum women in distress report that they relate to each other's stories and crave the endorsement and comfort derived from shared experiences. This desire for connectedness and desire to retreat into deep loneliness is a pervasive contradiction of emotions that can keep women silent and unmotivated. When possible, they should be encouraged to step toward their desire to connect and find community or family support. When they do, it can feel enormously validating. One mother from our support group said:

I wish mothers were more honest with other new mothers about what to expect. I like to be prepared. It was like jumping on a treadmill already at a sprint from the get-go! I would have appreciated it if someone told me that the first couple of months were gonna be this rough, and it's normal if you cry a lot. Maybe I wouldn't have felt so weird or scared.

What is disconcerting is that many women claim they feel unprepared, highlighting the sharp contrast between what women think motherhood will be and the reality of their experience. The unsuspecting shock of how hard it can feel makes many mothers perceive themselves as alone in their experience or impaired in some way. Idealized representations of motherhood, reinforced constantly by cultural expectations and social media distortions, make it difficult for mothers to express negative or conflicted emotions, especially to family, friends, or healthcare professionals who have their own expectations for this transition. Symptoms of postpartum depression and anxiety are complex and disheartening in a way that makes them difficult for loved ones to witness, but to a woman trying desperately to be the best mother she can be, symptoms can feel insufferable. Most women who experience these daunting emotions tell us they have never experienced any feeling like this before. They have never felt this bad. They have never felt so alone and isolated.

Recent research shows that the experience of loneliness is believed to play a primary role when perinatal women were asked to describe feelings associated with their distress (Adlington et al., 2023). Women described feeling alone, disconnected, and isolated from others. Fear of being judged by others and comparing themselves to others and wrestling pervasive feelings of not being "a good enough mother" appear to exacerbate feelings of loneliness. The researchers suggest that addressing issues related to stigma and providing culturally appropriate support measures are good attempts to ease some of the loneliness. Not surprisingly, feelings of loneliness were deepened by lack of support from partners or family, while feelings of loneliness improved when the mother felt validated from trustworthy healthcare providers, family members, and peers.

The Quintessential Paradox

Holding on for dear life. That's how one woman explained it, as she unwittingly embodied Winnicott's description of unthinkable anxiety, or "falling for ever" (Winnicott, 1965). Falling forever seems to perfectly express what postpartum women in despair describe: *It feels like I will never get better. I will go crazy. I will die.*

Here's how Alison described her experience:

I felt like I was spilling out of myself, that waves of pain and anger were knocking me over, breaking me apart, and that I was running around trying to collect all of the pieces of myself. My mind seemed to have no power to rationalize over my heart – my feeling took over everything and reduced me to a painful pile of liquid on the floor. I felt that I was every day, every moment, free falling through air. Other times, I felt I was hanging from a tree branch over the swirling sea. I was falling and suffocating at the same time.

I kept falling down and trying to pick myself up. I felt so out of control and it was that very out of control feeling that made me hate myself and want to fix myself. I realize now, looking back, how embarrassed and ashamed it made me feel because I couldn't overcome it on my own. I almost didn't want anyone to save me or catch me and I was so angry that I couldn't save myself that when someone tried, I felt like freaking out and screaming, I can do it myself! Like a toddler trying to buckle her own seat belt. And yet, I believe I wanted help more than anything else in the world.

Alison expresses the core paradox intrinsic to the treatment of postpartum women with symptoms of depression and anxiety: the legitimate yet collapsing desire for autonomy and control, in conflict with her very urgent need, and secret desire, for help.

The incompatibility between motherhood and a sense of control is apparent to most new moms almost immediately. It feels incomprehensible for moms to cling to a desire for control and autonomy while they simultaneously struggle to connect with and take care of their dependent infant. If motherhood temporarily robs women of a sense of independence it is reasonable that they would try to recoup this independence along the way, even though to some extent mothers do readily or reluctantly expect and surrender to this state. The timing and energy of this effort to reclaim a lost sense of self are different for each woman, depending on variables such as personality, history, current life circumstances, and environmental/social demands and support, for instance. The point is that postpartum women, whether depressed or not, are required to reconstruct themselves, to a certain extent, as a function of the demands of motherhood. It necessitates a practical, emotional, psychological, and extremely personal transformation. When depression and anxiety impose extraordinary distress, it can feel impossible to move forward. When depression hits, there is an abrupt disturbance that impedes the transition to motherhood. Mothers who trust the natural flow of life expect this adjustment to develop naturally, but instead are left feeling cheated, enraged, and misunderstood.

The current American culture reinforces the notion that women should anticipate a smooth and euphoric progression into motherhood, and until recently, this was the exclusive viewpoint depicted in the media. Even as healthcare-related advertisements and various promotions continue to portray new mothers as radiant, air-brushed, and unattainably blissful, some things are beginning to change. Public awareness campaigns continue to gain momentum, propelling healthcare providers and media channels to take a closer look at the prevalence of postpartum mood and anxiety disorders. Still, much continues to be misconstrued. Professionals and laypeople continue to misunderstand that postpartum depression refers to women who experience a clinical depression, with symptoms that meet diagnostic criteria of a major mood and anxiety disturbance. Not the blues, not an adjustment disorder, not, *oh she has a touch of the postpartum*. We are talking about serious symptoms that require serious attention. The good news is that postpartum women themselves are becoming advocates for their own healthcare, utilizing social media outlets to put a voice to their collective fears and frustrations and garnering more awareness than ever before.

Even with the promising national conversation and community participation, many postpartum women remain paralyzed by symptoms. What a cruel juxtaposition. Life's most precious experience set against a backdrop of unspeakable anguish. *All I've wanted my entire life is to become a mother. To have baby. And now this. It's so unfair. It's so scary. It feels unbearable. I'm not sure I can do this.* This is often what we hear.

An unfathomable contradiction. A contradiction that, ironically, compels her to pretend she is fine. She manages to tap into what little energy she has in order to create and maintain the illusion that everything is under control. After all, a mother who cannot adequately take care of herself certainly could not be expected to adequately take care of her baby, she thinks; thus, the pretense lingers.

One can only imagine how much energy it takes to sustain this pretense. With weariness at the center of this undertaking, if she's lucky, she musters enough strength to go through the motions while she braces herself in the face of crushed expectations and unforgiving symptoms. She twirls from one insurmountable task to another, unable to focus and unable to breathe. She rarely asks for help and seldom confesses her dark thoughts, lest she worry others or stir up suspicion that she is unfit to proceed.

It is this dance of duality that is the spirit of this book. Therapists who specialize in the treatment of perinatal distress are both challenged and honored to accompany a postpartum woman as she teeters on this precipice between her struggle to get through the day and her intermittent wish to give up. Sometimes releasing her grip and plunging into the abyss sounds tempting – suicide can feel like a better option than suffering. Surely, responding to that misguided lure is by far our most urgent call to action, but day to day, our job is to convince her that the journey back to her *self* is well worth the unimaginable effort. She wants to go home. She wants to return to her baby. Or her bed, or her aloneness. She wants to be well and be gone from anything, anyone, and any place that pathologizes her current state. She wants to return to her previous self. Before the baby. Or with the baby, or without the baby. She's not sure what she wants.

Most assuredly, she would prefer not to be in a therapist's office. Of course, some women *do* want to be in a therapist's office. They may be relieved to find a good therapist and are comfortable with the notion of therapy, in general or specifically related to the postpartum crisis. However, even women who are fans of therapy may prefer not to be going at this time when they expected to be home taking care of their new baby and family. Still, bad connecting with a caring therapist can feel like a lifeline.

Your greatest task, as you share the sacred space with her pain, is to preserve the integrity of her wishes while you gently lead her toward a more complete state of well-being. You do this in spite of her resistance. You do this whether she believes she will get better or not. You do this as she leans away from you, tempted by the darkness. You do this to help her breathe, whether she wants to be sitting there or not. This is why she has summoned the strength to be present with you.

Our appeal to you is that you become comfortable with this paradox. You must learn to refrain from seeking immediate solutions or quick fixes (to reduce her anxiety or yours); you must sit, and wait, and embrace her suffering. In doing so, you set in motion the possibility that therapeutic engagement will take place.

This is the essence of holding.

Moms and Therapy

After the birth of my first baby, I trained to be a lactation counselor, hoping it would be a good way to informally utilize my counseling skills while taking time off to spend time with my baby. That was where I met Janis, a 34-year-old first-time mom who was frustrated when her baby refused to suck. The three of us soon learned how to modify expectations in order to better meet the needs of both mama and baby, but it wasn't long before I sensed how unhappy Janis was a majority of the time. Like everyone else, I assumed she would be excited to be a new mother, because all was going well with her and her new baby. Still, each time we met or spoke on the phone, she expressed her disappointment and impatience. Nothing was turning out the way she thought it would.

Janis and numerous women to follow introduced me to the notion that new mothers do not always feel good about being mothers. Many do, of course, describing a boundless wellspring of mutually satisfying needs. In this role however, more often than not, I spoke with women who yearned for closeness with their babies and found themselves struggling to revise the inescapable illusion that new motherhood would bring infinite joy. In its place, they described a new level of consciousness. An acute awareness that sparked constant critique and unwelcome emotions. When I explored my observations aloud with Janis, she introduced me to the words that would later characterize the majority of women I would see throughout my career: "Something is not right. This just is not me. I do not feel like myself." When I suggested she might feel better if she found a professional to talk to about this, she smirked, "Right. Like I have time."

Reasonable Opposition

Resistance to therapy is as old as therapy itself. Karen remembers a professor in graduate school who declared that if one does not encounter resistance to therapy, it is not working. Too much resistance is counterproductive. Too little may be also. Either way, resistance is a well-known psychological phenomenon in therapy because, well, change is hard. People understandably stand firm against the prospect of learning new ways to think, behave, or feel.

Let us break this down further.

Postpartum women in distress often do not have the time, the energy, the interest, the wherewithal, the resources, the finances, or the motivation to go to even one more healthcare provider. Add a therapist to the mix? *You've got to be kidding me*. New mothers confront stigma against mental illness, distrust of healthcare systems, embarrassment, shame, and all-around protest against seeing a therapist. Particularly when she hasn't slept through the night in weeks, has a screaming baby at her breast or a colicky infant who relentlessly requires attention, or is simply trying to get through the day weighed down by piercing guilt and unrelenting grief. *Seriously? A therapist?*

If it weren't a matter of life and death, it would be preposterous.

Many postpartum women in acute distress know that something is wrong. These women are extremely in sync and sensitive to their own needs as well as the needs of their babies. Despite, or because of, their symptoms, and somewhat ironically, they are acutely tuned in when it comes to self-awareness. All systems are on high alert. In response to the needs of their babies, they remain vigilant and attentive. In response to their own needs, however, many deliberately or frantically rely on avoidance, afraid to face the intuition that something is not right.

- Some hope it will get better on its own.
- Some fear it's just how being a mother feels.
- Some worry that if others find out, they will be judged or labeled ill-equipped for motherhood.
- Some agonize that if they put words to how they are feeling, it will make it permanent or something catastrophic will happen.
- Some hope that if they ignore it, it will go away.

The idea of therapy in the midst of one of life's most challenging developmental responsibilities simply doesn't make sense to a new mother. She recently had a baby and now, without warning, she feels so bad that people who love her are telling her she should talk to a professional about it. This sounds absurd to women who are whirling from the absence of a good night's sleep and overwhelmed by a nagging inner voice preoccupied by alleged wrongdoings. Paying someone for a once-a-week reflective dialogue seems indulgent and impractical. Although therapeutic work with postpartum women is aligned with the standards of any good therapy, a few important distinctions set it apart:

- The consequences of untreated or under treated postpartum depression and anxiety are dire and run the gamut from suicide to a lifetime of self-doubt associated with one's role as a mother.
- Often mothers misunderstand or misinterpret their symptoms, minimizing the seriousness of the situation.
- An urgent need for mom to return to her previous level of functioning so she can attend to the needs of her infant.

These factors create a demand on the part of both the therapist and the postpartum mom to manage her symptoms without delay and resume her normal routine.

Quickness is not a concept that rests well with the tenets of talk psychotherapy. This is another of the many paradoxes inherent in this work. Therapists who are not skilled at recognizing this discrepancy between the need for a rapid assessment and the therapeutic value of sitting back and listening to her story will lose precious opportunities to secure the connection critical to her recovery. Put another way, if you swoop in prematurely, she may feel suffocated by the therapist's impulsive reaction to her description of how she is feeling. If you postpone your response to serious symptoms, however, you risk underreacting to a potential threat to her well-being.

Achieving this balance is key.

Postpartum women in distress present a rewarding challenge for therapists. New motherhood and therapy may be perceived as an oxymoron, reinforced by an abundance of interpretations and misinterpretations about therapy. Some women presume they just don't need the help and therapy is for people who are *really messed up*. Therapy is for people with *real* problems. Not new mothers of babies. Therapy is time consuming, expensive, and draining, the last thing a woman caring for a new baby wants to initiate. But she also wants to feel better. She wants to sleep and stop feeling guilt, shame, and self-doubt. She yearns to return to her previous level of function and wake up feeling like herself again. If postpartum women in distress are generally not in the mood for therapy, but desperately want to feel better and right now, therapists can find themselves in a precarious position.

- How do you respond once she does make it to your therapeutic space?
- How do you help her without patronizing her, without infantilizing her, without offending her?
- How do you convince her that what she is feeling is not what all new mothers feel and that her coming for help was a courageous, important step?
- How do you proceed with recommendations when she may or may not understand what's going on?
- What if she were coerced into coming in and not motivated to receive help?
- How do you help her if she believes that a couple of good nights' rest is all she needs to feel like herself again?

The Art of Holding Perinatal Women in Distress model offers a therapeutic response to these questions. Responding with specific techniques that can increase motivation, provide access to personal resources, and allow healing to begin.

The Urgency Is High

In spite of the disincentives, denial, and distractions, and due to a trending endorsement of the process, more and more postpartum women in distress *do* seek out therapists to help them during this difficult time. Reasons some women may decide to seek help:

- Because they are utterly exhausted and tired of feeling like they are doing everything by themselves.
- Because their symptoms are stronger than their resistance. Or their desire to feel better is stronger than their symptoms.
- Because they are terrified and need to know they'll get better and be okay.
- Because they truly want to feel better, more than anything else in the world.
- Because they have tried to feel better on their own and it's not working.
- Because they hoped this would go away by itself, but it is getting worse.
- Because no one seems to be listening or understand how bad they feel.
- Because they are afraid if they do not, they will feel worse and never feel better again.
- Because they are terrified by what they are feeling and thinking.
- Because they do not want to die.
- Because they want to be there for their baby and enjoy this special time.
- Because they want to be the best mother they can be.
- Because someone they trust has strongly suggested they seek help.

As clinicians, our task is to create the space in which postpartum women in distress can safely decompress and begin to cultivate a strong core self in the face of staggering challenges. Any time you hold someone in despair, whether it is a 4-year-old in the middle of a full-scale tantrum or an adult whose panic disables her ability to think clearly, you need to proceed lovingly but firmly, with intentional resolve and with affection for any and all opposition.

Is Empathy Enough?

The cornerstone of any psychotherapy experience is the therapeutic relationship. One of the most consistent conclusions in the psychotherapeutic literature is that the quality of the alliance is a powerful predictor of treatment outcome (Horvath & Symonds, 1991). Volumes have been written on this subject, and although there is no one-size-fits-all protocol, it is agreed that early stages of treatment techniques involving the relationship are central to fostering positive outcomes (Baier et al., 2020; DeFife &

Hilsenroth, 2011). The concepts of empathy, positive regard, and genuineness, based on the work of Carl Rogers (1957), continue to define the fundamental constructs of good therapy today. *Empathy*, a word that is practically synonymous with good therapy, is not uncomplicated. It is, as Rogers defined it, an evolving process rather than a state, which relies on entering the private perceptual world of another person.

> To be with another in this way means that for the time being you lay aside the views and values you hold for yourself in order to enter another's world without prejudice. In some sense it means that you lay aside yourself and this can only be done by a person who is secure enough in himself that he knows he will not get lost in what may turn out to be the strange or bizarre world of the other and can comfortably return to his own world when he wishes. Perhaps this description makes clear that being empathic is a complex, demanding, strong yet subtle and gentle way of being.
>
> (Carl Rogers, 1975, p. 4)

Empathy, a prerequisite for holding, is a mutual and collaborative experience and a primary agent of change within the postpartum treatment paradigm. The mutual and collaborative aspect, although essential for change and growth, is often postponed with postpartum women who first and foremost seek information and a more didactic experience. The requisite for immediate responses and specific answers conflicts with the early stages of traditional therapy, but there is nothing traditional about therapy with a postpartum woman. This entire subject of treating women with postpartum depression and anxiety would be easier if psychotherapy were a precise and predictable science, with standards of exact care applicable to each and every therapist. In reality, every time a postpartum woman walks into a therapist's office for the first time, neither she nor the therapist knows what to expect.

In contrast, when a woman meets a medical provider with a more basic physical condition, she has some sense of how that appointment is going to turn out. If she sees an orthopedic physician for a swollen ankle or a gastroenterologist for abdominal pain, she has a reasonable expectation that she can anticipate attention to her symptom and have hope for at least partial relief from her discomfort or a treatment regimen with that result. Likewise, the medical provider can reasonably expect that she has willfully sought treatment and is likely to comply with the prescribed treatment plan. It's a mutual agreement of sorts.

Not so with postpartum depression. Or psychotherapy, in general, for that matter.

Although we have theories to support our interventions and guidelines to direct our intentions, therapy can present as an abstract notion that is unimpressive to a bleeding, lactating, exhausted woman pleading for her life back.

Our empathetic response is a required first step.

The anatomy of a solid therapeutic relationship is difficult to teach if it is not something that comes naturally to someone in this field. Much of what defines the relationship is anchored in non-verbal interactions, making it tricky to articulate when teaching, supervising, or refining a therapist's style or effectiveness. Instructing a therapist to be warm, if it is not a natural tendency, creates a no-win situation. There will be zero therapeutic gain from warmth that is contrived or manufactured. The mere mention of this creates a contradiction that doesn't fit well within a therapeutic model.

One can see how the therapeutic liaison is compromised from the outset if the woman coming in is ambivalent or extremely symptomatic. When anxiety is severe, fatigue is pervasive, thoughts are distorted, sleep deprivation is all encompassing, and hopelessness is ever present, insight and ambitious goal setting is compromised. *I don't know what I need. I just need to feel better, and I need to feel better now*, you often hear. Some postpartum women are coming to therapy for the first time. Others, who have a history of depression, may have been in more than one previous therapeutic relationship. Regardless of the varying levels of experience with therapy, they all come needing the same thing. That thing, which is the thrust of this book, is hard to put into words.

There are no simple directives for how to provide postpartum women what they need and want, when they are in an emotional crisis. The intention of this book is to generate the groundwork and specifics that underlie the empathy, compassion, and skills necessary to guide a postpartum woman out of distress and provide a safe place for her to land before she moves forward. Therapists who are committed to this process will find that each woman's story carries a unique and complex map of instructions, sometimes subtle, sometimes painfully conspicuous, but always enlightening. She is hungry for attention and rest, whether or not she can articulate that. As she shares her story, you carry her pain and share the weight. It will become clear to readers that empathy provides access to holding, and learning to hold a postpartum woman in distress is a prerequisite for good therapy. Good therapy in this context refers to the process that enables her to experience symptom relief, to heal more completely, and to function optimally with her baby with greater self-awareness and confidence.

A Word on Behalf of Fathers and Non-Gestational Parents

As discussed earlier, The Art of Holding Perinatal Women in Distress model of intervention was originally inspired by the work of D.W. Winnicott, who first used the terms "holding environment" and "good-enough mother" to describe certain conditions that are central to the healthy emotional development of infants. Karen applied these concepts to the particular relationship between mental healthcare providers and new mothers. Thus, the use of cis-gender language in her work is reflective of her intentional response to Winnicott's work as the theoretical foundation of the art of holding perinatal women in distress. As referenced in the first edition. Winnicott says it best: "If I say, 'the mother' more often than 'the father' I hope that fathers will understand" (Winnicott, 1987a, p. 33).

Nevertheless, we strongly acknowledge the critical importance of intentional efforts to provide equitable treatment for all parents and birthing human beings, regardless of gender expression, gender identity, or sexuality. We are committed to expanding our work and theoretical foundations so that we may uphold our value of inclusivity and continue to provide leadership in the field of reproductive mental health.

When this book was first published, attention on depression and anxiety disorders that affect fathers after the birth of a baby was increasing, a topic that was discussed only briefly toward the end of the book. In this edition we feature the experience of both fathers and other non-gestational parents such as adoptive parents, parents who conceive via a surrogate or gestational carrier, and non-gestational partners in Chapter 13. We recognize this inclusion as an improvement but also acknowledge that further exploration of these topics is critically necessary, for the health of all parents, infants, and families. We encourage you to seek out training and information that is beyond the scope of this book in order to continue honing your skills as an expert, a holding therapist, and a healthcare provider.

Notes

1 Permission to republish quote granted by www.scarymommy.com/letter-sons-postpartum-depression.
2 Also referred to as postpartum mood and anxiety disorders, or PMADs.
3 Although the number of women who experience postpartum blues is high and many seek professional support – either because they are frightened and seek clarification, or they experienced a previous depression and now request supportive or prophylactic intervention – they will not be the focus of this book. Likewise, women with postpartum psychosis also fall outside the margins of our focus, primarily because their medical needs are extraordinarily urgent and always require aggressive intervention and, most likely, hospitalization. After stabilization, the principles reviewed in this book would be suitable and beneficial.

Chapter 2

Preparing to Hold

Jackie was 5 months postpartum when I met her for the first time. She had seen two previous therapists. One, she saw only once and decided not to return after the therapist said something like, "Oh, this is not postpartum depression. That's when you want to kill your baby. Do you want to kill your baby?"

The second therapist Jackie went to was "nice enough," as Jackie put it, but didn't seem to know anything especially relevant to being a mother or how the experience of motherhood influenced how Jackie was feeling. By the time I met Jackie, she was tired of looking for the right fit, tired of asking for help, tired of explaining what she needed, tired of hoping it would get better.

"I feel like a slimy deer." She told me. "It's all bullshit. Like I don't have anything better to do than slip in and out of people's offices while they read from some freakin' script, *oh you have this symptom, this means you should do such and such.*"

I couldn't resist. "You feel like a slimy deer? In what way do you feel like a slimy deer?"

I had my own vivid depiction, of course, engraved in the forefront of my brain.

"Yeah, I'm kickin' and screamin' and strangers are grabbin' at me, but nothing takes hold. I'm sliding all over the place. I just want to be myself again. I just want to stop all of this. I just want to go home." *Nothing takes hold,* I thought to myself as I listened to her description. We talked more about the deer, which didn't make sense to me at first, but evolved into an earnest cry for help when Jackie described an early memory of her dad assisting the birth of a baby deer on their farm property. She recalled standing behind the fence watching her dad straining to grab hold of the slippery fawn while its mother wailed and the baby desperately tried to run before it could stand. Her memory of this incident was both touching and terrifying, as she was around 8 years old at the time, intrigued by the miracle in front of her and equally disturbed by the chaos, the blood, the panic, and the primal cries.

DOI: 10.4324/9781003402145-2

This unsophisticated and random analogy of a slimy deer may not resonate for everyone. It did for me. Perhaps because the reference conjures images of a wild, wide-bellied mommy deer in the midst of a grueling labor process, leading up to the delivery of our precious, vulnerable fawn. What could this possibly have to do with postpartum women? Can you allow yourself a moment to think about this experience of trying to grab firmly in order to harness the mucus-coated, flailing limbs? Can you envision the grateful yet terrified animal sliding right out of your earnest embrace, despite your best intention? Can you imagine the mutual frustration of the baby deer yearning to be free, and you, trying to grab on and help but not frighten or restrict it?

Instincts to escape from circumstances that may ultimately be in our best interest are well known throughout the animal world and our understanding of human behavior. Feeling threatened by predators while in a vulnerable state not only makes sense, it is adaptive and, often, a sensible response. That is where my head went when Jackie described herself as a slimy deer. Right there, with limbs thrashing.

Postpartum women who are bombarded with symptoms find themselves a bit mistrustful. When the world as they knew it has turned upside down betraying lifelong fantasies, a natural reaction is to push back and desperately try to make sense out of things; try to regain control. Holding a postpartum woman in distress while she wrestles with her perceived loss of self and anxious ambivalence produces the dynamic that inspired this book. Her requirement for autonomy and separateness at this critical time can make connecting in therapy feel threatening to her and nearly impossible to us. Even so, her desperate need to return to normal functioning eventually fuels the holding process.

We must be ready to catch her and grab hold.

Standards of Readiness and Proficiency

Empathy and attunement, instinct and intuition, are legitimate and driving forces in psychotherapeutic work. Therapists who identify with their clients in this context, such as becoming mothers themselves, may feel, and *may be*, especially in tune with the experiences of their clients. However, we will see that these shared life experiences can also be a liability in this work. Readiness to engage in this intimate process with perinatal women in distress requires both the acquisition of applicable clinical skills and the management of personal vulnerabilities. To hold with confidence and success, you must learn how to suspend your reliance on tried-and-true, evidence-based interventions (which remain excellent resources), boundary the parts of your own experience that bleed into your therapy space, and begin to believe that, in addition to every bit of exquisite knowledge you have obtained along the way, *you* are your most essential resource.

Your belief in your own self, your experiences, your training, your compassion, your essence – when reinforced through the framework of holding – will be your greatest tool of intervention.

The Clinician's Experience and Self-Disclosure

We are witnessing a substantial shift in the workforce which now abounds with well-educated, trained perinatal specialists who, for many different reasons, are extremely motivated to provide a safe space for perinatal women in distress to express themselves, feel heard, and begin to heal. Our professional training program at The Postpartum Stress Center is filled with enthusiastic and highly qualified professionals eager to dig deeper into this specialized work. Therapists feel drawn to this work for a variety of reasons, some personal, some professional. Some say they feel inspired by virtue of their own personal reproductive journey. Some expound further and say they feel "destined" to do this work, or that helping perinatal women in distress feels like a "mission" which they are "compelled" to carry out with great passion. These driving forces have the power to galvanize the therapeutic alliance as well as cloud clinical interpretations. It is imperative that we take a closer look at what drives this work to ensure our work remains unbiased and in the client's best interest.

The cautionary question repeated throughout this book is in what ways does a therapist's individual journey impact this work? Whether you have a baby, want a baby, do not want a baby, lost a baby, are trying to conceive a baby, are planning to adopt, or are experiencing infertility or a perinatal mood and anxiety disorder, any birthing person who has at any point considered the pros and cons of having children needs to understand that these inner dialogues can insidiously and quite unexpectedly find their way smack into the middle of the therapy session. I remain particularly concerned about therapists who are driven to do this work as a direct result of their own personal experiences who may not yet be sufficiently healed from their own strong emotions or disruptive experiences. It feels crucial to me that perinatal therapists who are dedicated to this work make certain they make the time and effort to do their own work to secure their professional readiness.

Here are some preliminary considerations:

1 You may feel ready to do this work before you are ready to do this work. Make an honest appraisal of your own personal experience and the impact it might have on your work.
2 You may already feel like you are holding your clients. Perhaps you are. I suspect you will learn how do to this better after you pay close attention to the client-driven resistances that are getting in the way and the specific skills you will acquire to penetrate those resistances.

3 While understandably inspired, be extra careful if you presume that your personal reproductive journey automatically prepares you to do this work. In many ways, it might. Again, it might also create impossible temptations to share or overshare or misinterpret or make presumptions which can cause you to lose focus. Honor your personal experience, do your private work on your own time, and be especially prudent how you answer personal questions that might request or require too much self-disclosure.

4 Self-disclosure in any psychotherapy process is complicated. We have touched on potential downsides in this particular special area of practice, but clearly new mothers might want to know if you're a mother, or if you had postpartum depression, or if any other life experiences predispose you in some way to better understand their circumstance. This requires a delicate balance between being authentic and not saying too much. Of course, depending on your relationship with your client, you will be the best judge of this but when in doubt, take a breath and resist the impulse to divulge. You cannot take words back and you may have no idea how those words will be heard, interpreted, or perceived.

5 If you experienced a significant clinical mood or anxiety disorder during pregnancy or after the birth of your own baby, this work may become even more provocative. Again, you may believe that this gives you unique insight into her experience, but, of course, her experience is uniquely hers and it takes a great deal of fortitude and self-awareness to keep your experience separate from her narrative. This is what makes this work so meaningful as well as tricky for the well-intended, highly sensitive therapist. Do your work. Get excellent supervision or mentoring. Stay present with your client.

6 Constructive disclosure should be brief, focused on what meaning it has for the client, and shed light on her story.

As professionals we are obligated to continuously monitor our emotions and responses to keep them in check. Only then can we begin to have the objectivity when it comes to the pros and cons of self-disclosure. Managing our emotional regulation skills requires intentional control and balancing our authentic self with our best professional self. What makes our self-reflection distinctive is the possible intersection of personal, reproductively related experiences rendering the therapist highly vulnerable and less objective on a regular basis. Put another way, general populations in therapy do not inevitably raise personal issues for the therapist. That is certainly an occupational hazard, but it is not a given. While there is always a likelihood that aspects of our personal life will intersect with our client's story, our work with the perinatal population imposes a more consistent and likely parallel experience.

So then how best do we protect ourselves and our clients during this very personal, very sensitive, co-journey of perinatal mental wellness? One way is by applying holding techniques. You will learn in Chapter 6 that these techniques provide tools for keeping ourselves in check while we focus on tuning into our client. By doing so, we create a safe and attuned connection.

Does a Woman with Postpartum Depression and Anxiety Need a Therapist Who Specializes in the Treatment of Postpartum Depression and Anxiety?

I am often asked this question.

And while it feels less relevant today due to the plethora of perinatal therapists and trainings for all therapists, not only those who wish to specialize in the field, I do believe that it is worth examining.

Thirty-plus years ago, when I first envisioned a postpartum landscape where the presence of a depression and anxiety disorder would be accepted and understood as a very real and serious life crisis, my answer was *no, not necessarily*. I explained that what a woman needs most is a good therapist and second (preferably) someone who specializes in the treatment of women and depression.

I believed this for a very long time.

After decades of digging deep into this work and after coming face to face with private lives and tender stories of loss and transformation, I have reached a different conclusion. The following is a glance at the process that influenced this change of heart:

1 First, I took a look at our referral sources at The Postpartum Stress Center. The majority were initiated by obstetricians and pediatricians. Few referrals came from primary care physicians (unless they were especially attuned to this population or had been trained [scolded] by me directly). Some referrals came from childbirth-related disciplines, such as midwives, birth centers, breastfeeding groups, doulas, and hospital-based behavioral health programs, for example.

   I found it noteworthy that we rarely received referrals from other therapists, such as private practice family therapists or local psychologists/ social workers, or group practices. Are they working with women with postpartum depression and missing it? Or are they treating it? Did therapists who treat couples notice if a couple in therapy for marriage issues has a 5-month-old baby? Were therapists considering the possibility that, in addition to being exhausted and irritable, there might be other issues to consider? Are either of the two partners depressed, for example? Could the depression contribute to the discontent in the marriage, either by provoking or resulting from it? And, if so, how is this being treated?

I can hear the outrage now: *I've been a therapist for over 25 years! I'm pretty sure I know how to treat a woman with postpartum depression.* This may be perfectly true. After all, the definition of postpartum depression is the presence of clinical depression during the first postpartum year. It follows, therefore, that any good therapist, whether or not he or she has expert training, should be able to successfully treat postpartum depression.

Right?

Perhaps. Perhaps not.

2 Why was I seeing so many women come to our Center *after* they had a disappointing session with a previous clinician? Or two. Or more.

So I asked my clients:

Why did you feel you needed to leave your previous therapist? What did you feel was missing?

Their individual answers resounded with comparable disappointments:

"I didn't feel like she understood."

"They told me this was the best time of my life. That didn't help."

"I didn't feel like she realized having a baby had anything to do with the way I was feeling."

"I felt patronized. I was told I should just relax and enjoy myself and everything would work itself out."

"My first therapist told me I should start each morning with a bowl of oatmeal and never spend the day in sweatpants."

"I don't think he had any idea how bad I was really feeling."

"The therapist said I was fine. I was not fine."

The theme I heard repeatedly was that women felt misunderstood, even by very accomplished, seasoned therapists.

3 What was it that some of these therapists were missing? What is it that postpartum women need from a therapist when they are in crisis?

4 If we know that the combination of therapy and medication continues to be the first line of treatment for postpartum depression and anxiety and women get better as a result of that combination, why and when would they need more than that? Why isn't that sufficient for healing?

5 Did it or did it not really matter if a therapist had special training in, a comprehensive understanding of, or a personal experience with postpartum depression and anxiety? The unexpected conclusion I came to was: *It does matter.*

Women who seek help from therapists who do not specialize in this unique field of study/treatment can, and certainly do, get better. Still, women who receive help from therapists who have received specialized training, who have cultivated a deeper understanding of the impact postpartum depression and anxiety can have on a family, who have developed the precise skills to connect within the gravity of postpartum perplexities, well, they get better, *better*.

Foundational Concepts

While a strong desire to specialize in the treatment of perinatal mood and anxiety disorders is an important first step, it is a first step that is often characterized by intention, motivation, and inspiration, all admirable qualities. It is not, however, enough for the woman in distress sitting in front of you. Specialized training is a necessary next step in this process.

What Is Meant by "Specialized Training"?

1   Attend one or many continuing education program(s) from well-known and reliable training organizations dedicated to the treatment of perinatal mental health. A one-hour presentation as part of a general conference on maternal wellness is fine; it is rarely sufficient.
2   Read and study scholarly literature, research, and books on the subject written by experts in the field. Familiarize yourself with emerging self-help materials, such as books directed to moms and families, support programs, and nonprofessional interventions. The more, the better. Information is evolving at lightning speed.
3   Become acquainted with the names and affiliations of top researchers, authors, experts, speakers, and advocates of this distinct field of study. Today, we have access to both essential information and that which is not only unfavorable, but potentially harmful. Learn where you should go, what you should read, and to whom you should listen.
4   Stay connected to the maternal mental health community. Social media and the internet have merit as well as considerable pitfalls. No one disputes the value of communicating with moms directly, as well as staying in contact with the appropriate professional resources. Although this does not qualify as specialized training, it can supplement the information you have and keep you up to date with burgeoning needs and issues. Be discerning when gathering information originating from these resources.
5   Familiarize yourself with current political, legislative, medical, and psychotherapeutic campaigns and recommendations. Consider how much or how little energy you wish to invest in these movements toward improved awareness and protocols and how much direct relevance they have to the work that you do.

Can a therapist achieve a specialty in this area *without* participating in any formal, structured training program? I did, but I wouldn't recommend that today. Numerous excellent training opportunities are available in person, live online, and recorded as webinars. Decades ago when no such training was available, I listened intently to the voices of women who revealed to me, hour after clinical hour, what they needed. Times were different then; there were fewer advocates and far less awareness. Years later, some things have not changed. Becoming a specialist still requires a commitment and loyalty to this work and a hunger for all that is related to this population. It means reading, talking, researching, studying, and most importantly listening. Let your clients tell you what they need from you. Listen to what is being said. *Listen to what is not being said.* And yes, find a specialized training program that will help you synthesize previous and current research as well as expand your knowledge base and refine your clinical skills. Any therapist who aspires to specialize in this field should make certain they have access to the current best practices.

If we agree that a) there are exceptional attributes attached to the postpartum period, b) this is a time when women are most at risk for mental health issues, and c) there are distinct and complex biopsychosocial factors affecting the postpartum period, are we not obliged to take a closer look at how clinicians are treating women with perinatal mood and anxiety disorders? Shouldn't we be confident beyond any doubt that all clinicians who work directly with this population are equipped to meet the needs of each woman who presents in crisis?

I believe so.

Definitions and Conflations

It is important to pause in order to present definitions that will ensure everyone reading this book is informed with fundamental terms. At the time of this writing, it is estimated that one in seven women will experience symptoms of perinatal depression, anxiety, or other perinatal mood disorders. The incidence of these disorders is increasing, particularly in lower socioeconomic status communities and among non-Hispanic Black, Hispanic, Asian/Pacific Islander, and American Indian/Alaska Native mothers (McKee et al., 2020). If left untreated, postpartum depression can develop into severe and chronic clinical depression and, in tragic cases, it can lead to suicide. Suicide continues to be a leading cause of death in perinatal women (Chin et al., 2022).

The extent to which misinformation continues to be widespread within the healthcare community is alarming. This is said with no disrespect to dedicated providers and institutions working tirelessly to establish suitable, evidenced-based interventions. The pressure to pack patients into crowded medical-setting schedules is at an all-time high, and chat time during an office visit is severely limited. Unfortunately, the needs of post-partum women continue to fall through the cracks, as first mentioned in *This Isn't What I Expected* (Kleiman & Raskin, 1994), three decades ago. Why are so many of us in this field repeating the same discourse over and over again?

Here is the crux of our outrage: In *This Isn't What I Expected*, Karen and co-author Dr. Valerie Raskin Davis outlined the differences between postpartum depression and the baby blues. Some are subtle differences, as symptoms of postpartum depression can overlap with the early postpartum days. However, some parameters of the established definitions are not so vague. For example, baby blues is a mild and transient phenomenon that is characterized by feeling weepy, sad, forgetful, overwhelmed, emotional, anxious, and fatigued. The blues typically occur within the first postpartum days and can last a few days to a couple of weeks. Although reports of this phenomenon date back to the late nineteenth century, it was Brice Pitt (1973) who coined the term "Maternity Blues" in the 1970s, noting that the syndrome was organically driven and most likely a temporary imbalance between the hormones estrogen and progesterone.

While baby blues are recognized as a normal result of giving birth, experiencing baby blues is a risk factor for the development of perinatal depression (Tosto et al., 2023). Because the prevalence of the blues is so high, many providers normalize these symptoms in response to patients who present with tearfulness, exhaustion, and persistent sadness well beyond the first few weeks postpartum. Shockingly, women who are well into the first postpartum year still report being told by their healthcare provider, *Oh, you'll feel better. This is normal. It's just the blues.*

It is acknowledged and well supported in the literature that the time frame for baby blues is immediately following birth up to 2–3 weeks post-partum. After that period, if symptoms that resemble the blues persist, it is best practice to assess for the presence of depression. Still, blatant misinter-pretations of this definition persist with a resounding lack of clarity over what appears to be a straightforward designation.

To be clear:

- If a woman complains of symptoms that bear a resemblance to the blues and she is beyond the 3-week post-delivery period, it is not the blues.
- If this woman is mistakenly told she has the blues by a provider, she is being a) misinformed, b) patronized, c) dismissed, d) treated by a mis-guided provider, and e) put at risk for a continuing, untreated depres-sion or other mood or anxiety disorder.

Let's do what we need to do to make sure everyone in a helping position understands this.

Many new mothers are so overwhelmed and confused by the way they feel, it is difficult for them to know when they need help. It can be equally unclear to health professionals who are trying to sort out what symptoms may be a concern from those that may resolve in due course. Women are told to bring their concerns to their providers' attention, but as we have seen, even the most informed healthcare practitioner may not attribute these feelings to postpartum depression and may mistakenly presume her symptoms go with the territory of adjusting to motherhood. This mistake in judgment can be very costly. Although healthcare practitioners may be uncomfortable with the idea that their postpartum patients with depression and anxiety are at high risk for suicide, it is critical that providers determine the safety of each postpartum woman by asking if she is having any thoughts about hurting herself or dying or if it feels like life is not worth living. Inquiring about suicidal thoughts will help keep her safe and let her know she is in the hands of a provider who understands the seriousness of how she is feeling.

What Is Normal?

Pre-existing or new-onset medical conditions can confound a diagnosis during the postpartum period. For example, it is well known that extreme fatigue can mimic depression symptoms, such as low energy, decreased appetite, and impaired sleep. Physiologic causes could include thyroid disorders, anemia, chronic fatigue syndrome, and infections (Mayo Clinic Staff, 2023). Postpartum thyroiditis, which occurs in 5% of patients (Naji Rad & Deluxe, 2023), can mimic symptoms of postpartum depression and affect the response to therapies (Epp et al., 2021). Significant weight changes could also be a signal of a medical condition such as diabetes or hypothyroidism. Careful medical history taking and relevant laboratory testing by the healthcare provider are essential. Whenever behavioral or physiologic changes are noted, particularly by others, immediate attention should be placed on the well-being of the mother to determine what factors could possibly be contributing to those changes.

Mood and Anxiety Disorders: Diagnostic Tips

Women who have recently given birth who are experiencing distress over a period of time want answers. They want information and they want relief. Our culture has made it difficult for women to step up and ask for help and the medical community continues to tiptoe around diagnoses for fear of labeling and reinforcing the stigma. Nonetheless, many women tell us they want to better understand what they are going through. Medical providers could push this movement forward by having direct discussions with their patients about possible diagnoses and referring every single postpartum woman to local resources for support.

When considering classification or diagnosis, the term *postpartum depression* is still used, particularly in academic literature, as an umbrella term that encompasses several mood and anxiety illnesses that follow childbirth. At the same time, as noted previously, many experts now use the term *perinatal mood and anxiety disorders*, or *PMADs*. Due to some similarities in symptom presentation, it may be helpful from the outset to note some of the distinguishing features in order to secure your foundation of diagnostic knowledge.

- *What are the baby blues?*
  Baby blues are considered a common feature of postpartum adjustment. The blues are understood to be related to hormonal shifts following delivery, affecting 80% of new mothers (Balaram & Marwaha, 2022; Henshaw, 2003). Transient periods of sadness alternating with joy are typical. Other manifestations are frequent crying, anxiety, fatigue, and irritability. The blues are self-limiting and require no treatment. Symptoms generally appear within 3–4 days after delivery, peak on day 7 postpartum, and remit spontaneously within 2–3 weeks. For most women the blues are uneventful and fleeting. There is, however, evidence that suggests women who experience the blues are at risk for postpartum depression (Balaram & Marwaha, 2022).
  Differential Diagnosis Tip: If emotional vulnerability lasts beyond 2–3 weeks postpartum, it is not the blues. The blues do not typically interfere with maternal functioning. Severe, incapacitating symptoms that manifest within the first few weeks are indicative of a more serious postpartum illness.
- *What is postpartum stress syndrome?*
  Postpartum stress syndrome (Kleiman & Raskin, 2013, 2nd ed.) refers to an adjustment disorder specific to the postpartum period that falls between baby blues and postpartum depression. Postpartum stress syndrome is characterized by persistent low levels of distress that do not resolve with reassurance or self-help measures. Women describe having a hard time getting through their day (though they continue to function relatively well) and report going through the motions of caring for their baby and profess feelings of deep love and attachment. Women may feel consumed by feelings of anxiety and self-doubt and feel pressure during this major life transition from external stressors or internal pressure to be the perfect mother who is in control at all times. They frequently feel guilty and duplicitous as if they are imposters who are getting away with faking it and no one really knows how bad they feel. If left unsupported, postpartum stress syndrome can make a woman more susceptible to postpartum depression.
  Differential Diagnosis Tip: Symptoms of stress and feeling overwhelmed are pervasive but do not meet diagnostic criteria for a major

depressive episode or anxiety disorder and do not require treatment beyond professional or non-professional supportive interventions. Postpartum stress syndrome may be identified clinically as an adjustment disorder with or without anxious and/or depressive features.

- *What is postpartum depression?*
Postpartum depression, one of the most common complications of childbirth, is a major depressive disorder and typically occurs within 1 month to 1 year after delivery. Postpartum depression, while common and very treatable, can be severe and incapacitating for some women. Early-onset postpartum depression can present with symptoms similar to baby blues; however, symptoms of depression are more disruptive and persist beyond the first 2 weeks after delivery. It is characterized by a depressed mood most of the day nearly every day. To an untrained eye, symptoms of postpartum depression can be difficult to distinguish from "normal" postpartum conditions associated with being a new mother. Symptoms might include insomnia; significant change in appetite; moderate-to-severe anxiety with scary, ego-dystonic obsessive thoughts of harm coming to the infant; weepiness; feelings of inadequacy; irritability; anger; hopelessness; suicidal thoughts; difficulty functioning; difficulty concentrating; and loss of pleasure. It should be noted that a high number of women report feeling depressed and anxious during pregnancy, which is now believed to be a powerful factor in predicting postpartum depression.

It is worth noting that the risk of postpartum depression to birthing parents, their infants, and their families has increased since COVID-19 and the rate of perinatal mood and anxiety disorders rose significantly during the pandemic (Bajaj et al., 2022). These statistics make it imperative that all medical and mental health providers be aware of current best practices for screening and treatment options so the huge number of women at risk get the help they need (Usmani et al., 2021).

Differential Diagnosis Tip: Symptoms meet diagnostic criteria for a major depressive episode. It is worth repeating that one defining diagnostic criterion is that the symptoms fall outside the 2–3 week postdelivery time frame. A feature that can distinguish postpartum depression from other depressive disorders is that it is often marked by prominent and pervasive anxiety. It is not uncommon for women with postpartum depression to have comorbid symptoms such as panic attacks, obsessions, compulsions, or even psychotic features.

- *What is postpartum anxiety?*
Postpartum anxiety is comparable to generalized anxiety disorder, or GAD, which is marked by excessive worry.[1] It is often diagnosed as a result of the degree to which it interferes with a woman's ability to

function and how much distress her symptoms cause her. Women with postpartum anxiety report feeling tense and irritable, nervous in social situations, feelings of pending doom, and preoccupied with uncontrollable worries related to the physical well-being of self and other, particularly the baby. Frequently, there is an increase in attention to physical symptoms such as nausea, shakiness, insomnia, fatigue, restlessness, racing heart, and shortness of breath.

Differential Diagnosis Tip: Although some worry is normal, women with generalized anxiety experience excessive, uncontrollable worry more of the time than not. This experience of worry is pervasive and associated with emotional distress.

- *What is postpartum obsessive-compulsive disorder?*

Postpartum obsessive-compulsive disorder, or OCD, is an anxiety disorder characterized by obsessive, intrusive thoughts, images, or urges that are accompanied by compulsive activities or mental actions. Intrusive, unwanted thoughts characteristic of OCD may be triggered by a stimulus or may appear "out of nowhere." Either way, they are highly distressing. Compulsions may present as outward, such as repeatedly checking the baby to alleviate anxiety about whether the baby has stopped breathing, or internal, such as saying a prayer a certain number of times in a row to alleviate this anxiety. Women with postpartum OCD report feeling overwhelmed by anxiety and depression. Estimates vary, but OCD is reported to affect about 3–7% of pregnant or postpartum women (Pereira et al., 2022).

In postpartum OCD, it is common for mothers to experience intrusive thoughts associated with their baby and that involve very scary or graphic content (Fairbrother & Abramowitz, 2007). Mothers with OCD may imagine themselves dropping the baby down the stairs accidentally or even intentionally hurting the baby. These mothers may fear being alone with the baby and may avoid certain activities that trigger scary thoughts, such as bathing the baby or picking up kitchen utensils. Typically these mothers fear themselves and experience thoughts like "I must be a horrible mother to have thoughts like these" or "I must be a danger to my baby and should stay away."

What distinguishes these mothers from mothers with psychosis driven intrusive thoughts is a clear awareness that any actions taken in response to these thoughts would endanger their babies, a recognition that causes extreme agitation for mothers. Reassuringly, research shows there is no correlation between negative intrusive thoughts and women taking action in response to these thoughts and that despite this upsetting symptom their infants are not at an increased risk for harm (Collardeau et al., 2019) This is a crucial piece of psychoeducation that may need to be repeated and repeated to a mother in high distress.

With postpartum OCD, obsessions typically focus on the baby. There may be ego-dystonic obsessive thoughts about the baby getting hurt, contaminated, sick, stolen, lost, or dying. Thoughts or images that are particularly disturbing to a mother involve obsessions that are sexual in nature. Women may be extremely reluctant to share their obsessive thoughts or images with others, even those closest to them for many reasons, including fear they are psychotic, will be hospitalized, or have their baby taken away.

Differential Diagnosis Tip: The boundary between excessive worry and obsessive thinking can be indistinct. The diagnosis of OCD is made based on the intrusive thoughts that are accompanied by compulsions. Postpartum OCD is characterized by a swift onset, as contrasted with typical OCD, which tends to manifest gradually (Forray et al., 2010). Postpartum OCD can be confused with postpartum psychosis, as both might involve thoughts about harming the infant. Women with OCD are terrified of their thoughts and images and try to avoid the thoughts or make them go away. The ego-dystonic nature of these thoughts is characteristic of OCD. Women with psychosis believe their hallucinations and delusions to be reality.

- *What is postpartum posttraumatic stress disorder?*
Postpartum posttraumatic stress disorder, or PTSD, may occur following a threat of death, serious injury, or sexual violence to the mother, her infant, or someone close to her. Women with PTSD experience intrusions such as nightmares or flashbacks, avoidance of triggers or reminders of the traumatic event, changes in thoughts and mood like increased anger or fear, and changes in arousal and reactivity, difficulty sleeping and/or concentrating, helplessness, and/or a sense that they may lose control (American Psychiatric Association, 2022).

Examples of traumas that can lead to PTSD after childbirth are history of previous PTSD or trauma, birth trauma related to medical complications or injury, birth loss, and neonatal intensive care unit (NICU) experience. For women with histories of abuse, the pain and perceptions of helplessness associated with childbirth can cause women to re-experience the original trauma. An important note of clarification here is that anxiety and trauma attached to the event are contingent upon the mother's perception of whether or not a trauma affected her.

It is estimated that 9% of birthing women are diagnosed with PTSD (Akik & Batigun, 2020). More women will experience posttraumatic stress symptoms, or subclinical levels of posttraumatic stress (Heyne et al., 2022).

Differential Diagnosis Tip: Though intrusive memories of the trauma are key to a clinical presentation of PTSD, the majority of people who experience traumatic events do not meet full diagnostic criteria for

PTSD (Kendall-Tackett, 2014), but may experience anxiety and depression that features some of the symptoms of PTSD.

- *What is postpartum panic disorder?*
Postpartum panic disorder is an anxiety disorder that manifests as distinct periods of intense fear and typically involves physical symptoms such as palpitations, sweating, claustrophobia, chest pain, shortness of breath, dizziness, lightheadedness, numbness, and a fear of dying and losing control. Most of the time, panic involves a catastrophic misinterpretation of bodily sensations. Women state that symptoms of panic sometimes wake them up, and they frequently report no identifiable trigger.

  Differential Diagnosis Tip: With GAD, many women hyperfocus on the object of their worry. With panic, women tend to become preoccupied with the panic itself; they fear having a panic attack and may change their behavior due to their fear of having an attack. Mothers with primary panic disorder may or may not describe a depressed mood.

- *What is postpartum bipolar disorder?*
Childbirth is a strong trigger for mood and psychotic episodes in women who have bipolar disorder. Bipolar disorder during the postpartum period is characterized by periods of extreme highs (mania) and lows (depression). There may be need for less sleep, heightened irritability, more energy than usual, evidence of poor judgment, grandiosity, delusions, overconfidence, racing thoughts, pressured speech, and hypersexuality. Any irregular response to the initiation of antidepressants, including treatment-emergent mania, hypomania, or unusually rapid or poor response, should be reported to the patient's psychiatrist for immediate follow-up. It is essential that providers take a careful history of mood, sleep, and activity levels and inquire about the history of bipolar disorder or psychosis in a close relative.

  Bipolar I is primarily distinguished by the presence of *manic* episodes, whereas bipolar II is characterized by *hypomanic* episodes. Although postpartum hypomania, which is a persistent elevated or irritable mood, may not be associated with major impairment in functioning, it is common for it to be linked with a subsequent, significant depression. Bipolar II disorder may be misdiagnosed as major depression if hypomanic episodes go unrecognized or unreported.

  Women with a history or family history of bipolar disorder are at an increased risk of experiencing an episode during pregnancy and postpartum and should be carefully monitored. Present symptoms of bipolar disorder or a history of bipolar symptoms also increase a woman's risk for postpartum psychosis.

  Differential Diagnosis Tip: A woman with a bipolar I diagnosis may also have hypomanic episodes, but a woman with bipolar II cannot ever have had a manic episode. If a woman diagnosed with bipolar II experiences a manic episode, her diagnosis will change. Misdiagnosis of postpartum depression is more likely in cases of bipolar II because symptoms may be more subtle than bipolar I. Understandably, it may be difficult to differentiate normal postpartum elation from abnormal mood elevation. This is why screening is so important. Women should be asked if they feel as if their mind is racing or if they have an unusual increase in energy despite a lack of sleep. They should be asked if they feel a decreased need for sleep or have experienced an abnormal surge of goal-directed energy, such as cleaning in the middle of the night, or if they are spending more money than usual, or if they are feeling hypersexual.

- *What is postpartum psychosis?*
Postpartum psychosis is the least common, most serious, and least understood postpartum psychiatric illness. Symptoms of postpartum psychosis are distinctive and unique from other primary psychoses. The onset is typically abrupt, occurs within the first 2–3 weeks postpartum and affects 1–2 per 1,000 (0.1% to 0.2%) of postpartum women. The presence of psychotic symptoms, such as delusions and/or hallucinations (often involving the infant), avoidance of the infant, loss of touch with reality, extreme agitation, confusion, disorganized thinking, inability to sleep for several nights, significant irritability, racing thoughts, rapid speech, rapid mood swings, and paranoia with suicidal and/or infanticidal thoughts, necessitates immediate medical treatment and hospitalization.

Psychosis is strongly associated with bipolar disorder; therefore, women with a personal or family history of bipolar disorder should be carefully assessed. Contrary to women with OCD, women suffering from psychosis are at an increased risk to act on their delusional thoughts due to their disorientation and disconnect from reality. Despite its severity, with early intervention and professional support, the overall prognosis for most women who experience postpartum psychosis is good.

Differential Diagnosis Tip: The clinical presentation of postpartum psychosis is abrupt and usually occurs soon after childbirth. Severe presentations of OCD, anxiety, or depression may be considered, but be mindful of any symptoms of psychosis or bipolar disorder as well as any personal or family history of psychosis or bipolar disorder. Bear in mind that unwanted, intrusive, scary thoughts, which are common in postpartum anxiety, depression, and OCD, are anxiety driven and perceived as inconsistent with a woman's view of herself. In psychosis, these thoughts are rooted in symptoms and manifest as hallucinations (seeing bugs crawling on the baby's skin) and/or delusions (*My baby is not safe, someone is coming after him*).

Women at Risk

There is substantial evidence that maternal depression and subsequent poor maternal–infant interactions adversely affect the developing child. This is why healthcare providers, therapists, partners, parents, siblings, or friends must all work together to make sure each postpartum woman who experiences significant distress gets the support and treatment she needs. Given the inconsistent information and unpredictable support she might receive, we should not be surprised by her confusion. When she walks into our offices, we must make certain she knows she is in the right place and she will receive the appropriate care she needs and deserves.

The factors that contribute to postpartum mood and anxiety disorders are currently the subject of debate. What we do know is that there is no single cause. Most studies point to hormonal fluctuations, biologic and genetic vulnerability, and psychosocial stressors as the largest contributors. Still, the specific etiology remains unclear. The stress of pregnancy, childbirth, and the postpartum period are enough, in some cases, to make a woman vulnerable even in the absence of any predisposing or confounding factors.

Experts agree numerous theories combine to help us understand the nature of postpartum distress. To mention briefly, the medical or biological model confirms that hormonal changes during pregnancy, childbirth, and the postpartum period, in addition to the neurotransmitter fluctuations, contribute to the emergence of mood and anxiety disorders. Lazarus and Folkman's (1984) stress and coping model gave rise to the understanding that stressful events that occur following childbirth and the way they are interpreted may contribute to depression after delivery. Additionally, how women cognitively appraise these events and the availability of social support are extremely pertinent to this picture. Also, the feminist model suggests that the postpartum mood changes, including negative ones, are normal affective responses to the complicated physical and emotional changes and profound losses women endure. Nicolson (2001) believes that our attempt to label the feelings of a new mother as depression pathologizes what she deems a "normal and rational reaction to what is happening" (p. 27).

While the literature is mixed regarding some variables associated with postpartum depression (e.g. sex of the infant), the list below highlights those factors which have been well-established in the literature as strong predictors of postpartum depression (Beck, 2001; Bradshaw et al., 2021; Guintivano et al., 2018).

- History of prenatal or postpartum depression or anxiety
- History of depression or anxiety not related to childbirth
- Family history of depression or anxiety

- Social support
- Environmental stressors
- Marital dissatisfaction

Additional risk factors are current depressive symptoms during pregnancy, low self-esteem, infant temperament, childcare stress, and obstetrical complications. Ideally, contributing factors should be ascertained during pregnancy, as potential risk factors and women identified at risk should be followed closely, both in your clinical practice and by her medical provider. It is prudent for therapists to regard all factors and interpretations when considering the distress of any single postpartum woman.

As mentioned, postpartum depression is best thought of as having multiple contributing factors. Consequently, even in women who are more susceptible to hormonal changes or are genetically predisposed, the role of environmental or psychological stressors in the development of the illness should not be overlooked. In some cases, you can flush out probable risk factors and better understand what has made her susceptible to depression. In other cases, you are left to share her dismay that there is no obvious cause or explanation. Inadequate treatment of postpartum depression and anxiety puts women at risk for chronic, recurrent, and/or refractory depression.

While we are often left in a position to disappoint our client with few precise and acceptable answers to the universal question: *Why am I feeling this way? Or, what made this happen to me?* – even so, our understanding and exploration of her risk factors enables us to better understand her vulnerabilities which can help put her experience into context. It is incumbent upon all dedicated postpartum therapists to review the multitude of factors that put each woman at risk and incorporate them into our understanding of the woman who sits before us. In doing so, you create an environment that welcomes and respects her unique experience as you set the stage for holding.

Note

1 For an extensive discussion on postpartum anxiety, see *Dropping the Baby and Other Scary Thoughts* (Kleiman et al., 2020).

Chapter 3

Theories Behind the Concept

When Winnicott teaches us, "It appalls me to think how much deep change I have prevented or delayed in patients, by my own personal need to interpret" (Winnicott, 1969, p. 711) – he reminds us to wait. To sit. To listen. When I am otherwise tempted to fix, to hurry, to rescue. Ah, but that is the problem. Many of us were taught in graduate school to settle back in reflection and allow the client to inform us; in time, they will express what they need and what they know to be true in order to repair the hole in their soul. However, this is where traditional therapy and holding postpartum women in distress come to a crossroad.

The postpartum period, by definition, obliges us to consider the abundance of biopsychosocial influences that bombard each woman, whether or not she is or becomes depressed or anxious. Having a baby is a game changer for both the mother and her therapist. It shifts the therapeutic process into high gear. Sitting back and focusing on active listening techniques may be appropriate for a time, but her symptoms are likely to dictate a rapid assessment strategy. Because symptoms can feel like life or death to her, you do not have the luxury of time when an agitated mother of a newborn gasps for air and cries for help.

Theoretical Orientation and Options May Matter, May Not

A postpartum woman who – willingly or under duress from others – arrives at a therapist's office, is not necessarily in the mood for therapy. She may want help. And she most certainly wants to feel better. She may appreciate the value of therapy, perhaps in less pressing circumstances. Still, a woman who recently had a baby is preoccupied with distractions that take priority over making time to meet with a therapist. Holding a postpartum woman when therapy may be the last place she wants to be constitutes one of our greatest therapeutic challenges. She wants answers and she wants them fast. Providing direct answers to her questions is a response that smacks in the face of everything you learned in graduate school: Active listening.

DOI: 10.4324/9781003402145-3

Mirroring. Reflecting. Interpreting. However valuable these interventions are, *and they are*, they are not always in sync with her restless plea for symptom relief.

Learning how to provide her with the answers she seeks along with skilled management of her symptoms while mastering the holding environment can challenge any therapist. As you sit and listen carefully you prepare to respond with repetitive and consistent words of support at regular intervals. Her quest for immediate and unwavering relief is often apparent. You tune into and evaluate her distress and at a rapid pace, hoping your presence, your training, your preparation for this encounter can provide some preliminary comfort. Although each therapist's theoretical foundation will inform their clinical inclinations and actions, it will not preclude successful holding practices. We see early on how our primary holding posture can frame the therapeutic relationship as a safe and encouraging place for her to reclaim her lost self. In the short run, it reassures her that she is in the right place, which may provide immediate comfort. This will become clearer when we delineate the how-to steps through the holding points in Chapter 6.

Homesickness

Although the impact of clinical depression and anxiety is hard to convey objectively, people who have endured the inexplicable pain describe it with eloquence and the powerful truth of their personal experience:

> I don't want to see anyone. I lie in the bedroom with the curtains drawn and nothingness washing over me like a sluggish wave. Whatever is happening to me is my own fault. I have done something wrong, something so huge I can't even see it, something that's drowning me. I am inadequate and stupid, without worth. I might as well be dead.
>
> Margaret Atwood, *Cat's Eye* (1988, p. 408)

> The sun stopped shining for me is all. The whole story is: I am sad. I am sad all the time and the sadness is so heavy that I can't get away from it. Not ever.
>
> Nina LaCour, *Hold Still* (2009, p. 185)

When clinical depression descends during the postpartum period, the anguish burns a hole into everything a new mother thought she knew and thought she wanted. As therapists, we ask ourselves, what can we possibly do with so much pain? How can what we say or do even remotely make a difference? To begin finding answers to this question, we turn our attention to the therapeutic relationship, an exercise that will, and should, challenge our intentions and dedication to this work.

How *can* you effectively help a young mother who is suffocating from self-loathing and agony that others have misunderstood or dismissed as normal or temporary? How *do* you hold the putrid guts that spill into our sacred therapeutic space? What an oxymoron to reflect upon. If you represent the intersection between her desire to disappear and her wish for a return to her previous self, what is your role exactly? Are you simply a vehicle with information and resources? Surely you can help her find the right physician, the right medication, if indicated, and the right support network, if available. But of course, this is not your only role, and this is not her only expectation of you. She looks to you for reassurance that she will feel like herself again and that you can lead her back to herself. This is your greatest task, but how do you do this?

I had not heard of Dianne Connelly when I serendipitously came across her book, *All Sickness Is Home Sickness* (Connelly, 1993). Connelly is an acupuncturist who explores human suffering and healing with poetic elegance. The moment I fell in love with her book was in the early pages when she referenced a beloved book of her children, *Are You My Mother?* by P. D. Eastman. It catapulted me to my own childhood, when I first found myself worrying about the baby bird who, upon breaking out of its egg-womb, begins searching for his mama who had ventured off to find food for her baby. The baby bird calls for his mama. "Where is my mother?" begins the search. Along the way, he finds various animals as well as boats and planes and wonders aloud, "Are you my mother?" "Where am I?" asked the frightened (or so I projected) baby bird. "I want to go home. I want my mother." For years beyond an appropriate age to do so, I would find the most opportune moments to interject that question into any dialogue with my own mother. "Are you my mother?" I would ask, with my best squeaky rendition of my child-self. It always made us giggle.

What Connelly says at this pivotal point is: "Eventually he finds her and in finding her, he is home" (Connelly, 1993, p. 22). Home is an expression she uses to refer to one's whole self and healing. Connelly writes:

Home is the place from which I have come and to which I return. Home is where I always am. All circumstances call me to new steps in the dance. All sickness points me there. All sickness is homesickness. All healing is homecoming. Sharing moves me homeward.

(Connelly, 1993, p. 25)[1]

Symptoms manifest to bring individuals home, Connelly claims.

Symptoms of postpartum depression and anxiety serve to speak on behalf of a silenced mother, to call attention to her helplessness, to call out in support of her vulnerability. "This is the wisdom of illness," Connelly writes, "It is a call to come home to the ground of being." This is where we begin to understand early connectedness and empathy a bit differently than we have been taught in psychology books. If we believe ourselves to be the conduit through which postpartum women can find their way home, back to themselves, we need to recalibrate some of what we've learned and envision ourselves as monitoring a pause in the postpartum chaos. If healing is the process of coming home, per Connelly, and sharing moves a person homeward, then therapy is the ideal context for a postpartum woman in distress to find relief. You represent that space where she can sit and share, without fear of judgment, without shame, and with hope.

When you listen to a postpartum woman in distress, what do you hear? You do not always hear the names of the symptoms, or the problems identified with a clear understanding of what the matter is. Sometimes you hear weeping. Sometimes you hear a frantic cry for help. Sometimes, you hear the soundless throbbing of a weary heart or a surrendered soul who has nothing left to give. You have to sit with palpable sorrow that is, though unexpressed at times, conspicuously crowding her mind, her thoughts, and her desire to sleep forever.

Lessons from Winnicott

When defining the therapeutic process in general, experts refer to support and unconditional acceptance through the creation of a safe and non-judgmental space. Winnicott's concept of the *holding environment* was introduced to describe the biopsychosocial context in which babies are lovingly tended to by their mother or anyone providing primary care to the infant (Winnicott, 1965). Winnicott unveiled the intricate notion of imperfect parenting. He taught us that only through failing in amounts tolerated by the infant (then repairing or compensating for the failures) can mothers offer the best possible care by providing an honest representation of human connection. This idea of adaptation through failure is embodied in his concept of being good enough and encourages the merit of tolerating failure, a crucial lesson integral to our work with perinatal women.

When we apply his concept of the holding environment to our therapeutic practice with postpartum women in distress, we consider his description of the patient and her therapist as moving "from absolute to relative dependence and on to independence" (Winnicott, 1965, p. 65). Though clearly an oversimplification, the therapeutic purpose of the metaphor has the therapist functioning as the good-enough caregiver, containing but not confining her experience as is, with no opinion rendered. This is paramount.

To further explore this metaphor and parallel experience of the infant/mother and client/therapist relationship, let's look at anxiety. According to Winnicott, anxiety in the earliest stages of the parent–infant relationship directly relates to the threat of annihilation (Winnicott, 1956). In Chapter 1, we saw how he uses profoundly descriptive words to describe "unthinkable anxiety" (Winnicott, 1965). His depiction of this as it pertains to infants is striking:

1 Going to pieces
2 Falling forever
3 Having no relationship to the body
4 Having no orientation

Postpartum women in distress often experience these same or similar sensations. For example, severe anxiety can be associated with feelings of dissociation from self and body, and this experience for a woman with an infant to care for can feel impossible to tolerate. It can feel immobilizing and ultimately cripple moms who experience it. When symptoms feel unendurable, holding is called upon.

When working with the postpartum population, the holding approach, grounded in wisdom supported by theory, is made accessible by our fundamental understanding of the vulnerability of the postpartum period. Thus, you respond with attention to the raw emotion and unique neediness of the new mother as a mother does to her infant.

Consider the primary elements of Winnicott's concept of holding (infant/mother) and see how closely it resembles the therapeutic relationship (client/therapist):

1 A child is held when the mother is preoccupied ("maternal preoccupation" Winnicott, 1992, p. xxv) with the infant's needs; at first, body needs, but later, ego needs. Preoccupation with the infant creates a mutual space and significant exchange that enables her to consider the impact of her own reactions and emotions on the child. Winnicott refers to this as adaptation to a child's basic needs. I love how he elaborates on this: "and this happens to be something that cannot be done except by a human being" (Winnicott, 2002, p. 52).
2 A child is held when the mother provides mirroring by responding appropriately to the baby's primitive affects (Winnicott, 1967).
3 A child is held when the mother thinks of her baby as a person rather than an extension of herself.

Let's take this one step further. Winnicott says, "The mother is needed as someone who survives each day, who can integrate the various feelings, sensation, excitements, angers, griefs, etc. that go to make up an infant's life but which the infant cannot hold" (Winnicott, 1987b, p. 183). In this environment of holding, Winnicott explains, the child develops the freedom to move from dependence to independence.

Isn't that, essentially, what we are working toward on her behalf?

In Winnicott's holding environment, the mother's ability to meet the emotional needs of her infant is instrumental to her baby's development of a healthy self and, inevitably, his individuation. She responds to his needs, thereby protecting him and reducing initial anxiety. Similarly, when you respond to the primary and urgent needs of postpartum women, you personify Winnicott's good-enough mother. In your therapeutic holding environment, you recognize and respect all that is generously shared within that space. This holding environment for postpartum women is further interpreted as creating a sacred space between who she was before (prior to pregnancy/baby/motherhood), who she thought she would be (fantasies/expectations), who she is now (loss/grief), and who she will be (acceptance/resilience/transformation). This in-between state can feel unsettling and unacceptable. Yet this intermediate stage of being is where you are positioned to help her carry her pain, and in doing so, give rise to an early whisper of hope and recovery.

Do not forget that postpartum women in distress may not present for therapy (predominantly) seeking help for, as examples, social anxiety, low self-esteem, career disappointment, dysfunctional family-of-origin issues, or any number of presenting problems that might propel non-postpartum individuals into therapy. Although these and other issues might factor into her current depression and anxiety and play a role in her therapy and recovery, they may not be part of her presenting problem at this time. In the minds of postpartum women, they are coming to therapy because they recently had a baby. Certainly, issues that predate the events of childbirth can be exacerbated by delivery. Regardless of the pre-existing psychodynamic issues or long-standing risk factors, experts agree that the states of pregnancy and the postpartum period make some women more vulnerable than others to experiencing significant distress. In fact, postpartum depression and anxiety are the most common complications of childbirth. We often see women who manage well for many years without interfering symptoms who are then bombarded during the perinatal period with major episodes of depression and anxiety. Whether or not this is a recurrence of depression, an exacerbation of underlying pre-existing symptoms, or the emergence of an original psychiatric event varies on a case-by-case basis.

The current emotional state of a postpartum woman in distress is one that is jarring to her and not at all in harmony with her expectations. It represents irreconcilable discord for her. Trying to talk her out of that will be a waste of breath. This is where many loving family members, friends, or healthcare practitioners slide off course. Their attempt to normalize or minimize the difference between what she expected and what she experiences with an outpouring of platitudes ends up invalidating her suffering and alienating the support efforts.

In Support of Supportive Psychotherapy

Treatment for postpartum depression and anxiety commonly includes psychotherapy, which has shown to be effective for mild-to-moderate depression, and pharmacotherapy, which has shown to be effective for moderate-to-severe postpartum depression. A combination of psychotherapy and medication is considered the first-line treatment option for postpartum depression. Most women with postpartum depression and anxiety prefer psychotherapy over taking medication (Battle et al., 2013; Boath & Henshaw, 2001; Simhi et al., 2019; Whitton, Appleby, & Warner, 1996a, 1996b). Many mothers worry about infant exposure to the medication if they are breastfeeding and the potential for side effects, as well as their personal philosophies toward taking medication in general. Nevertheless, it can be difficult for mothers to follow through with recommendations or referrals to psychotherapy. Research shows that symptoms, personal and social stigma, access to care, and the approach of her healthcare providers all influence mothers' decision making related to follow-up (Canty et al., 2019).

Whether or not medication is used adjunctively, well-established psychotherapies have shown to be effective treatments during the postpartum period with significant decreases in symptoms. Cognitive behavioral therapy (CBT) and interpersonal therapy (IPT) are both well-studied and effective treatments for postpartum depression and postpartum anxiety. Also worth noting is that pregnant women who received CBT treatment were less likely to experience postpartum depression (Sockol, 2015).

IPT is a time-limited treatment for depression, which focuses on the association between interpersonal problems and mood, framing it as a medical illness occurring within a social context. IPT is a manual-based, structured therapy that has proven to be applicable to a wide range of client populations with strong evidence to support its use for the treatment of mild to moderate postpartum depression. Typically, it involves 12 to 16 weeks of therapy in accordance with the IPT manual (Klerman et al., 1984) with accommodations made regarding the postpartum context. Studies show that women who receive IPT treatment experience significant reduction in symptoms of depression and anxiety as well as improved social relationships and systems (Bright et al., 2020). New parents seeking therapy together can benefit from participation in couples-based IPT, a treatment approach that can result in significant reduction in depressive symptoms of both partners and improved relationship quality (Ngai & Gao, 2022).

CBT is another short-term, well-studied treatment for major depression. It is based on the notion that thinking and behavioral patterns are linked to one's mood. CBT focuses on modifying distorted patterns of negative thinking and making behavioral changes that improve coping skills while reducing stress levels. Evidence has shown CBT interventions result in significant reductions in symptoms in postpartum depression and anxiety (Li et al., 2022). In our book, *Cognitive Behavioral Therapy and Perinatal Distress* (Wenzel & Kleiman, 2014), Amy Wenzel and I adapted a CBT protocol to be more postpartum friendly, noting that homework and logs are not always easy to incorporate into a new mother's schedule.

One challenge with CBT is that it relies on the left brain, which focuses on rational cognition (Field, 2014). If arousal is too high, emotions take over and executive functioning can weaken or shut down. When that happens, the cognition we depend on to regulate high states of anxiety may be more difficult to access. While the neuroscience is fascinating and regardless of our theoretical predilections, our job is to balance these dynamics, assess and sit with her current mental and emotional state, and engage accordingly. The premise of this current book is largely based on the principles of supportive psychotherapy, which is a conversation-based, unstructured, strengths-oriented, and non-manualized therapy that relies on a strong therapeutic alliance (Grover et al., 2020). The practice of supportive psychotherapy focuses on helping clients adapt to their current circumstances via the processing of internal and external barriers to achieving this goal (Appelbaum, 2005). This book applies tenants of supportive psychotherapy specifically to treatment of postpartum women, taking into account the theoretical concept of Holding and clinical pearls collected over decades of work with both pregnant and postpartum clients (Kleiman, 2009; Kleiman & Waller, 2023; Kleiman & Wenzel, 2017; Winnicott, 1987a).

If you do an online search for supportive psychotherapy as a treatment for postpartum depression, peer reviewed, academic references are sparse. Short of having rigorous data to satisfy the scholarly community, the question that is woven within the pages of this book is this:

> Once a postpartum woman makes the difficult decision to enter the therapeutic alliance, can she expect to achieve the positive outcome of relief and recovery as a result of the supportive psychotherapeutic relationship and interventions?

Although we have an impressive collection of evidence-based support for the use of IPT for the treatment of postpartum depression and tons of rigorous research on the efficacy of CBT for the treatment of depression and anxiety in general, the majority of mental health therapists in the perinatal community do not rely solely on these two interventions. Many therapists who treat postpartum mood and anxiety disorders refer to their theoretical foundation as "eclectic," borrowing salient principles from both IPT and

CBT manuals, which are then infused with a fondness for supportive psychotherapeutic practice. This leaves our profession with a therapeutic conundrum. Even though there are sufficient data to strongly support the use of IPT and CBT for perinatal depression, and far less attention to supportive psychotherapy in the academic literature, it appears that most therapists who practice in this field lean heavily on supportive psychotherapy.

Although it may be desirable for the academic community to seek evidence-based protocols by means of randomized controlled trials and statistically significant differences, those variables appear less relevant to those of us on the front line. The constructs of supportive psychotherapy are not easy to operationally define. It is difficult to analyze and evaluate the experience of giving and receiving emotional and psychological support. It is similarly difficult to measure a construct such as holding. We must consider then whether these empirical challenges render the concepts less valid? If we do not have robust studies to tell us something is true, is it less true? Can we, ultimately, uphold the power of the individual and thereby endorse the experience as legitimate, with or without the support of evidenced-based inspection?

As you continue to explore the nature and application of the holding approach, consider the possibility that you may (and probably should) choose to incorporate elements of IPT and CBT into your work, if you are not already doing so. The integration of more than one therapeutic approach seems reasonable and appropriate. Therapists who have classic CBT training, for example, may find harmony between that orientation and the supportive nature of holding points, which will be elucidated in subsequent chapters. There are strengths in many theoretical frameworks from which we all draw. Consider this carefully as you move forward through the following chapters and begin to exercise or enhance your holding skills. The bottom line is that it may not matter which therapy is most effective; rather, achieving a healing experience may hinge upon which therapeutic intervention you are most comfortable with and feel most confident engaging in.

Narrative Influences: Her Story

Postpartum women have elaborate stories to tell, sometimes with few words.

Narrative therapy, developed by Australian therapist Michael White, encourages therapists to take a collaborative, listening approach, as therapists should always do, and to view the client as the author of their own unique history, separate from cultural narratives that may have been imposed upon them. As White defines it, "The person is never the problem. The problem is the problem" (White, 1997).

Yes. This makes perfect sense in our work.

Narrative therapy is first and foremost about *de-centering* the therapist (Morgan, 2000). This means that although the therapist is always influential, there is less emphasis on advice giving, resolutions, or opinions. In fact, there is a clear de-emphasis on the therapist as an expert or one in a position of authority. Maintaining this collaborative stance encourages clients to "become the primary authors of their lives" (Morgan, 2002, p. 86). Narrative therapy puts the client's perspective, desires, hopes, and expectations at the center of the process to increase personal agency and understanding about the self.

The Art of Holding Perinatal Women in Distress honors each woman's unique history, struggle, viewpoint, and personal resources, as well as her compelling need for immediate relief. While her journey must guide the course of her treatment, she looks to you for answers. Though therapy is not designed to give simple answers to complex questions, trust and rapport can be established by presenting yourself as someone who will help her find answers. If you fail to convey this important message, she may decide not to come back. Presenting yourself as an authority in this context does not mean you speak instead of listen. Nor does it mean you should have the final word on what transpires in the session. Being the expert entails an intricate balance between believing you can help her feel better and listening to her story. As you listen with an impartial ear, you are careful to contain any emotional response you may notice resulting from your own desire for a quick fix. You resume a state of calm presence. You must simply *be there*. It is not simple, of course, but that is what you do, or learn to do.

Be There

Your ability to be present, with confidence and caring, whether or not words are spoken or "work" is being done, is central to the concept of holding. Consider this notion of *being there* as presented to a new father, for example:

> Sometimes, the best thing you can do for someone who is suffering is just to *be there*. His hesitation is a reasonable retort to such a seemingly ambiguous statement and very loving husbands are often left feeling as though they speak another language with absolutely no comprehension of what it means to just *be there*. A new father, who is trying his best to support his wife, may respond with, "What do you mean, I should just 'be there' with her? What do you want me to do?"

The concept of *being there* is vague and hard for many partners to grasp. You coach a partner by saying *sit close, without judging, without words.*

Do not try to fix it. Be yourself, be present, be there. This is often met with a resounding "huh?" but in time, most partners do develop impressive skills in the face of depression and anxiety and learn how to faithfully attend to the needs of their depressed partner. The command of the moment that a partner emanates when they are able to *be there* mimics the command that a well-trained postpartum therapist embodies. This strength is conveyed through a belief in the relationship, in the expertise, in the communicated conviction that somehow things will be tended to and contained.

As her therapist, your ability to sit with, listen to, and shelter the turbulent insides of a perinatal woman in distress is a prerequisite for holding, and when accepted by the client, will endorse the relationship and permit holding to proceed. Being accepted by the client refers to the choice she makes to entrust her vulnerabilities in your capable hands.

As postpartum specialists, we are granted an esteemed position of expertise; one that entitles us to speak with authority, and, at the same time, create an environment that is conducive to psychic comfort, change, and personal growth. This can be accomplished by our secure hold of a new mother's vulnerability and all the imperfection that entails (Kleiman, 2009, p. 280). The capacity to be there with your client is what enables her to share her story, whether it is her birth story, her symptom story, her marriage story, or her story of panic and despair. It is also what tells her that she is safe, and this, in turn, sanctions our position to offer support and guidance with respect to the restless nature of postpartum distress. Although there are subtle variations with respect to the role of the postpartum therapist, all psychotherapeutic techniques merge when it comes to the basic collaborative consultation that takes place between the therapist and the client. For our purposes, the role of the expert comes into play as a necessary function on behalf of what makes the postpartum period so unique. Regardless of your theoretical training or practice, postpartum work distinguishes itself with biological, physiological, and psychological facets that require special attention with unique therapeutic perspective.

Externalizing the Problem

A basic premise of narrative therapy is the view that problems are separate from people and individuals have the ability and competency to change their relationship with a problem they are having. Ostensibly, each narrative conversation is guided and directed by the interest of the client, while the therapist helps her construe the problem as an entity outside of herself.

Postpartum women have a difficult time with this concept. There is a proclivity toward self-blame and internalization of each symptom: *I am depressed. I am a bad mother. I am useless. I am worthless. I am a chronic worrier*. Women tend to possess characteristics of depression as an established fact and find it outrageous to even consider any alternative. "It's just who I am right now," you might hear. "I am a piece of shit. I am worthless. I am so depressed." Any attempt to explain to her that what she is expressing are in fact symptoms and not who she is, is met with either skepticism or downright belligerence. "These are not symptoms," she contends. "I know what symptoms are. This is about me being a bad mother. This is about me not being able to do this. This is about me making the biggest mistake of my life."

Consistent with narrative theory, one of the best ways to externalize an internalized problem is to invite the client to reflect on alternative possibilities, not unlike a principle of cognitive behavioral therapy, when you ask the client to insert corrective thoughts. When working with a postpartum woman in distress who is likely to overidentify with each misappraisal, I remind her that these feelings may *feel like who she is*, but they are *symptoms*. When the symptoms are treated, she will no longer feel this way or think this way. It is also helpful to objectify the feeling, name it, or identify it as separate somehow by referring to it as apart from her: *This worry, it is with you all the time?* Or, in one case, a client named her the anxious part of herself *Anxiety Kid*. When feeling overwhelmed, she would tell me that Anxiety Kid would think that something terrible was happening. Together, we would carry on a conversation with Anxiety Kid to explore the nature of her worry and by externalizing her, enable the client to find solutions within herself. By actualizing a problem in this way, clients are better able to separate themselves from the problem and are more apt to discover a way out or, as narrative therapy teaches, an alternative story for dealing with their relationship to the problem. In this way, the problem is viewed as having an influence on her, rather than reflecting the essence of who she is.

Without this ability to objectify a symptom or problem, a postpartum woman in distress may feel destined to identify with her symptoms permanently. She believes the refrains, *I am anxious. I am hopeless. I am a bad mother. I am out of control.* When these conclusions about oneself take hold, she may believe and reinforce this distorted version of herself. When one woman's baby did not stop crying when she picked him up to comfort him in Karen's office, she remarked: "See? I told you I was a bad mother." These misinterpretations obscure the larger picture and sometimes make it impossible for a mother to see herself as separate from these troubling symptoms or emotions.

As you utilize the techniques of holding, you will notice that in time your therapeutic dialogue will help assemble her previous skills, strengths, and competencies that will challenge her symptomatic self, reconnecting her with personal resources she is unable to access when symptoms loom large.

A Universal Separateness

The postpartum experience is generally understood as a phenomenon surrounded by and embedded within numerous social structures and forces. It can feel like a conspiracy of sorts, as women describe intense feelings of isolation and abandonment of impressive proportion. Susan Maushart describes her daunting experience of childbirth in *The Mask of Motherhood*:

> My sense of abandonment, of exile, really, was nevertheless overpowering. I felt exactly as I had felt the time I nearly choked to death on a piece of steak in a dark, noisy and incredibly crowded room, in which, even if I'd been able to scream, no one could possibly have heard me. I had the same sense then, as I did in labor, that I was going to die, and that everyone around me was too busy partying to notice.
>
> (Maushart, 2000, p. 95)

Exile. A big word for an experience acknowledged as natural and, ideally, uncomplicated. An exile into motherhood. This is indeed how many postpartum women describe their new status, with its unfamiliar, indefinable mind-set, forcing unprepared women to muster the courage to sort it out by themselves. Much has been written about the shift from once common multigenerational support systems for new mothers to the siloed motherhood of present-day. If good social support is recognized as strongly protective against the development of perinatal mood and anxiety disorders (Feinberg et al., 2022), it should not be surprising that women, who both ache for help from others and feel encouraged, or forced, toward independence by others, wind up feeling so bad.

Holding is a construct that originates from this paradox, the recognition that new mothers do, in fact, need nurturance as badly as they need their independence. In the strictest sense, social support can encompass various degrees of communication, empathy, behavior, information, advice, or practical assistance – all of which can be beneficial to the new mother. Conversely, any of these forms of support can easily feel unsupportive or be ineffective and, in the worst scenario, compromise recovery. Interestingly, studies show that a mother's perception of social support is also an important factor in mitigating perinatal distress (Jamshaid et al., 2023; Yang et al., 2017). Thus, not only are the accessibility and presence of support relevant, a mother's *perception* of her support is pertinent as well. For example, while it might sound generous of a mother-in-law to offer to move in temporarily to ease the burden after childbirth, if the new mom would find her presence to be intrusive or agitating rather than helpful, all the social support available to her in that scenario may not lead to a positive outcome.

Here's a familiar scenario:

A postpartum woman feels overwhelmed and isolated. She worries about her scary symptoms. She refuses to discuss the details of how she is feeling for fear of judgment or condemnation, reinforcing her isolation. Her family hopes she finds the strength to do what she needs to do to feel better, but they are not sure what to do or how to help and so they wait for her guidance. But she does not know exactly what it is that she needs. The home-cooked meals and offers for help from her friends begin to wind down. Her doctor tells her she will be fine once she gets some sleep. Her inner critical voice tells her she is not cut out for motherhood. In short, postpartum women can quickly feel disconnected or dismissed from the very community from which they seek belonging.

As a therapist on the front line, when you practice holding you create a safe space from the pressure she feels to ask for what she needs. You are present, quite literally, and, perhaps more cherished by her, you are patient. You allow her space to discover what she needs from others and what she needs to find within her *self*. You affirm for her that this is the work of a new mother in therapy, finding the balance between strength and vulnerability, finding strength within vulnerability. You provide a sanctuary for imperfect mothering. One can imagine that this might feel both comforting and anxiety provoking for her.

By All Means, Bring on the Silence

When holding a postpartum woman in distress, you ride together on this journey, holding her truth, her story, and her interpretations. It requires a condition of complete openness to any possibility. She may not say what we expect her to say. You may not hear what you imagine you will hear. It requires listening to the voice of a heart that has been broken, to words that may or may not accurately reflect the seriousness of the moment.

When Connie came to see me, she was 2 months postpartum with her first son. At that time, she said, "It's so physically hard to talk when you feel this bad, the words don't come out. It is easier not to say anything at all." She said she wished she could slip into a coma and wait out this time of her life, which had been shattered. She said the sun had stopped shining. The darkness and the sadness were so heavy she could not escape it. Not ever. I remember how it felt for me to sit in that space with her. I recall sitting with the weight of her words and the thick stillness in the air. I remember listening to her while observing my own desire to dive in and make it all okay for her again.

As a therapist, it is as easy for me to stay silent as it is for me to spew forth my very opinionated opinion if I think something is blatantly amiss or if someone is in danger. I never (ever) stop wishing I could make the pain go away as magically as she would like me to. This urge to assuage discomfort is an occupational hazard for empathic souls who commit to this work, as we constantly work to reconcile our desire to ease her suffering with our ability to tolerate it.

We learned about the therapeutic use of silence in psychotherapy 101 courses. Its merit is indisputable. In our years of teaching perinatal mental healthcare providers, we observe that, in general, they tend to be a more proactive, more instructive, and more outspoken group of therapists compared to therapists who work with a more general population. Many therapists tell us it is unnerving to sit in silence when the woman sitting across from them is in high distress, waiting for an answer, a tool, a prescription, a book, a magic potion, a remedy for despair. The use of silence with glaring agitation and agony feels like an oxymoron of unachievable proportions. Still, we are her greatest teacher at those moments. There will be times when the very best way for us to inspire her while she stands on the edge of life is to sit there, as mentioned earlier in this chapter, to be with her. Without fear. Without judgment. Without words. Her pain is a compelling invitation to those who can sit in that space. We do so with tacit strength and reverence worthy of that moment.

It is tempting to allow our own anxiety to interrupt this process. Jumping in with empty words is not only counterproductive, it can derail her present moment and set the session off course. Allow the process to take hold. Staying silent in therapy enables us to catch the chaos, to hold what feels so uncontrollable to her. The power of silence is defined by the ability to manage without "doing anything." Containing through silence is holding magic. It is how we use our *selves* as our best tool. It is what connects us to any opposition to this process and ushers in early stages of empathy. As overwhelming as this work with postpartum women in distress can be, *and it can be*, it is also enormously gratifying.

- Resist thinking that you have nothing to offer this woman sitting in front of you with soul-crushing wounds.
- Do not be afraid to sit in that silent space shared between the two of you as long as you remain attuned to the process.
- Do not think that *who you are* isn't enough to help her heal. *It is.*

When you believe you are enough, you will be on the road to lead her home, as Connelly teaches us. Connelly's portrayal of herself as a health practitioner coming to the aid of a client in pain superbly describes who we must be in the eyes of our client.

If we are willing to take another human being with us to our secret places, to the places where we deny or do not recognize ourselves, then in the moment of arriving to our "secret" we enter ourselves newly. The person we allow to come with us, the intimate traveling companion, comes without adding anything or taking anything away, comes silently, empty and following exactly. The healing is the discovery of the self. It is the homecoming, the returning home, the restoring of all lost parts.

(Connelly, 1993, p. 24)

The person we allow to come with us. You are that person. Each postpartum woman you see ultimately determines whether or not she will allow you to come with her on her journey home. Home to where things do not hurt as much. Home to where she can feel in control of her life again. And feel safe. And feel joy.

Note

1 Permission granted from Dianne M. Connelly to republish her quotes.

Chapter 4

Postpartum Mamas

The crusade to find meaning in her changing self-identity is an evolving and demanding endeavor for any new mother, depressed or not, whether in therapy or not. The inability to lessen the day's load or find purpose in the endless rounds of laundry and vomit can make the most dedicated mother intermittently doubt her decision to have a baby in the first place.

Motherhood, even when it is everything one hoped it would be, is fraught with burdens of ambivalence and echoing uncertainty. When we move aside the rewards and profound possibilities built into this life-altering and exhausting role, we make room to understand the other side. The darker side. Whether depression is part of her experience or not, many postpartum women do acknowledge the presence of feelings that are deeply difficult to reconcile with their strong desire to become a mother. Unexpectedly, motherhood drives women to confront aspects of themselves they may neither have known nor noticed. This can be a shocking discovery to make during such a highly anticipated time of life. Personal reactions to competing emotions (coupled with the biological impact of this period) are as varied as the women themselves and range from mild discomfort to a full-blown psychiatric crisis. The complex set of emotions rarely leads to resignation without an earnest and dedicated effort.

The dichotomy of motherhood and loss is well recognized to those who study and work with postpartum women, distinguished by grief over the prevailing loss of self (Mauthner, 1999). At various times in a new mother's world, the experience of joy and pleasure may alternate with feelings of sadness and anxiety. Although this is perfectly normal, it can be upsetting and confusing to the woman who is unprepared for the presence of negative emotions during this time. When a major mood or anxiety disorder descends upon a postpartum woman, the negative emotions swell exponentially and settle into the cracks, creating a landscape of loss and

DOI: 10.4324/9781003402145-4

perceived personal failure. Loss is a predominant theme that alerts our holding response. When we describe holding as a loss-informed, strength-based approach, we begin by understanding the layers of grief that accompanies the postpartum period.

A Fine Mess and Other Postpartum Paradoxes

I hate myself sometimes.

Like those times my sweet angel is mesmerized by my very presence. My eyes burning with tear-stained sleeplessness. He doesn't seem to notice as he sucks vigorously on the synthetic nipple I kindly substituted for my own more obvious option. I am simply too tired to move. Too tired to offer any more of my flesh – not a single drop of my being – to my hungry child. No more, my darling. Mommy has nothing left to give. I am weary. I must rest. Or, surely, I will die.

Sheri, 2 months postpartum

There is little room for harmony when anguish and elation occur simultaneously. When intense enough, the opposing emotions can effectively cancel each other out, resulting in a numbing response, a disconnect, a disengaged spirit, of sorts. A mother struggling with conflicting emotions might describe the detachment as a defense against herself, believing that, in some way, this protects her baby from what she perceives as her "not good enough" self. Women dealing with uncomfortable emotions surrounding motherhood often work hard to figure out a way to try to make sense out of the unsettling feelings in an effort to normalize their experience and adapt as best they can.

We imagine motherhood to be somewhat easy, natural, predictable, at least in our fantasies. After all, women have been having babies since the beginning of time. We hope to experience the same rite of passage that we have read and dreamed about. Many women, however liberated and feminist their ideals may be, confess they yearn for, and may even expect a storybook childbirth and motherhood experience. It is an enduring and deeply personal desire. Though there may be layers of intrinsic fears and social mandates that obscure this desire, it remains a secret and powerful hope for many pregnant women. However, it is this very entrenched belief that ultimately sabotages a woman's transition into motherhood. Her private vision, reinforced by our worn-out cultural scripts, can leave her unprepared to cope with the profundity of her situation and the potential onslaught of complicated emotions.

Winnicott teaches therapists to hold ambivalence, hers and ours. To tolerate our own personal failures. In the therapeutic relationship Winnicott describes gentle failures in attunement as opportunities to convey reliability of love from the therapist:

As analysts... we are all the time failing, and we expect and get anger. It is the innumerable failures followed by the sort of care that mends that build up into a communication of love, of the fact that there is a human being there who cares.

(Winnicott, 2002, p. 76)

The metaphor of Winnicott's original concept of a holding environment has been a part of psychoanalytic therapy for decades. Applied to the therapeutic environment, the metaphor of a mother holding her child parallels the way the therapist ideally holds their vulnerable clients. Holding became conceptualized as a safe place created by the therapist where the client could rest comfortably in the trusting presence of the caring mother/therapist (Winnicott, 1960).

Holy Crap, I Have to Sit Where?

Early in my career, I was listening to a radio show featuring a local psychologist discussing the fundamentals of psychotherapy and some common misperceptions. He said people often think that going to a therapist means sharing their mess with the hope that the therapist will help them clean it up. That makes sense to most, he said. But here is the real deal. You decide to go to a therapist when your life is in chaos. Imagine this scenario, in all its glory: bringing all your shit to a stranger's domain. Shit stinks. Feces. It's messy. It can be downright disgusting to some people. It is not something most folks are comfortable talking about or sharing with others, unless they are telling a joke. There can be shame associated with it. Embarrassment? Humiliation? The product of a natural human, animal physiological system, a bowel movement, is accompanied by strong negative emotions. Still, you decide to take all this embarrassing, shameful shit with you to a therapist. You hope the therapist will clean it up, or at the very least, help you clean it up. What we are there to do, however, is something quite different. The message we convey is this:

It is okay. You can bring your shit in here. I don't care how much you think it stinks or how messy it is. It is okay if you are embarrassed and self-conscious. I can tolerate the mess. I can endure the smell. I will not grimace or wince. I will remain neutral despite your declaration of repulsiveness, and I will convince you that sitting here together, in this mess, will feel like a safe place for you. I can sit in this shit with you. In time, we will take steps to clean this up.

It's like holding someone's hair back while they throw up. It is not a particularly comfortable position for either person. Once you get past the awkwardness that we as a culture impose upon it, it boils down to a bodily function. Sensory responses, like how it smells, how it looks, how it feels, are often social versions of a civilized nation, which makes total sense to those of us who prefer to remain civilized. Nevertheless, if you take a deep breath, you can, amid social or personal constraint, sit in her shit. If you have children, you have done this with them. You can do it with her.

So you ask yourself, *Am I ready to do this? Is this really different from the other therapy I've been doing successfully for years?* Again, what makes this area of work unique is a) the context of childbirth and the transition to motherhood, b) the urgency of symptoms and symptom relief, and c) the therapist's own identification with childbirth-related experiences. To be clear, volumes can be written about these three variables that uniquely affect perinatal mental health work. Do not underestimate the force of these contextual issues and the impact any one of them can have on a woman's sense of self and subsequent despair. Therefore, we are obliged to respond with swiftness and unwavering control of the situation.

Perinatal-Specific Distinctions

Therapists who specialize in the treatment of perinatal mood and anxiety disorders understand that there are aspects of this work that differentiate it from non-perinatal populations. It is precisely these differences that we highlight in the holding model as we address and respond to the unique and urgent needs of a mom in distress.

The Pretense

Postpartum depression is not always what it looks like. We hear this phrase often within the postpartum community. We use it in public health announcements. We attach it to our outreach efforts. Still, many in a position to help intercept postpartum women and lessen the suffering continue to miss the message. Women who are severely ill can present well and look good. They can look really good. At first glance, they can present so well that many skilled healthcare practitioners and therapists are easily convinced that everything is fine. If providers and clinicians aren't reading between the lines at all times, they might miss the fact that serious and relentless symptoms of a clinical depression may be lurking just beneath the surface. Do not assume if she looks good that she is okay; do not underestimate the extraordinary power a postpartum woman achieves by maintaining her illusion of control.

The massive energy and effort many postpartum women put forth to present the appearance of looking good to the rest of the world can, ironically, keep them feeling worse longer. It is the most classic postpartum paradox. Seemingly, it can help a bit if women take the time to care about how they look. No one would argue that self-care interventions, such as taking a shower, brushing hair, and putting on a pair a jeans or even makeup, can help lift spirits, albeit temporarily, and are worthwhile distractions when battling depression.

How does a postpartum woman reconcile the intense contradiction of feeling so out of control with the equally intense need to maintain control?

One way she does it is by looking good.

Make no mistake about it; postpartum women are *extremely* good at this. They can convince the best of us, as well as every member of their family, that they are fine. They can sit in your office for an entire session and leave without you knowing how bad they feel. This is not only an occupational hazard for the novel therapist. This is a remarkable phenomenon that postpartum women carry off with amazing finesse, and the risk is high that something essential could be missed by any treating therapist. Some postpartum women in severe distress are driven by desperation to summon their innermost shred of strength so they look *fine*, so they look like everyone else, like everyone expects them to look. They then manage to carry this right into the therapy office for fear that any break in character will fracture their delicate fortress.

This can work for a while. It can feel good to her that she can pass as the image of the mother she hoped she would embody. Eventually, however, as symptoms of depression sink deeper, systems weaken and the pretense of control crashes around her. When this happens, women are left vulnerable and feeling excruciatingly helpless.

Life is messy. Life with a baby is really messy. Life with a baby and symptoms of depression and anxiety is out-of-control messy. She feels like she must hold tightly. She doesn't want to let go of this shield she has set up to protect her. The last thing she wants right now is to feel vulnerable. And letting go feels extremely vulnerable.

So she pretends.

She hides.

She denies.

She disallows.

This leads to an elaborate dilemma, the one in which she is most invested: what remains and takes center stage, when she retreats into silence, is shame. As shame is correlated with depression, it becomes our most formidable challenge. If you do not address the shame, you only scratch the surface. Shame corrodes the soul. *I am a terrible human being. I should never have had this baby. I am a disgraceful person for having these thoughts.*

A good mother would never think these things. Mothers in our culture have been socialized to believe they can do it all, do it perfectly, and never let anyone see them sweat, or complain, or whine, or, God forbid, ask for help. This leaves them with massive unobtainable and conflicting expectations. Of course it would. Secrecy, most often arising from a fear of judgment, is an inevitable consequence of shame. To insist that women divulge the nature of their thoughts, or worse, their shame, illuminates the paradox.

Vulnerability is not new for a postpartum woman. She has most likely opened her heart, she has opened her mind, and she has opened her legs to various levels of invasive inspection. She has learned how to bleed, discharge, defecate, and lactate in front of strangers with little regard to judgment or consequences. I'm not saying that is easy to do, but she does it. It goes with the territory of giving birth. However, the vulnerability that comes with admitting you don't feel like being a mother, or you regret having your baby, or you have thoughts of harming your baby, well, that is a state of nakedness that is simply too hard to bear.

Postpartum women are very tuned in to what feels good and what does not. Their sensibilities are often on hyperalert, and most of the time – not always, but much of the time – they are right about what they need and what they want in order to heal. We need to hear that part, even when it is shrouded by agonizing symptoms. Still, exposure takes courage. It's hard to find the energy when you are bone-tired and weakened by symptoms. Our job is to help postpartum women in distress strengthen their resolve to acknowledge their suffering and talk about how they feel.

We do this through holding. When therapists and healthcare practitioners begin to understand this masquerade of perfection, they will be in a better position to accurately assess the emotional state of the women they treat. If we can challenge the cultural myth of the perfect mother, we gain insight into how easily some women are tempted to beat themselves up with secret thoughts. The shame attached to perceived failure or weakness is often reinforced by social pressures, relentless comparisons, and shaming contests. It's hard to remain untouched by the all-encompassing drive toward idyllic motherhood. It is also exhausting and counterproductive.

The paradox informing our therapeutic task at all times is that this loss-driven shame strengthens her charade of perfection. Holding a postpartum woman who is determined to manage her emotions by clinging tightly to her defensive posture creates a complex therapeutic issue. To repeat, this is not to imply that all postpartum women resist therapy. Certainly many postpartum women in distress readily seek therapy for support. Still, there is often a knee-jerk self-protective response to high levels of distress marked by a considerable effort to preserve what is familiar. Staying in control is paramount for postpartum women. This is what can manifest as resistance, despite their most sincere desire for help.

The Proverbial "Why Me?"

Affective incongruities are at the heart of postpartum suffering and can result in the difficulty women experience asking for help. A sense of well-being and hopefulness has suddenly been replaced by a peculiar disconnect that causes her to wonder whether she is or is not a good mother.

"I don't think I should have had this baby. I mean, I love him, like I'm supposed to, but I really don't think I have the right instincts. I don't even think he likes me much."

"What makes you think he doesn't like you?" I asked Jamie during our second session.

"I don't know. It just doesn't feel right. Nothing feels right."

"Are you surprised by how you are feeling right now, Jamie? How did you hope you would feel?"

"Um, fireworks of some sort? How does maternal bliss feel? Flooded with magnificent elation, destined to get better and deeper? Profoundly touched by the smells, the coos, the essence of it all. I honestly thought that would happen like that. But I sit here, tired and fat and wishing I had my life back. I wish I could kick my ruby shoes together and go home to the life I had before."

Home. The pre-baby state of (perceived) balance and a (perceived) sense of being in charge of her own life. Research has shown that although one's actual available amount of support does matter, a woman's perception of her circumstances matters as much, if not more (Inekwe & Lee, 2022). In other words, a woman's response to her new circumstances can have a direct impact on her ability to cope and move through them. It is natural to yearn for previous states of being when one is overwhelmed by change. Wanting to go "home" to what is familiar and safe is a natural response to feeling thrust into the unknown. Accommodation to this abrupt transition does not come easily, even without depression in the picture. Still, part of our therapeutic response to this is to help her adjust to her perceived loss and move forward through the uncertainty. It is a delicate balance to honor her sense of loss and her desire to return to her previous self, while we sit with her distress and lean her in the direction of well-being. As we return to Connelly's (1993) work, within the context of holding, a client's home-sickness is often at the heart of our work with her.

Symptoms and the Death of Her Former Self

A constellation of losses during the postpartum period is a hallmark feature of postpartum depression. Symptoms can quickly lead postpartum women to define themselves by an overidentification with perceived and pervasive loss, worsening the depression. When discussing the postpartum period with groups of moms or healthcare providers, I often pose the question: "What are some of the losses associated with early motherhood? Not just for moms with postpartum depression, but any mom." It is easy to call upon a list of the joys and fabulousnesses that come with a new baby, but discussions of the downside of new motherhood have been off the mainstream radar for generations. Understanding that losses are a normal part of the transition to motherhood is vital as we strive to normalize areas of deprivation associated with new motherhood. If we fail to recognize that losses can provide a gateway for growth and healing, we risk minimizing or missing completely the full experience and story of the postpartum woman we are sitting with.

Consider the litany of losses related to the transition to motherhood: sleep, finances, alone time, former self, couple time, self-identity, body image, adult conversation, predictability, calm, spontaneity, freedom, friends, her previous body, career, leisure time, privacy, intimacy, sexuality, confidence, self-esteem, to name a few. Many women recognize that these losses come with the territory of parenthood, and, by and large, are transitory. Even so, the individual sacrifices made by women are huge and rarely acknowledged. Sacrifices come with a cost and for the most part, moms perceive their surrender to self-denial as an expectation of motherhood. When a woman forgoes her own needs with a healthy dose of ego strength, depletion can be lessened as she experiences her sacrifice as valuable. If, on the other hand, yielding to the all-encompassing needs of early motherhood carries resentment or an expectation of accolades that never come, bitterness and disappointment can increase.

In the 1950s, a woman was expected to sacrifice all on behalf of her children and to do so without resentment or sadness. As reported in *McCall's* magazine in 1957:

> She must alter her life completely – rise with the cold dawn, sniff without disgust the sour odor of spit-up milk, adjust to changing relationships with her husband and relatives, and adjust to a new personality – her baby.
>
> (McGowan, 1957, as cited in Held & Rutherford, 2012, p. 111)

During that era, women who expressed sadness or disappointment related to motherhood were viewed as adjusting poorly to their new role of being a mother. We now know that it is normal for women to experience intermittent negative emotions as they transition into motherhood. It doesn't feel good, but it is normal. It seems that if mothers were given adequate preparation for this and knew to expect some degree of negative feelings, there would be less self-criticism, blaming, and shaming across the board.

The negative emotions in the list that follows flood the space between the therapist and the postpartum woman. These primary symptoms that are often associated with depression and anxiety in general take on new meaning when they are understood within the context of having a baby. Again, these strong negative emotions are *symptoms*, but they are experienced as *self*. A woman with postpartum depression does not understand (or believe) that she has an illness with symptoms. The mere attempt to explain this to her can drive her impulse to retreat even further into her private hell. *No one can possibly understand me*, she may think. Her anguish becomes both the reason to hate herself and the punishment for doing so. Her desire for relief can be side-tracked by a premature interpretation if too impersonal.

First and foremost, she needs to tell her story.

The emotional states below are loss-informed features of postpartum depression and anxiety, and are pervasive during this period: because of their ubiquitous nature they make up a large part of the holding landscape. Keeping them in mind and in context, when working with a postpartum woman in distress, will arm the therapist with an entry into her suffering. Helping them articulate these early strong emotions can provide an initial release. Note that these are complicated emotions, worthy of deep study; here we mention them briefly in an effort to outline their foundational position in the art of holding.

Grief

Postpartum women may outwardly mourn the loss of their former self, or they may be unable to articulate why being in their own skin can feel foreign and unfamiliar. Women often yearn to reconnect to their former self, clinging to something familiar during this deeply jarring time. This longing can lead to sadness and inexplicable weepiness. The sorrow that accompanies a woman's journey through the early days of motherhood can feel as if it disrupts the very flow of life. *It's not natural*, women say, *to feel this way when you have a baby. Something must be terribly, terribly wrong.*

When women feel they can no longer trust the natural order of things, it is hard to know what to do or where to look for help. Suffering feels easier.

Helplessness

While some mothers express feeling both empowered and powerless simultaneously, often women with depression and anxiety convey feelings of helplessness and immobilization. Feeling ineffective from the outset and struggling to relate to the overwhelming unknown, postpartum women with depression and anxiety reel from states of denial, anger, and rage. An onslaught of unpredictability and chaos make it feel impossible to keep up, impossible to gain control, impossible to help oneself. Feelings of inadequacy and failure replace any hope that she could adjust or one day feel capable in the face of the intrinsic uncertainty that comes with parenthood.

Winnicott's holding environment may be interpreted as a transitional space in which a feeling of helplessness on the part of the baby (or our client) gives way to their personal agency. This idea applies well to most psychotherapeutic models. It follows, then, that if therapists are mindful of their capacity to accept and tolerate clients' feelings of helplessness, and any other negative emotions, this gives way for the client to also accept and tolerate them and, ultimately, to feel less helpless.

Anger

Some women with postpartum depression and anxiety feel perpetually frustrated. Although they may express an overwhelming sense of responsibility toward their baby, as well as a desire for all to be good again, they are periodically or incessantly pissed off and irritated. *It's not fair,* we hear. Feelings of aggression and even rage may ensue.

Postpartum women in distress repeatedly state they feel cheated. They say they have been robbed of the maternal joy they expected. They may resent the fact that their partner goes to work as if nothing in their lives has changed, while they are left to fend for themselves and their dependent newborns. They are angry at their partner for not understanding or rearranging their lives to better meet their needs. They are angry at the medical establishment for failing to take their condition seriously. They are angry at society as a whole for expecting so much from mothers, while providing such insufficient support. And they are angry at themselves for feeling ill equipped to deal with so much sudden anger and disappointment. They describe an unfathomable pressure to redefine themselves to existential proportions while their babies protest for instant attention.

It is quite understandable that some women will respond to such extreme losses with resentment and rage.

Ambivalence

The conflict of intensely loving your baby and wanting to flee as far away as you can from the sound of his cry is insufferable. Though maternal ambivalence has graced the pages of many psychological writings and has been accepted as a universal phenomenon, it remains a taboo subject that many moms wrestle with silently. There remains great humiliation surrounding any confession of negative views of motherhood, within both our cultural and personal accounts. Images and distorted beliefs of the "perfect mother" abound and continue to thrust new mothers into a frenzied attempt to meet such idealized expectations. Ambivalence toward one's dear baby is hard to swallow and nearly impossible to admit. Daphne DeMarneffe, in her book *Maternal Desire*, writes,

> Even if a mother derives satisfaction from taking care of her children, it is hard for her not to feel ambivalent about having rearranged her life to take it all on, especially if her partner doesn't acknowledge or value the effort involved.
>
> (DeMarneffe, 2004, p. 128)

Guilt and Shame

The crushing guilt that many women with postpartum depression and anxiety experience often stems from a belief that they let themselves down. They struggle with the belief that they have failed to live up to societal expectations and certainly to their own expectation, that new mothers should bond instantly and bathe in the joyous glow of motherhood. Instead, they feel that they have failed. They wonder if they made a colossal mistake. Mothers drenched with guilt may isolate themselves in fear of judgment or criticism, further alienating themselves from some of the very people who are in position to help them. Extended guilt can lead to a considerable decrease in self-esteem and self-confidence. If shame is present, it can be accompanied by self-loathing. One way to think about the difference between guilt and shame is that guilt often refers to something one did or didn't do, feeling remorseful about behavior that is considered wrong, even if that behavior is only imagined or misperceived. Shame refers to her core self: who one *is* and how they believe they are perceived by others. For example, a mother with shame may find herself believing that she is, in fact, a bad mother.

Distress

We have seen that postpartum depression is an agitated depression characterized by significant anxiety. Because anxiety is a normal part of mothering, determining whether one's anxiety is indicative of a perinatal anxiety disorder can be confusing to new mothers. Postpartum women can sustain enormous levels of nervous worry. While some degree of anxiety goes with the territory, it can also be a signal that extra support is needed, especially when anxiety manifests as scary thoughts. Distress is a term that encompasses the experience of both anxiety symptoms as well as depressive symptoms.

Postpartum dysfunction as a consequence of depression and anxiety marks the collapse of all that was previously known. Moms tormented by the belief that the world is now a scary and dangerous place for her and for her baby begin to experience unbearable anxiety that can make them feel that they are truly going mad. The authors of one study described depression as not something that you simply *have* while the rest of yourself is left unaffected. Instead, depression is something that you experience, that you live and breathe. It affects everything you do, everything you think, everything you are. This is why, they elaborate, it is not sufficient to tell depressed people that they perceive the world incorrectly, because how they perceive the world is an accurate reflection of their illness and how they experience life right now (Roseth et al., 2011).

The emotions mentioned earlier – grief, helplessness, anger, ambivalence, guilt and shame, and distress – are most notable for their prevailing and problematic nature. Other symptoms of postpartum depression and anxiety are no less troublesome, both from a mother's perspective and a clinical one. Understanding and accepting these symptoms as representing losses is critical for any postpartum woman's emotional recovery. Interventions aimed at enhancing a person's sense of self should instill hope and foster positive but realistic appraisals of her *self*. At the same time, treatment should include identifying, supporting, and developing her existing strengths Tapping into her strengths can help stabilize her experience of loss.

Barriers: Everything Gets in the Way

Postpartum women in distress express an ongoing need to be heard.

My husband is trying to understand. I mean, he's wonderful, really. But how can he possibly understand? My doctor says I will feel better soon. She says this is normal for new moms, and I shouldn't worry. My friend says she knows just how I feel and she felt that way too and I should go exercise. The therapist I went to, who supposedly specialized in this area, said something like, well, it's hard to have a baby. Oh my god, yes, I'll be back to pay you hundreds of dollars to tell me that again. No thank you. I am so tired of trying to explain how I feel. So tired of asking for help. I just want this to go away. I just want to feel like myself again.

Unfortunately, there is a universal lack of clarity when it comes to what is a "normal" emotion and what's not a "normal" emotion during the postpartum period. Understandably, many women and healthcare providers alike have difficulty with the distinction between expected postpartum adjustment challenges and impairment in functioning that justify seeking help:

> I was exhausted and anxious all the time, like I couldn't do what needed to be done, but everybody says, "Oh, that's normal. You've just had a new baby." I was scared and I knew something was not right, and then I thought I must be insane if I am the only one thinking something is wrong.

Complicated by fact that most healthcare professionals have been taught to expect a certain degree of emotional upheaval during the postpartum period, this gap between what is an acceptable emotion and what is problematic deepens. Normalizing distress in this life stage, however, with a worn-out cliché such as, "Oh that's normal, you've just had a baby," is a lackadaisical response, at best, and a serious mistake, at worst. If we are aware that symptoms of normal postpartum adjustment overlap with symptoms of a major mood or anxiety disorder, it makes more sense to refer any woman in question to a competent mental health provider rather than dismissing it as par for the postpartum course. The risk is too high to assume this laissez-faire posture. Still, most women and healthcare providers alike have difficulty with the distinction between normal postpartum adjustment difficulties and impairments in functioning that justify seeking help.

This confusion over what is normal and what requires further attention is a constant barrier to seeking and receiving help and can delay treatment. As we've seen, many women suffering from postpartum depression do not seek professional help, despite frequent contact with health providers. Many mothers tell us they failed to recognize symptoms of depression and presumed their symptoms or experiences were simply part of being a new mother.

Another major barrier to help-seeking is the stigma associated with depression. Depression is sometimes viewed as a private failing, particularly within the context of the transition to motherhood (Jones, 2022). New mothers worry that disclosure could lead to abandonment and lack of support (Zauderer, 2009). The stigma associated with mental health issues in general is profound, but when attached to the heart of a new mother, it takes on extraordinary proportions of shame and personal disgrace. A consequence of this shame is that mothers may isolate themselves, refusing to talk about their feelings or experiences.

At odds with going to therapy, postpartum women express their concerns with resigned determination (Kleiman, 2009):

- It's a weakness.
- It's too much money.
- It means I'm crazy.
- It means I'm not a good mother.

- It means I'm not doing something right.
- It means I'm not in control.
- It is inconvenient.
- I don't have time.
- I don't have childcare.
- I don't have transportation.

The list of barriers that interfere with a postpartum woman's ability to commit to therapy, or other self-care commitments, is outrageously long. Just ask any postpartum woman. She will rattle off 10 or 20 reasons why she cannot make that happen. To further complicate things, these obstacles are real, energy is low, and resources are scarce.

It is understandable that women find it difficult to take the time and energy to face how much they are suffering. In addition to the logistical overwhelm it presents, therapy requires that she take a close look at the very emotions she is trying to ignore. Why would she want to do that? Unless this is understood with compassion for its origin, therapists may risk misinterpreting the opposition to therapy as confrontational or provocative in some way. Appreciating this resistance in general, as well as each obstacle that may impede her connection to the process, is crucial to the early stages of holding a postpartum woman who is hard-to-hold.

Holding Neutralizes Barriers

When we talk about barriers to treatment for postpartum distress, we typically review them from two perspectives: the mother's and the healthcare providers.

Expanding our discussion of resistance to therapy, review some of the barriers that affect a woman's decision to seek help and how she might express her need for support. Be mindful that what we hear her say will influence our holding response.

1 Mother's denial.
   I'm fine. Really.

2 Inability to mobilize.
   I cannot breathe. I cannot think. I cannot move.

3 Unsupportive spouse.
   My partner says I just need to be strong.

4 Wonder what other people think.
   None of my friends had to go get help when they had a baby.

5 Desire for quick fix.
   I cannot feel this way anymore.

6 Social/family pressure and expectations.
Everyone said this would be the best time of my life.

7 Financial burden.
I cannot afford to pay that much money to go talk to someone.

8 Geographic isolation.
I have no idea how I will get to those appointments.

9 Failure of women and physicians to recognize symptoms of depression.
I had no idea being a mother would be so grueling. My doctor says this is normal.

10 Symptoms resemble postpartum "normal changes" (fatigue, loss of sleep and sex drive, appetite changes).
I'm just tired. It's probably normal for me to feel this bad all the time.

11 Avoidance of the stigma of mental illness or having depression.
I just had a baby. Now all of a sudden there is something wrong with me?!

12 Association of depression with severe pathology or dysfunction in her family history.
I am stronger and healthier than my father. I cannot be sick like he was.

13 Fear of being labeled a "bad mother."
If I tell anyone the thoughts I am having, they will not believe me or they will think I cannot take care of my baby.

14 Belief that there is a benefit to not getting treatment, based on hope of spontaneous remission.
If I wait long enough, this will go away by itself.

15 Prior negative experience with treatment.
I am not seeing another therapist who doesn't know how to help me.

16 Depression is not viewed as an Ob-Gyn issue or not knowing that the Ob-Gyn or another doctor can help.
My doctor's job is to care for my physical well-being.

17 Confusion between clinically significant symptoms and normal maternal adjustment difficulties.
Don't all new mothers feel this way?

18 Fear of having her baby taken away.
If I share my deepest fears, someone will call the authorities.

19 Fear of being rejected.
No one will take this seriously.

20 Feeling that it is inappropriate to discuss self-care or mental health issues.
It's so personal; it feels awkward to admit this out loud.

21 Concerns about confidentiality.
Who knows what my doctor will do with the information I share?

22 Uncomfortable disclosing feelings in general.
I don't think it's right to talk about private issues outside the community or family.

23 Somatic expression of symptoms masks clinical presentation of depression.
If I could just sleep, everything will be fine.

24 Typical symptoms of depression (fatigue, amotivation, apathy, despair) interfere with help-seeking behavior.
There's nothing anyone can do for me.

25 Poor access to mental health resources, shortage of providers.
I cannot find anyone to help me.

Here is where maternal mental health therapists can assume a more suitable stance to support the urgent needs of a postpartum woman. One way to hold postpartum women even before they enter your office is the inclusion of appropriate marketing and promotional efforts that align with your greater mission. Providing psychoeducational support for healthcare professionals should be a component of a therapist's decision to specialize in this field in response to the paucity of good, accurate information. Despite years of frustrating door-to-door strategies and my personal expedition to improve a medical community of bad attitudes, resistance to the facts in hand remains ubiquitous. A comprehensive commitment to the treatment of perinatal mood and anxiety disorders incorporates sharing pertinent information with your clients' circle of healthcare providers.

Provider Obstacles

Barriers that are provider oriented are equally impressive in that they, too, can mean the difference between a woman feeling comfortable enough to disclose or choosing not to relate how she is feeling.

Provider barriers typically fall into these categories:

- Time constraints.
- Belief that mental health is not part of their job description and reluctance to discuss emotional issues with patients.
- Uncertainty regarding how to refer to mental healthcare effectively.

Although healthcare provider barriers are not the focus of our discussion here, the solutions are clear:

• Screen routinely.
• Mental health *is* part of your job.
• Education and specialized training are *key* to providing the proper information and reliable mental health resources for your patient.
• Provide psychoeducation and create supportive environments.

The reason to specify the barriers might be obvious, but unless we understand the myriad and complex variables each mother carries with her into your session, we have not distinguished ourselves from the many therapists who believe that treating postpartum women is the same as treating any other client with depression and anxiety. The barriers are what keep her staying sick, longer. They are why her depression is worsening instead of getting better. They are why she is spending so much energy just getting through the day and not taking steps in the direction of recovery. They are what is standing in the way between her and early intervention with optimal treatment outcomes.

Disclosure is painful. When you, as her therapist, understand the barriers that thwart her desire for help, when you can articulate for her what she is unable to articulate for herself (e.g., *I know it's hard to get here. I know this is the last thing you feel like doing*) and praise her for gathering her resources to make this possible (*It is good you are here. It is so important for you to take care of yourself by coming here; I know it may not feel that way, but it is good that you can do it*), you hold her. Sometimes against her better judgment. Sometimes while she's kicking and screaming, but you hold her, nonetheless. In doing so, you communicate to her that she has come to the right place and she will begin to feel better.

Screening Recommendations

Depression is very treatable, especially when identified during pregnancy or early in the postpartum period before symptoms become protracted. Early identification of mothers who are at risk for prenatal and postpartum depression and anxiety augments treatment, which can prevent problems for both the mother and baby. Thankfully, the organizations that develop best practices for healthcare providers are working hard to improve mental healthcare screening practices within a variety of medical settings. The United States Preventive Services Task Force, The American College of Obstetricians and Gynecologists (ACOG, 2018), and The American Academy of Pediatrics (Walsh et al., 2020) are among the groups advocating for providers to take a more proactive role in identifying women in distress and educating all women about perinatal distress.

Still, maternal depression goes undiagnosed and untreated. If one out of every seven (or more) women who walk into doctors' offices is experiencing symptoms of depression or anxiety that meet diagnostic criteria for a major mood or anxiety disorder, which includes the potential for suicidality, should providers ever wait for it to simply call attention to itself?

- Would it matter if they knew that their patients took time to meticulously put on makeup and look presentable so their doctors would think everything is fine but left the office in despair believing that no one can help them?
- Would providers change their policies if one woman in their practice decided she could not take this deception anymore and could not sustain the pretense of looking good against the dark thoughts invading her mind and acted on her suicidal thoughts?
- Would they modify their screening protocol if that woman who was suffering was their sister or their wife or their daughter?

The push for improved screening is excellent. But it is not enough. The stigma is huge and remains one of the biggest obstacles standing in the way of a woman's disclosure. If healthcare providers do not change their attitude about perinatal mental health risks and realities, women are not going to take the risk of exposing how they feel even if screening does take place. Medical providers should confront the issues of maternal mental health with the same seriousness with which they approach a physical crisis. Adding this to the litany of personal and medical questions and assessments should be a requirement.

Attitudes notwithstanding, screening is a straightforward method to help identify women whose symptoms interfere with functioning. The increase in advocacy among governing bodies, individual providers, and also patients themselves are giant leaps forward. Following up with universal screening recommendations and protocols and enabling the smooth implementation of these programs seem to be our biggest hurdles. The practical application of the recommendations on a local level will require scrutiny and ongoing assessment. Mandates do not ensure proper execution. Again, screening is only effective if it leads to the appropriate referral to mental health professionals and/or proper medical treatment. And if women feel safe enough to reveal how they are really feeling. We know that with effective treatment, women with postpartum mood and anxiety disorders recover. We can be hopeful that recent developments in the right direction will contribute to the consolidation of consistent screening, assessment, and treatment practices.

Chapter 5

Mother and Therapist
On Being Good Enough

Rebecca was 4 months postpartum when she described how she was failing:

> I am the worst mother in the world. I have no idea how to do this. This depression has stolen my joy and my ability to think. Women say they don't compare themselves to others, but they do. We all do. We say we want to stop the mommy wars, but we are them. We embody them. We are all watching each other. Competing with each other. We cannot win. No matter what I do, someone tells me I'm doing it wrong. Being depressed doesn't feel like an accident. It feels like an appropriate response to all of this pressure.

In the United States, culture has redefined expectations for motherhood over decades. We have navigated women's liberation, the sexual revolution, and national conversations regarding the role of women in the home and in the workplace. Within psychology we have learned that there are biological components to depression, which took some of the blame off mothers for a while. We have learned that there is a link between a mother's mental health and her pregnant and postpartum state, which both validated and marginalized mothers. Along the way, we have gained insight into the heartbreak that often co-exists with the joy of becoming a mother, opening up a whole new and complex notion of conceptualizing the transition to motherhood (Held & Rutherford, 2012).

The term *matrescence*, first coined by Dana Raphael (1973) is used currently to normalize the emotional, physical, and psychological adaptations that take place during the transition to motherhood. Identifying this important this complex transition as a major biosocial life event highlights the need for social recognition and support during this time (Orchard et al., 2023). Many contemporary writers focus on this term as an explanation for so many of the expected and profound changes throughout the motherhood journey. The caveat worth mentioning is the potential

DOI: 10.4324/9781003402145-5

confounding of variables when we try to normalize maternal distress. While we would love to get away from over-pathologizing new mother stress, we certainly do not want to miss symptoms or developmental crises that warrant close attention and perhaps treatment.

Today, the pressure to succeed at mothering remains at an all-time high. Succeeding at mothering means different things to different people. To some, it means just getting through the day. To others, it means doing so with ease, with grace, and with outcomes that reflect positive emotions and accomplishments. The urge to compare to others is pervasive. Moms perceive themselves as surrounded by neighborly supermoms characterized by exaggerated and romantic portrayals of what motherhood should look like. Complicated by the immeasurable stress created by the pandemic and the ensuing lack of sufficient support, mothers struggle whether or not clinical depression and anxiety are part of the picture.

In Search of Excellence

Despite decades of rich discussions on the making and meaning of motherhood and a vast collection of poems, articles, books, film, and various other media on the subject, mothers are left with one enduring irony above all: our contemporary society continues to consider the notion that a woman can be a loving mother and experience devastating feelings of loss and sadness directly related to her childbirth or mothering experience taboo. To those of us in the trenches, the juxtaposition of new motherhood and distress is poignant and obvious. To new mothers who are experiencing an identity transformation still in its infancy, the dichotomy of new motherhood and distress is overwhelming and may be shocking, guilt provoking, or shameful. The absence of consistent understanding and confirmation that a new mother can indeed feel joyfulness and loss simultaneously fuels this precarious paradox. Reinforced by ever-present and sometimes unforgiving social media, this generation of women who have been raised to believe they can find solace on the internet or in a text message feel increasingly lost.

When Valerie Raskin, MD, and I revised *This Isn't What I Expected*, almost 20 years after its original publication, we were surprised to discover how much had *not* changed for postpartum women in distress. Deeply moved by the ongoing push to keep postpartum depression and anxiety in the public eye to ensure accurate portrayals and proper treatment, we were equally dismayed by how much of what we had written was exactly the same. The shame, the judgment, the misinformation, the barriers to treatment, and the stigma. All persist to this day. As mentioned in the introduction of the second edition of the book, we were astounded by how relevant the book's original messages remain to this day.

Women with postpartum depression and anxiety continue to wait apprehensively in the dark corners of their lives, fearful of judgment, stigma, ridicule, and misdiagnosis. They wait, hoping this will go away by itself, hoping they will not go completely mad, hoping they do not have to let anyone know how they are really feeling.

(Kleiman & Raskin, 2013, p. x)

This quandary, women continuing to feel bad and surrounded by a medical and public community of contradictory messages (*I care about your well-being, I may be misinformed*) seems to be a primary reason that postpartum women seek therapists who specialize in this field. After all, if she is holding on to dear life, as Alison described in Chapter 1, she herself needs to be held by someone who knows how to help stabilize her loss of footing. She does not need another professional or layperson telling her what she should or should not be feeling. She is slipping.

A well-trained postpartum expert response is to therapeutically hold her so she can find her own answers by finding her way back home, to her *self*.

Good-Enough Is Enough

As we look closer at this concept of the good-enough mother and its application to therapy, we return to Winnicott. He writes: "...success in infant care depends on the fact of devotion, not on cleverness or intellectual enlightenment" (Winnicott, 2005, p. 14).

When teaching perinatal therapists, this notion resonates for most and is a belief that I emphasize adamantly: the heart of the therapeutic relationship and your client's journey toward wellness lies within *you*, who you are, your devotion to this work and to her. Your own *cleverness and intellectual enlightenment*, as Winnicott says, and your clinical skills are an added bonus (Winnicott, 2005).

For the new mother, however, it is not always this clear. Winnicott's concept of devotion and making adaptations translates into the mother's ability to read and respond appropriately to her infant's cues. This can be daunting to the mother who fears she is unable to respond properly, leading to constant worry that good enough can't possibly be enough.

"Look how upset he always is. Ugh. I'm not good at this."

"How do you know he's upset?" I ask.

"'Cause he's so fussy. Look at him. I changed him; I fed him right before we came here. I know he's not hungry. I don't know what's wrong with him."

"I wonder if he is making that little noise for another reason. Maybe he is fine. Maybe he's talking to us," I propose, unconvinced his whimper signified distress. "Maybe he loves it in here and he doesn't know how to express himself yet," I quip.

She smiles. "Well, I don't know much but one thing I know for sure is that I'm going to have an anxious baby. Every time he squeaks, I worry that he needs something that I'm not giving him."

"Maybe. Maybe not. You've thought about all of his needs and we're still not sure what he is trying to say. That's okay. Let's let him squeak for a while, talk about something else, and see what happens. If he needs something beyond just hearing himself squeak, he will surely remind us! Let's give him a chance to tell us."

Helping a mother endeavor to be less perfect than she is inclined to be and accept this as her best and healthiest choice is a grand undertaking. One that may be met with opposition, perhaps to the point of feeling misunderstood. Being less than perfect feels wrong to many moms. It feels like they are letting their guard down, like something really bad could happen if they don't hold tight and keep everything in order the way they think it's supposed to be.

So we remind her to breathe. As we dig for tools, we remind her of a water balloon. Perfectionism is compared to clutching a filled and wobbly water balloon, trying not to let it burst or plop onto the floor. The harder she grabs it, the less control she has and the more she increases the likelihood that it will burst or pop out of her hand. The only way to maintain control is to release her grip and let go. Clutching tight, *holding on for dear life*, is a natural response when losing control.

Good enough, to a mother, can feel like a reference to a minimal effort, as if anything less than perfect is substandard. But most postpartum women in distress who come for relief are seeking that message: that good enough is good enough. No more. No less. That is exactly what we communicate to her both implicitly and overtly. She needs to hear it. She needs to begin to believe it.

Again, we reinforce that *good enough is good enough* by sharing holding gold nuggets. These statements might appear trite at first glance, but when inserted at the right time, with the appropriate use of holding skills, and repeated to a mom with a broken spirit, any one of these can ground her and help her feel heard and safe, when offered by someone whom she trusts to provide feedback, someone she trusts to safeguard her:

- You are good enough.
- You don't have to work so hard.
- You are a good mother.
- Everything is okay.
- Nothing bad is happening.
- You do not have to do this alone anymore.
- You are not your symptoms.

- You will feel like yourself again.
- You can learn to let go and hold tight at the same time.
- You will not always feel this way.
- You are doing a great job.
- You are stronger than you know.

Is a Good-Enough Therapist Good Enough?

The concept of "good enough," as a mother, a parent, a spouse, or a therapist, poses the idea that we need to conduct ourselves skillfully and mindfully, but that every interaction may not occur in perfect harmony with our child, partner, or client. If we apply this principle to our attempts to hold a postpartum woman in distress, we recognize that being good enough means both:

- Honing and utilizing our skills so that we can effectively sit with suffering, contain uncertainty, and create interventions to reduce symptomatology

and

- Learning how to recover both the therapeutic relationship and our own self-esteem when interventions fall short, or even fail.

When therapists master these skills, they begin to role model that good mothers make mistakes and that good enough is enough.

The comparison between a mother and her baby and a therapist and their client has been made by many psychodynamically oriented psychotherapists. It is tempting to draw a parallel between these relationships and their objective from the outset, as each of them desires to establish a primary connection of trust and security. A baby learns to trust their mother as the mother works to enable that. A client hopes to trust her therapist as the therapist works to facilitate that. Setting aside any oversimplification of this parallel, let's consider some of the reasons that a client may report dissatisfaction with a previous therapist and their likeness to Winnicott's interpretation of mom and baby and his classic reference to mom as a transitional object necessary for healthy development and autonomy (Winnicott, 1963).

1   Client reports that her previous therapist over validated, seemed fake, or cared too much. The therapist appeared inauthentic.
    If the mother is too intrusive (too good) her child may feel suffocated; Winnicott theorized that this would interfere with the child's separation and development of self.

2 Client reports that her previous therapist *seemed cold, didn't know much about postpartum depression and anxiety or could not tolerate her emotions.*

Winnicott teaches us that when the mother is too distant, anxiety can manifest in the infant. Confronted with outbursts of infantile rage, Winnicott suggests that the good-enough mother remains attuned to the emotions and needs of the infant. She waits, then contains the rage in a gentle but determined manner. We will learn in the next chapter that these are holding points of intervention.

After containing intense symptoms and crisis in early sessions, the holding therapist fosters a sense of control and comfort through increased attunement. In time, the mother will begin to rely on the strength of the therapeutic relationship to redirect and encourage the development of self, a new self, as she advances through her new role. Keep in mind that creating a safe holding environment for a good-enough mother in response to her unbridled anxiety may present in stark contrast to what she is hearing in her day-to-day world. She may not know how to respond to the unfamiliar invitation to come here exactly as you are with all of your emotions in tow. Over time, the environment you create, fortified with attunement and compassion, will provide a welcome respite.

Therapist as Good-Enough Mother

Postpartum women suffocating under judgment, opinions, decision fatigue, and the needs of others suffer from unforgiving and parched air. When they find you, they have found a restorative oasis. When offered an environment that values unconditional acceptance, including for the parts of themselves they perceive as terrible, postpartum women feel cared for and valued. They may find it hard to believe that a person who invites them to be fully themselves could still like and care for them. At this early stage they may begin to view you as their good mother, the person in their life who knows exactly what to say, seemingly at all times.

How do we, as a culture and as individuals, designate what it means to be a good mother? This question is provocative and is a topic far more extensive than this book allows. Nevertheless, it is worthy of brief discussion here as it raises the issue of cultural humility. We must be mindful that the definition of a good mother can differ across cultures, religions, and generations. Anecdotally, when asked to list characteristics of what it means to be a good mother, trainees of The Postpartum Stress Center often describe an idealized good mother who says and does the right things all the time, just like in a storybook.

In many ways, however, the focus of our work is to help mothers relinquish these exact expectations of perfection. Thus we are best positioned to do this if we assume and embody the good-enough mother in our presentation to our client. This can be an incredibly difficult task, particularly because at home, we might struggle alongside our clients as we navigate unchartered territories with our own growing children. Therapists often believe that carrying out our professional role and responsibilities leaves little room for error. Although we might falter at home and cringe with each life lesson learned, we may not allow ourselves this luxury at work with our clients.

Remember, taking on the role of good-enough mother doesn't imply that you should let down your professional guard and bring a boundaryless version of your authentic self into your sessions. In fact, arguably assuming the role of good-enough mother requires increased boundaries and vigilance as you work hard to attune to the complex and unique distress of each perinatal client. The holding techniques are designed to increase our attunement to our client's needs, to help us remain regulated and differentiated, and also to provide a path for repair when our imperfections feel triggering to our clients.

The Therapeutic Relationship and Postpartum Clients

Many therapists aspiring to specialize in this field may be peers of their clients. There may be some clumsiness when a 31-year-old therapist attempts using Holding skills to comfort a 40-year-old mom in distress. Do not confuse expertise with self-importance or you will skid off course. Postpartum women in distress are not interested in spending time with a therapist unless that therapist conveys confidence in their knowledge and offers the anticipation of symptom relief. Early false impressions or conclusions about your expertise or life experience may tarnish her early connection to you, which is why first impressions are so meaningful. If she feels patronized by you, she will believe she is in the wrong place. One way to offset awkwardness in the early match between you and her (e.g., age difference, racial difference, cultural difference, she has four children you have none) is to address it directly. "You might be wondering if I can help you since we may have different life experiences." Practice with a colleague, a friend, or in the mirror responding to her in a way that communicates, "Yes. I can help you." Being transparent about potential stumbling blocks displays humility, builds the therapeutic relationship, and helps focus the session.

Here are some relevant preliminary holding dos and don'ts:

1 Avoid coming across as cavalier or parental, which could reinforce feelings of dependency or insult her. Be aware that this style of caring might offend her. Alternatively, it could inadvertently force her into a regressed state.

2 Avoid contrived sympathy at all costs. She can tell.
3 Do not underestimate the healing power of helping her restore her physical health.
4 Do not contradict her self-report. Her story is her story. Inquire beyond her report to navigate the nuances.
5 Always balance her pain with *your* hopefulness, her suffering with *her* strengths.
6 Always honor and acknowledge her decision to come to therapy, whether or not she is in crisis.

What distinguishes the relationship between a postpartum client and her therapist is that women who have recently given birth often crave support and attention from their own mothers. They may be receiving it from their mothers, or they may be yearning for the love of a mother they have lost. Or they may be ambivalent about their impaired relationship with their mother. Regardless of the psychodynamic influence, some transference and counter dependent issues are likely to transpire in that space between the two of you.

Postpartum women may be of two minds when it comes to understanding the clash of their need to care for their infant and their need to be cared for themselves. This can arouse a profound inner conflict.

> As our client sits awkwardly, in this state of imposed dependency, she finds herself reluctantly clinging to the desire for comfort (symptom relief) and nurturance (compassionate expertise). This is not to suggest that she has reverted to an infantile level of functioning. It does suggest, however, that in order for her to successfully re-enter her mommy-baby world, which is often contaminated with negative thoughts and feelings that repel her, the postpartum woman must first sit with her ambivalence, anxiety, and symptoms of depression, forcing her to confront her simultaneous need for caretaking. When she acknowledges, on some level, this state of vulnerability, she enters the holding environment and allows us to care for her in manner that is compatible with an optimal therapeutic outcome.
>
> (Kleiman, 2009, p. 39)

As a therapist working within the Holding framework, you are encouraged to acknowledge that the presence of these conflicting states could disturb her. Although your role as "caretaker" can agitate this conflict, exacerbating her intolerance, as always, your best response is to understand what this is and to accept it by not reacting. Your holding skills will demonstrate that you can tolerate her emotions, no matter how powerful or uncontrollable they feel to her. In a holding environment, we respond to strong emotions in a gentle but firm manner. You sit with her. You let her feel.

Boundaries and Breaking Rules

Therapists working with perinatal clients may occasionally (or often) find themselves moved to make accommodations for clients, adjusting rules along the way. This is understandable given clients' unrelenting symptoms, coupled with the presence of an infant. Depending on how long ago you learned to adhere to the rules of good therapeutic technique, you may or may not feel obliged to strictly follow those rules. Professional guidelines are created for a reason and must be respected. Even so, the Holding model calls upon therapists to remain authentic and reliable; if/when you make the concerted decision to maneuver off a well-traveled course, you need to know exactly what you are doing and why.

In general, breaking some of the traditional rules of therapy on behalf of postpartum women emerges from the conviction that their emotions are unpredictable, their egos are fragile, and their needs are urgent. There is an uncommon overlap here between medical and psychological acuteness, one that spurs us to act swiftly on our client's behalf. We must take our client's well-being into account and sometimes acting on behalf of her urgent need takes precedence over following standard procedure. For example, most practices follow a tried-and-true procedure for the initial intake session. There are assessments to complete, releases to review, and data to collect. It can be very difficult to check all of these boxes when a mother in distress finally feels able to let down her guard and to experience expressing her emotions in a safe space. Interrupting her tears and confessions with questions about her health history can feel awkward or insensitive at best, or may interfere with her feeling seen, heard, and safe at worst. Many of us will choose to balance collecting essential information in this first session with allowing her to share, even if our time runs over or we need to schedule a second session to complete the initial intake.

Why would our instincts trump what we have learned from scores of scholars and/or well-established protocol? It depends, but sometimes it is to prevent prolonged suffering. Or ease her anxiety. Or save her life. The scenarios and the justification for intuitive actions are variable. But they are always in support of her well-being, with an eye on her recovery process.

Boundaries frame the therapeutic relationship and exist to protect both the therapist and the client. Therapists in all fields of study continuously reassess the value of boundaries and how they adapt their standard of care depending on the needs of the client. There are times when adhering to certain boundaries makes more sense than at other times. A home visit, for example, may be appropriate for a client who is confined to bed rest and unable to travel. However, it does not feel appropriate if that were an able-bodied borderline client who had expressed sexual feelings for the therapist. For decades, therapists have been instructed to follow a "hands-off" model which discourages touching a distressed client, refusing gestures of gift giving, bartering, dual relationships, meetings outside the office, and self-disclosure (Zur, 2007).

There is no justification for a strict boundary violation. This is when a therapist breaches the line of decency and integrity and misuses their power to exploit a client for the therapist's own gain (Gutheil & Gabbard, 1998). Even when it is inadvertent and not as sinister as the definition makes it sound, it must be avoided at all costs. Over time, we have seen both rigid overreactions to boundary concerns and an increasingly flexible acceptance of minor boundary transgressions. As far as boundary rules go, your good instincts coupled with ethical decision making are your best tools. You must always be mindful of the subtle enactments within your relationship with your clients and the implications and ramifications of choices you make. It should go without saying that first and foremost it is your duty to protect your client from harm or exploitation. You must always consider whether your actions are in the best interest of each particular client with their particular needs, at a particular time, and within a particular context.

Though the behaviors outlined next have traditionally indicated soft boundary crossings, I confess I experiment with each of them, given a particular client and her circumstances. Occasionally it backfires, forcing me to re-examine my decision, which is a critical component of maintaining ethical practice when boundary breaking goes awry. Most of the time the traditional rules of therapy that follow work for postpartum women and occasionally I bend them ever so slightly.

Ways We Might Bend the Rules if We Are Careful

1 *Giving Advice*
   This is tricky because postpartum women ask a lot of questions and want a lot of advice. Why? Partly because, as previously mentioned, they are beset by many contradictory opinions and long for clarity or validation. Things can feel black and white during the postpartum period. *I'm having a good day or a bad day. I either slept last night or I did not. I am panicking or I am good. I suck as a mother or I do not.* But many of the questions have no such black and white dimension, no single answer: *Am I a good mother? What should I do to get some sleep? How do I stop panicking?* She wants a definitive answer to each question right now. Or, she could be obsessing. Which means, even if you were to answer her question with what you thought was a reasonable response, it may not come close to satisfying her need for reassurance and may undermine her need to develop confidence in her own judgment.

After burning symptoms begin to ease, sessions can unintentionally slide into "Parent Education 101" if one is not careful to stay focused. While practical matters are certainly relevant, such as helping a new mom structure her day, develop a sleep schedule, or set limits on well-meaning but intrusive family members, be mindful of your reaction when she asks, "What do I do?" You may need to abruptly regulate your response to make sure you are responding in a way that will be most valuable to the management of her symptoms and building of her self-esteem as opposed to offering an ultimately irrelevant opinion.

2 *Revealing Personal Information*

Discussions of self-disclosure date back to the early years of psycho-therapy. Way back in 1912, Freud emphasized that "The physician should be impenetrable to the patient, and like a mirror, reflect nothing but what is shown to him" (Peterson, 2002, p. 21). Through the course of many years, we have witnessed an interesting shift toward a desire for more information and more transparency from our practitioners. The internet and social media fuels this. So do reality shows and 24/7 non-stop, uninhibited exposure to anything and everything. Consumers exercise their right to know what they want to know. They can search online to see what they can find about their treating practitioner. Or, they might choose to ask their questions directly while being treated. This applies to their medical concerns as well as their desire for information about their specific healthcare provider. In response to this, healthcare professionals may feel compelled to include personal information on their website, in their brochures, or in discussion with their clients.

When it comes to personal self-disclosure with a postpartum woman in distress, this is not without its complications (as discussed in Chapter 2). Remember, postpartum women are vulnerable and they are hungry. They are scared and they are eager for answers. Until you know who she is and what she needs, the rule here should stand firm: *when in doubt, do not disclose.* It is better to err on the side of curbing an urge to reveal personal information. If you wonder whether you should say it or not, you should not. At least, not at that moment.

Over the years postpartum woman have commonly asked "Do you have children?" and "Did you have postpartum depression?" I usually reveal that I do have children and I did not have postpartum depression, and we follow that with a discussion of why she asked and what it means to her. I answer it because I think it helps her connect, regardless of what the answers are. Are these questions a test of sorts? Perhaps. When deciding whether to trust us and the process of therapy, mothers want to know who we are and if we are going to be authentic with her. I think, within the confines of our working principles, we should be. But being authentic does not mean telling her everything she wants to know.

Authenticity does not mean you must express blatant details about your own experiences even if there may be morsels that would be helpful or meaningful to her. When discussing the implications of self-disclosure, content is only part of the issue. The content of your disclosure is subjective. Built-in biases are attached to what you say and how it is perceived and interpreted. It is another balancing act, one that insists that you put her first, always.

3 *The Value of Chitchat*

Sometimes (and that is a big *sometimes*), it does feel therapeutically pertinent to introduce a diversion. This should always be done with intent, and although it may feel a bit chatty to her, your clinical motive is to check her reaction, to monitor her connection to the outside world, to assess her ability to relate to something outside of herself, or perhaps to see if she can laugh or say thank you. I might compliment my client at some point and tell her I like the way she cut her hair. Or, if I notice she has something new with her, I will comment on it. I am not averse to breaking the therapeutic frame for a brief fashion critique if I believe that is important to her. Praise, admiration, self-esteem, and self-worth cannot be underrated in this setting. Most likely, her self-esteem is at an all-time low, and although she may not feel worthy of a compliment (it might irritate her), if it is genuine and stated with the purpose of connecting with her, it can settle in nicely until she is ready to hear it.

Many of us were trained to keep free-flowing conversations to a minimum in therapy. Although we constantly process and interpret, we have been instructed that we should not, necessarily, comment in response to the material our clients present to us.

I am a great fan of spontaneous conversation. Within the confines of this sacred therapeutic space, accidental gems can emerge in dialogues that may not feel particularly therapeutic at the moment. There will be times when the content of what you talk about is not always as valuable as how you do it and how it makes your client feel. As stated earlier, there can be great significance in the exchange of seemingly superfluous details or silly references to things that may mean nothing beyond the fact that it made her smile for the first time in a very long time. I am all about making her smile. It has tremendous repair value. Although it may appear to be chit chat to an outsider, some informal exchange of less weighty topics can be highly engaging for some women, enabling them to connect to the process with more ease. It is also a great way to gauge affective responsiveness. Many times she will react with more authenticity when she tells me where she bought her shoes and why she loves shopping at a particular store than when I ask her to tell me how it feels to be a mother. When you access that affective realness, you engage her. There is meaningful information in almost every interaction.

I am careful to study how she responds to the tone of the session and do my best to adjust respectively. If I am taking too much of the lead, I back off. If she is lost and seeking direction in the session, I step in. If she is therapy-wise and can carry the session in the direction she needs it to go, I surrender to her lead. Much of the time, a postpartum woman prefers you to guide the early sessions and may let you know this through her silence, through talkativeness, or through any number of symptom-driven digressions. You take charge with your agenda and your plan to help her feel like herself again. You are proactive, you are positive, and you believe in your ability to help her.

4 *Touching*

Touch is important to healing. Although no one would disagree that inappropriate touching is damaging and forbidden, a rigid avoidance of touch can also deprive our clients of much needed human contact and relatedness. This is an area that requires intense scrutiny on our part in determining the Who, When, and Why variables in this scenario, and again, if in doubt, do not do it.

Within the context of therapy, there may be many tempting moments when touching feels like an appropriate response, particularly when emotions are raw. I limit touching to my greeting hold or handshake and sometimes our exit, depending on the client and our relationship (while keeping a close eye on any resistance due to a possible fear of contamination, for example). Any impulse to touch in an effort to console or soothe should also be discouraged, as this can interfere clinically. Rushing to physically comfort a client is never a good idea. It can send the message that you want her to control her emotions and that you are unable to tolerate the emotional expression. Be wary of instances that make you want to reach out in this way and check in with your own emotional state.

5 *Pursuing an Uninterested Client if They Disengage from Treatment*

Postpartum women are drowning in ambivalence and are often side-tracked by numerous obligatory priorities. Therapy is not one of these obligatory priorities. It is fair to say that although I may be far less concerned than she is about some postpartum symptoms (that is, I may not be clinically concerned about her high level of anxiety even though she feels so bad), I may be *more* concerned than she is about others. For example, if she is flat, disconnected, and feeling despondent, she may find the energy to call for an appointment out of compliance but may not return our phone calls when we try to follow up.

At The Postpartum Stress Center, whereas we may leave one follow-up phone message for a non-perinatal client, we will call a postpartum woman back two to three times, asking her to let us know how she is or to make sure she is in good hands with another therapist. In such cases, we often hear back from them eventually, telling us that they appreciate our follow-up and that either they are feeling better or they have found another therapist in their insurance network or closer to home. There have been times that our follow-up has led us right into the anxious vortex of her inability to make a decision, in which case, we find ourselves with another opportunity to discuss options and help guide her toward treatment options. Understanding the barriers that interfere with help-seeking behaviors will help you determine when and how to follow up in individual cases when symptoms make it difficult to connect, despite a desire to do so.

6 *Spending Time on the Phone Discussing What You Can Be Discussing in a Session*

After the initial meeting, it is neither feasible nor advisable to attend to each anxious request for reassurance between sessions. Though that may be an occupational hazard, it will do neither of you any good if you do not set limits on that behavior and explain basic therapeutic protocol. However, you must also learn to differentiate the anxiety-driven need for kind comfort in between sessions from symptoms that signify greater clinical concern, such as excessive agitation that may indicate anything from panic to mania. Postpartum women may call more and need more than non-perinatal clients, due to their heightened degree of anxiety, their urgency to return to normal functioning for the sake of their baby, and their extremely compromised physiological state of exhaustion and hormonal flux. Your task is to understand that this is associated with behaviors that may demand attention while they simultaneously challenge us to set appropriate boundaries and contain her symptoms.

7 *Am I Enough?*

This is a question that all good therapists might reflect on from time to time, regardless of the population they work with. Within a perinatal context, it seems that therapists are particularly susceptible to merciless self-scrutiny as they work hard to keep their own issues from spilling into the work with their client. Any and all reproductive events that directly impact a therapist can threaten boundaries and reinforce the dreaded notion that good enough is not good enough as a therapist. The therapist might be currently dealing with issues that are identical in many ways to those that their client is focusing on, such as cultural pressures, lack of support, or reproductive trauma. In such cases, the therapist might understandably feel unequipped to provide problem-solving solutions as this might feel hypocritical or ungenuine.

A good-enough mother must learn to balance her earnest desire to provide perfectly for her child's every need with the recognition that she will inevitably make mistakes. Similarly, a good-enough therapist must learn to balance their earnest desire to provide urgent symptom relief to postpartum clients with their client's need to be heard, validated, and understood. This concept requires authenticity from the therapist, including a willingness to relinquish anxiety about one's own capability in order to guide the therapeutic relationship toward a positive outcome. Identifying your own tendency toward perfection is not easy to do, and letting go of perfectionism is an important part of modeling self-awareness. The balance you achieve by presenting your most authentic self, your best self, breathes life into Winnicott's always relevant ideas and gives you both permission to be good enough and assurance that good enough is good.

Chapter 6

The Practice of Holding

Years ago, The Postpartum Stress Center distributed an informal survey online in an effort to establish a better understanding of what postpartum women are looking for when seeking therapeutic support. The good news is that many women reported satisfaction with their therapist, even those whom they said were not specialists in the treatment of postpartum depression. Although at first glance, this result seemed to defy my premise that it would be better for the postpartum client if she went to a therapist trained in treating perinatal mood and anxiety disorders, I realized that what postpartum women need more than a specialist is someone who is good at holding.

One woman wrote "I was so looking forward to being a mother that I couldn't handle the admission that now that I was actually a mother, I hated it. That was so hard. I felt so bad at this mothering thing. It was like my whole being had cracked and I couldn't snap myself out of it. When I finally found a therapist, she was very kind, spoke softly, and never made me feel like I should be ashamed."

Another said "It didn't matter that she wasn't an expert. She seemed knowledgeable and totally validated my feelings and experience. I'm not sure if she had specific training in postpartum depression, but I felt very comfortable with her and she reassured me that I would feel better."

A third woman wrote "I felt so disrespected because the therapist did not believe in postpartum depression. I wanted reassurance and some direction, but I didn't get much for my money! It was like I was talking to myself; I didn't really need to pay someone for me to do that. I thought I would have gotten more specific guidance."

Approximately one-half of the respondents felt that their therapist was qualified to treat their symptoms of depression and anxiety, whether or not they were aware of any specialized training in that area. That was a wonderful discovery and a higher percentage than anticipated. This also, however, reinforced the concern that postpartum women continue to engage in

DOI: 10.4324/9781003402145-6

therapeutic relationships with professionals who may, even inadvertently, contribute to their feeling worse when they leave the office than before they went in. This can happen with just one misstep, one bad sentence, as recounted by one woman who said she did not return after her therapist glibly asked: *You don't feel like killing yourself, do you?*

Holding Fundamentals

The Art of Holding recognizes that the role, the essence, and the self of the therapist represent an essential component of the therapeutic connection in the face of profound resistance to the process. Yet, paradoxically, this crucial role can be compromised by the potential for the therapist's own reproductive journey becoming a template which can complicate and jeopardize the therapeutic dyad. Awareness and competence of the holding skills allows space and containment for distress that feels unendurable. When the holding therapist attunes to this discomfort, the skills described in this chapter are used to stabilize the client while concurrently checking in with their own nervous system.

Central to developing skill in The Art of Holding is mastery of the six holding points. The six holding points infused into the remaining chapters of this book should be incorporated into every moment when working with postpartum women. As we delve further into holding specifics, always keep in mind how her symptoms, her state, her plan, are touching you and any biases you may be leaning into.

The Six Holding Points:

1 Grounding
2 Current state
3 Expert
4 Design
5 Presence
6 Safeguarding

Given that there is no validated protocol for this intervention, the application and timing of each point is reliant upon good clinical interpretation and judgment. Within each interaction with a postpartum woman in therapy, you are likely to utilize or consider all six facets simultaneously. They are not separate points. They are tied together seamlessly. In practice, you will find that this model of intervention will continue to inform your work with a client over the course of several weeks or months. Your awareness and ability to apply these holding points within each therapeutic moment are what will set you apart from a good therapist who does not specialize in the treatment of perinatal emotional illness. While each holding point has its own objective, all intermix to inform our responses and interventions. At the end of this chapter you will find a table outlining the specific objectives of each holding point.

Consider a brief overview of each holding point.

Point 1: *Grounding*

Effective treatment for women with postpartum depression or anxiety incorporates knowledge of the context of childbirth and the transition to motherhood with a woman's unique history and life story. Above all, therapists must appreciate how difficult the first outreach for support and initial session are for many postpartum women. Again, the difficulty is not necessarily because she is opposed to therapy or because she doesn't want help. It is because it is hard to settle the disparate emotions that have arisen within this sacred realm, and it is not easy to know where to turn or what to do.

The initial objective of grounding is to reinforce her decision to seek support, validate her range of emotions and create an environment that is conducive to safe disclosure.

Example opening statement: *It's hard being here. I'm hopeful that you will feel a little bit better by the time you leave today.*

Grounding is your skilled response to the symptomatic expression of everything she feels she has lost and now feels disoriented by. Grounding conveys the message that you are in position to help and while you normalize her dysregulation, you offer hope that you can calm her unruly symptoms and help her regain control of the way she is feeling. Grounding techniques are used frequently in therapy to reduce excess emotional energy. In the same way that a grounded wire secures physical safety, grounding in therapy can help a client feel less agitated and more secure. Often, therapists employ physical and gravity-related strategies, such as telling clients to plant their feet firmly on the floor or perform a breathing exercise. These suggestions can help stabilize high levels of distress. Another useful exercise is the 5 × 5 practice. This is when the client is instructed to take note of her senses and name five things she sees, smells, tastes, feels, and hears.

Well-established grounding techniques will work in the postpartum context, too, but within the holding environment grounding energy comes from *you* and your energy. Her body and her experience of distress and dysregulation will find balance when you can lead her through your own embodiment of balance. Your voice, your tone, your eye contact, your words, your knowledge, and your confidence, combined with your resources and tools to contain her symptoms and model regulation, will keep her in the present moment so she can focus and begin to believe that she will not always feel this way.

Point 2: *Current state*

The primary objective of the *current state point* is to elicit the client's self-reported perceived level of distress as well as our observations and interpretations of her reported and presenting distress. This will allow us to assess the degree to which her distress is interfering with her ability to function regardless of where she is in her recovery process. Due to the unpredictable nature of circumstances and emotions during this time in her life, assessment of her emotional state should take place throughout the course of the therapeutic work.

Example opening question: *Can you put into words how bad you feel?*

The current state point involves the clinician's ability to conduct a rapid evaluation of the client's immediate circumstances, which includes determination of physical safety. In the earliest sessions, a thorough history is taken in order to evaluate the total clinical picture, but there will be times when acute symptoms supersede history taking, pressing you to concentrate on symptoms and stability. When that happens, priorities are reorganized and the process shifts. This process of *listening to her symptoms* is when you pay attention to whatever is calling out for immediate consideration while embracing the broader perspective at the same time. In this context, listening to her symptoms obliges us to observe and begin to understand what her symptoms might be telling us, even if her words may not. This is discussed further in the following chapter.

Various emotional states will necessitate different interventions or treatment tracks, which is why it's important to review her current emotional state carefully and at regular intervals over the course of treatment. As the sessions proceed, evaluating her current state remains a primary task as it sets the stage for subsequent therapeutic decisions and interventions.

Point 3: *Expert*

The objective of the *expert point* is to present yourself with confidence to convey that you are equipped to help provide symptom relief.

Example opening question: *What is worrying you the most right now?*

This question, when asked with a confident, soothing tone, can communicate that you invite and are able to tolerate whatever she needs to say to you at that moment. Within the context of the holding environment, the term expert refers to the embodiment of the words, posture, and tone the therapist chooses to convey competence and a belief in their ability to help the client. When a client enters the therapy space and is met by this steadfast energy, distress can begin to settle as she quietly wonders whether it is possible that *everything will be okay* and that you will know how to facilitate that. While it will not be possible for a therapist to establish precise expectations of any treatment trajectory, therapists are encouraged to use phrases such as "the distress you are experiencing is a symptom of your depression and anxiety and as we treat your symptoms you will start to feel better, more like yourself again." You may be the first healthcare provider to look her in the eyes and express with assurance that you hear her and care about how she feels. Do not underestimate the subtle yet forceful energy this entrusts to her. If she feels that she is in a safe place, she can begin to connect with your confidence and feel more secure with herself. This transfer of energy from the therapist to the client is best achieved through intentional practice and a strong sense of professional and personal self. It is not your extensive knowledge that makes you an expert. It is about your belief in yourself and in your ability to help her.

Point 4: *Design*

The objective of the *design point* is to determine the most immediate course of action to provide symptom relief and to problem-solve in response to her expressed concerns.

Example opening statement: *What were you hoping we might come up with to help you get some relief?*

The design point encompasses your shared motivation to mitigate interference from her symptoms. Therapist and client collaborate, using a combination of your therapeutic resources and clinical judgment and her expectations and preferences. Treatment options may include any or many of the following: psychotherapy, medication, non-pharmacological interventions, alternative/complementary therapies, group support, and self-help options, such as sleep, nutrition, and exercise, for example. But at the early stages of connection, more important than the treatment itself is the prospect of a plan. The genuine intention of the therapist, presenting a clear and endorsed treatment track, can captivate even the most negative critic of the therapeutic process.

Point 5: *Presence*

The objective of the *presence point* is to understand her narrative as her unique experience of loss as a primary means of therapeutic connectivity. In doing so, the therapist remains focused on the nuanced language, expressions, and experiences that bind the therapeutic alliance.

Example opening statement: *Let's talk about how hard it is to get through the day when you feel this bad.*

The ability to establish and sustain a meaningful connection with a postpartum woman can be initially and continuously challenging for the therapist. To reiterate, there is an emptiness and rawness that is so flagrant and obvious but still, so irreconcilable. This fifth point incorporates the therapist's response to the screaming symptoms with the embodiment of the holding environment. When you can represent the good mother with kind-hearted realness, you bring your client closer to home, as in Connelly's reference, and create a space that makes it possible for her to express herself and feel what she needs to feel. Providing this calm, attuned attention for a client who brings a hurricane of emotion into the therapeutic space can feel professionally demanding, to be sure. However, presence presupposes authenticity. Here we offer her our best professional self. This is where you sit with suffering. Where you tolerate her chaos. Where you endure the discomfort she personifies. Remaining present in this way enables you to further demonstrate how to contain her big emotions with the power of your stillness.

Point 6: *Safeguarding*

The objective of the *safeguarding point* is to protect her at all times, including her life, her baby's life, her partnership, her level of distress, her physical health, her social network of support, as well as her connection with the therapeutic process.

Example opening statement: *Are you okay?*

Safeguarding, as all the holding points, should be implemented during and beyond the first few sessions. As you proceed through later phases of treatment, again, with all holding points, you never lose sight of how exposed she may continue to feel, even as she begins to heal and feel stronger. Safeguarding, in particular, implies that we are continuously on guard to monitor her vulnerabilities, whether or not they are expressed openly to us. Keeping her feeling safe requires that we intermittently tweak the therapeutic space to ensure transparency and authenticity in order for us to successfully protect her perceived areas of weakness. If we presume she may be withholding to some extent, due to her fear of disclosure, we are obliged to listen hard to what is not being said.

Safeguarding involves her implicit and/or explicit understanding that you are always on the lookout for signs of relapse or breakthrough symptoms so that you can help lessen the risk of this occurring. She doesn't trust herself yet. One way you accomplish this is to honor her emotional pain as you lead her toward her own personal resources that have proven to be helpful in the past. This interplay between her pain and her areas of strength is where she begins to access areas of resilience, which will protect her, from herself and from her symptoms. Finding resilience in the face of perceived emotional collapse will enable her to begin to believe that she will be okay.

Holding Opportunities

While certain clinical moments call out to you and yearn for attention, this should not obscure the fact that other, more subtle needs also inform your work, sometimes catching you off guard. There are relational aspects of each interaction which set the stage for holding throughout the course of your work together.

If you aren't paying attention, you might miss them.

Phone Intake

I am not a fan of scheduling online unless phone contact is also involved. Although The Postpartum Stress Center does offer an option for scheduling through our website, it is not a direct link to schedule. Rather, it is a request for an appointment. We follow up with an intake call from one of our therapists, recognizing that if we miss this first opportunity for voice contact, we potentially miss the chance to connect prior to the appointment and to assess for urgent situations that should not wait.

A therapist's first phone contact is an excellent opportunity to utilize the holding points. Many therapists agree that any initial contact with a client, including a phone call, provides an opportunity to build therapeutic trust. Any opening that lends itself to personalization, where you can begin to connect on an individual level, will help facilitate the connection. Attaching names and individualizing her experience grounds her. It can reduce the potential awkwardness of this first contact and make it feel more caring to her.

Consider this exchange:

"Hi Suzanne. This is Karen from The Postpartum Stress Center returning your call."

"Oh. Hi. Thanks for calling back. My doctor told me to call you."

"I'm glad you called. Is your doctor concerned about the way you are feeling? Are *you* concerned about the way you are feeling, Suzanne?"

"I'm just not feeling like myself at all since I had my baby 6 weeks ago."

"I'm sorry you are feeling bad but it's good that you called. Let's see what we need to do to help you feel more like yourself again."

Her voice cracks, "Okay, good. That would be great." She sighs heavily, gasping for a full breath.

"I'd like to ask you a few questions first, would that be okay?"

"Sure." She whispers in compliance.

Holding positions you to instill a sense of trust from these first moments of this first phone call. This initial contact is when I ask her what worries her the most about the way she is feeling so I can determine the degree to which her distress is interfering with her ability to function and how it might be affecting the way she is thinking. Listening to her words, her voice, her ability to express herself, her story, and her symptoms provides meaningful information regarding her perception of the problem. It may or may not be as problematic as she feels it is, but her insight and her appraisal of her current state is relevant. Put another way, it may or may not coincide with my subsequent clinical assessment, but her awareness and judgment of how she is doing are directly linked to her level of distress, whether or not there is an acute clinical concern. This is where we gather preliminary information about her current state.

As we briefly chat about her personal and family history of depression or anxiety, I also seek to determine any critical risk. I will ask her if she is having any thoughts that are scaring her and whether she is experiencing suicidal thoughts or negative intrusive thoughts about harm coming to her baby. If she denies suicidal thoughts but reports the presence of scary thoughts about her baby, I employ the expert holding point by offering a brief psychoeducational explanation about how common scary thoughts are during the postpartum period. I am cautious not to over-reassure and hope to gain clarity when I can look her in the eyes and complete a comprehensive evaluation. I attempt to reduce her anxiety by letting her know in a soothing voice that I am familiar with this high level of agitation, and by saying this, demonstrate that I am not as worried about her high anxiety as she is. Maintaining a calm tone and even cadence to my voice can help ground and comfort her.

I make sure to explore her support network to further assess the level of urgency and available resources. Is she isolated? Does she have a partner? A family? Good friends? Community of support? Does she perceive her support network as helpful? Does she feel cared for? Is she open to additional types of support? Is she experiencing intense emotions such as rage, irritability, anger, hopelessness, or despair that can make this support less accessible to her? I am learning about her life, her environment, her resistance, and her preferences; I am beginning to consider the design for her treatment.

If she has a partner, I will explore the nature of this relationship, insofar as that is feasible in the few minutes that we have:

"Suzanne, are you in a relationship?"
"Yes. My husband wanted me to call you too."
"What's your husband's name?"
"David."
"Does David know how bad you are feeling?"
"No."
"Why do you think that is?" (There are many reasons why she responded that her husband does not know how bad she feels. Perhaps a) she has difficulty expressing the extent to which she is suffering, b) he doesn't listen, c) he is in denial of sorts and wants her to return to her previous level of functioning, d) they had pre-existing marital issues and she is hurt and angry and feels abandoned by him, e) he has difficulty hearing and handling emotions, f) he cares very much and is listening to everything she says, but his ability to process deep emotions is limited

by his own personal history or symptoms of depression or anxiety, g) she doesn't want him to know... this list is endless. This is why I ask, "why not?" when she said he doesn't know how bad she is feeling. Another reason I ask is to personalize the discussion so she can begin to feel that she is connecting with someone whom she perceives as caring, who feels real and presents as invested in her.

"He tries. He just doesn't understand. He's been wonderful, really; I know this is hard for him. He's not very good at emotional things."

"I'm glad he is trying and that you can say he has been wonderful; that is good to hear. For now, that's enough. This is hard for him, too. You and I can help him get better at this after we meet, okay? (I smile through the phone, hoping she can see/feel/understand my early attempt to join with her.)

"Yes." She returns my smile. (We can hear that, can't we?) "That would be great."

"What is your baby's name, Suzanne?"

"Gracie."

"What a beautiful name. Gracie. I love that." Here again, the attempt to join by personalizing her experience. To me, it feels maternal. It feels friendly. It feels complimentary. It feels approving. Depending on her personality and/or her symptoms, she may or may not like that, or it may or may not go by unnoticed.

Can you feel the difference in the following responses?

"Oh, thanks. Gracie is unbelievably adorable. She so sweet." She starts to cry, "I feel so bad that I can't be the mommy that she deserves. I love her so much."

As opposed to:

"Thanks," Spoken in a soft, barely audible, monotonous tone.
Or nothing at all. Silence.

I have noticed that when I ask and respond to the baby's name, it can unlock a woman's outermost layer of defense, making it possible to contemplate her readiness and willingness to engage in this process. What is revealed in this minute dialogue is a peek into her relationship with her partner and her baby. If you tune into to the words she chooses and the tone she uses, you will hear clues regarding how she is feeling and what she may need.

After assessing immediate risk and briefly discussing her relationships and support, you discuss whether coming in would feel good to her at this point. If she is ambivalent, I will pitch it as "I'm thinking it would be help-ful for you to come in one time. If you felt bad enough to make this call, and I know how hard it is to make this call, why don't we meet one time? That way, I can take a look at you and together, we can decide what you need to worry about and what you do not need to worry about. How does that sound?"

My pitch to gently nudge her in the direction of therapeutic support demonstrates my presence, by identifying and validating her suffering. I am careful to support her ambivalence, respect any resistance, assuage the bur-den of worry, and place a boundary on her fear of entering into an unknown process with unknown parameters. This way, we present the possibility of relief and help her make the decision at a time when decisions feel impossible to make. Moreover, this effort to encourage her to get pro-fessional help and support is actually our earliest effort to safeguard her, since we are only too aware of the potential danger lurking behind untreated symptoms.

I may reinforce this presence and safeguarding with a statement such as, "I know this feels terrible right now. And I know that waiting to come in feels like forever. But I am just a phone call away and soon, we will be on track to getting you some relief. In the meantime, you can... (*offer sup-portive interventions*). You do not have to go through this alone anymore."

Many women have told me they felt better after that first phone call.

In addition to earlier assessment questions regarding safety and scary thoughts, I typically include a review of additional assessment items for depression, such as appetite, sleep, pleasurable activities, concentration, and anxiety. It is then recommended that a plan of action be discussed for the time between your phone contact and first appointment. In an ideal world, this would only be 24 to 48 hours, but the real world doesn't always accommodate this, and, most likely, she will need to endure several more days of discomfort before she can get in to see you. Therefore, it is sug-gested that this first phone contact ends with these suggestions:

- Make yourself available to contact if her symptoms worsen. Let her know the best way to reach you if anything scares her or if her symp-toms intensify.
- Tell her to let her partner and/or family know how to contact you if anyone is worried about what they see or hear.
- Remind her to eat even if she is not hungry and rest if she is not sleeping well.
- Give her permission to engage in good self-care and to increase her access to rest until you see her and to try to let go of guilt about disen-gaging from social activities for a bit.

- Reinforce the importance of letting others close to her know how she feels and what she needs.
- Praise her for taking this difficult help-seeking step and let her know that this bodes well for her longer-term well-being given that she is able to advocate for herself.

As a result of this initial contact, I have, in a fairly short amount of time, skimmed the six points of holding.

1 I have **grounded** her by encouraging this initial contact and helping her feel comfortable by personalizing her loved ones and commenting on any strength in those relationships. Further grounding comes from her feeling listened to by someone who does not patronize her or prefer she focus on feeling grateful and positive. This first phone contact can make the difference between her getting help or not.
2 I have acknowledged her **current state** by discussing her symptoms and responding with an impartial, non-reactive reflection of her experience. Early assessment of her experience should always rule out emergency situations and, ideally, prepare her for a first office visit.
3 I have employed my **expert** self with words of comfort and assurance in my ability to help her.
4 I have put forth a **design** for an early plan of action between now and our first appointment so she can renounce her diminishing control and agree to let me help her.
5 I have established my ability to remain close to her distress and stay **present** with her pain and reinforced it during the dreaded void between this initial contact and her first appointment.
6 I have demonstrated my intent to keep her **safe** by not overreacting and recognizing that this high level of distress is a common feature of post-partum depression and anxiety, by honoring her opposition or fear, and by gently guiding her in the direction of recovery. By attending to her distress in this way, I am reflecting my confidence in her ability to cope as well as my ability to help her manage her acute symptoms.

Holding Refined

It will soon become clear that most of your current practices align with holding principles. When considering your current practice through the specific filter of the holding points, however, you will discover a mechanism for structuring and monitoring those interventions that can be otherwise difficult to define. Let's see how this works.

One of my favorite interventions for shifting negative thinking is based on mindfulness-based cognitive therapy (MBCT). MBCT combines aspects of cognitive therapy and mindfulness practice to help clients isolate their upsetting automatic thoughts and view them as separate from the actual present moment. Elisha Goldstein, PhD, describes a quick and easy intervention in his book *Uncovering Happiness* (2015), where he talks about steps to take to free oneself from negative thought cycles. In his work, Goldstein refers to four steps which are useful to help our clients cope with distorted thinking traps such as catastrophizing, blaming, obsessing on the negative, and ruminating.

The practice begins like this: Tell your client to notice when a negative thought first enters her mind. Next, she is instructed to stop, take an intentional deep breath, and move through the next four steps.

1 *Name it.* Tell your client to name the distorting thinking (e.g., catastrophic thinking, excessive worry, ruminating). By labeling the thinking style, she creates awareness by interrupting the negative cycle. This has also shown to increase activity to the part of the brain that regulates emotions. By doing this, she externalizes her painful thought process and can begin to see it as separate from who she is and what the problem actually is or is not.
2 *Feel it.* This part is hard because no one wants to choose to feel the feelings associated with negative thoughts. But experiencing it in the body and expressing it help her stay in the present moment and provide access to making a choice going forward. It's like pressing a pause button to help her see that she can decide if she wants to continue to feel this way.
3 *Release it.* Tell your client to repeat this phrase along with breathing in and out: "Breathing in, I acknowledge the feeling that's here; breathing out, I release it."
4 *Redirect it.* Finally, she is instructed to shift her attention, distract herself to something that feels better, healthier, or more important. In doing so, she is again making a choice, and that is empowering when she feels out of control.

This exercise may be used in the holding environment as a **grounding** technique that serves to reduce distress and help manage how she is thinking and feeling. It is, simultaneously, attentive to her **current state**, illustrates your confident, or **expert**, interpretation of her experience, and **designs** a step-by-step tool on which she can rely. Introducing a soothing exercise in response to her high distress reflects your **presence**, your ability to tolerate her distress and intervene on her behalf and **safeguards** her from the shockwave of her constant negative thoughts. In this way, you can see how a technique you likely are already using can be redefined through a holding lens. When you execute and monitor interventions via holding principles, you offer the exercise with more precise attention to her by paying more attention to *you*. This enables her to engage more completely, heightening the potential for connectivity, and building the relationship with you that can sustain her through the process of gathering her strength during these early stages of her treatment.

Holding her brings you into that process. Think about this. A doctor will hand out a prescription with instructions. A physical therapist will provide a picture of the workout with a detailed step-by-step protocol. Another healthcare provider might give her a list of things to avoid, things to do, ways to improve her current state. What you give her is you. For now. Until she is stronger.

Single-Session Holding

You cannot assume your client is coming back after the first session.

If you treat every new client as a possible single-session intervention, you might be surprised to discover how helpful you can be in such a short period of time. Did you know that almost 20% of patients drop out of treatment prematurely (Leichsenring et al., 2019)? However tempting it may be to take therapy drop-outs personally, most of us who practice in the field of psychology learn to reframe such events as preliminary treatment failures with some reference to the client's inability to connect with our awesomeness. The truth is, some people want or need only one session. This would not be the case when a postpartum woman is immersed in symptomatology of a major depressive disorder. But it could very much be the case if she has postpartum stress syndrome and seeks support and validation. There have been a number of postpartum women who have come to The Postpartum Stress Center for one or two sessions, never to return. These are generally women who come seeking reassurance that what they are feeling is within normal limits and perhaps a discussion of coping strategies. On the whole, these women do not have a history of significant depression or anxiety and state they feel supported in their relationships.

From the outset, you might tell a postpartum client that your goal is to get her in and out of here as quickly as possible. *As soon as you feel better, you will be done here*, I tell her. I want to dispel any hidden bias she might have about therapists persuading clients to do work they are not interested in doing, such as family-of-origin exploration. I also want her to know that I am fully aware of what an imposition this is and that I am on her side.

The potential downside to this notion of a single-session intervention is the obvious, *what if I miss something? What if she needs more than this and just never comes back?* Of course this is an occupational hazard that can emerge at any time with any client. The point here is that we should do our best to engage any perinatal woman who contacts us so we can at least introduce her to the prospect of her finding relief from the support. Ultimately, if she isn't interested in ongoing support or resists our suggestions, the decision is up to her. But if we suspect we may only have one or two opportunities to meet with her, we might want to arm her with some super-holding and make sure she knows we are here in the event that she changes her mind or needs something going forward.

Breaking Down the Hyperbole

Exaggerated descriptions of one's symptoms is expected at the outset of therapy. It is natural to magnify one's experience of distress when over-come by mental, physical, and soulful discomforts that are all-consuming. When performing an early assessment, whether on the phone or in a first session, you might hear:

I haven't slept in months.
I haven't eaten a single thing in days.
I don't remember the last time I took a shower.

Sometimes, these statements are said with exasperated humor or sarcasm. Sometimes, however, they are said because they feel accurate to her. Our S.E.L.F. acronym, first presented in *Dropping the Baby and Other Scary Thoughts* (Kleiman et al., 2020), is used to remind moms to make them-selves a priority. This directive is often met with frustrated opposition, but still, you say it and repeat it often. It stands for a) Sleep, b) Exercise, c) Laughter, and d) Food. If these four conditions are adequately attended to, even minimally, it increases the likelihood that she will feel better than she does in her current state of distress.

No one would argue that it is difficult to exercise when you are depressed. It is also difficult to laugh. If both of these things feel impossible to her, it is still helpful, with the right timing and language, to acknowledge their importance while offering her permission to postpone this directive for now. You could say, "You will find that your sense of humor returns as you begin to feel better."

However, with some women, you might want to provide just a small entrance into the world of possibilities. If she enjoyed exercising prior to her depression, for instance, you might suggest, "When you feel better, it will be easier for you to exercise again, and enjoy it, even though that might feel unlikely right now. Until then, I wonder if you might be able to spend a small amount of time outside in the sunshine; perhaps walk your dog around the block and see how that feels?"

Black and White Thinking

Clients with a tendency to inflate the presence and impact of a symptom may be associated with perfectionistic or black-and-white thinking. *Either*

I am okay or I am not. Either I am anxious or I am not. Either I am sleep deprived or I am not. There are not a lot of gray areas in this way of thinking.

Let us look at how you might respond to overstated declarations about sleep and eating in a manner that employs the holding points in a way that benefits her and enables you to determine the degree of distress with a bit more accuracy.

SLEEP

When asked if she is able to sleep when her baby sleeps, a client replied:

"Honestly, *I haven't slept at all in weeks.* I'm so tired I can barely move. I don't think *I'll ever sleep again.*"

"I know you are very tired. It is hard to get through the day being so tired. How much sleep were you accustomed to getting before you had a baby? How many hours is a good night's sleep for you?"

"I used to get 8 or 9 hours. And on Saturdays, I could easily get 10 hours or more."

"Okay, that gives me a good idea of what your baseline is. Let's talk about what it looks like now. Can you describe a typical night for me? When do you go to sleep? When do you wake up through the night? How long do you remain awake? Are you awake because the baby keeps you up or do you have trouble falling back asleep? Can you describe what it looks like from when you start to go to bed until you get up for the day? For instance, how many times are you getting up? How long are you up for? What is waking you up? Lots of questions, right? Why don't you tell me what last night looked like?"

"Well, I got in bed at 10. I probably fell asleep at 10:30 or so. I woke up around midnight and fed the baby. She wouldn't go back to sleep, so I'm not sure exactly what time it was, but I'm pretty sure it was like 2 in the morning before I fell back to sleep. Then she woke up again at 4:30; I think I fell asleep around 5:30 and slept until 7:00."

"Okay, so if my math is correct, I figure you got approximately five and a half hours of broken sleep. Does that sound close?"

"Yeah."

"So what that says to me is that it's only about half as much sleep as you would love to get, so we definitely want to work on creating more sleep opportunities for you. It's no wonder you feel tired. However, I am relieved to hear that you are sleeping somewhat and are able to fall asleep when you have a chance to do so. While we surely want to augment your sleep so that you feel well, I am impressed that you are functioning pretty well with much less sleep than you are used to getting. We will discuss strategies to enhance your sleep, but in the meantime, I'd like to help you decrease your anxiety by talking this through a little differently. Let's talk about your tolerance for tiredness. It's okay to be tired, especially right now. Do you notice a shift in your anxiety when you think about yourself as feeling tired instead of thinking about sleep as a hopeless endeavor?"

EATING

When asked about her appetite, the conversation went like this:

"I have no appetite at all. I cannot eat a thing."

"Were you a good eater before you had the baby? Did you enjoy food?"

"Oh yeah. Too much, if you know what I mean."

"What are you feeling now that makes it hard to eat?"

"I'm nauseous. I have this thing floating in my stomach, like butter-flies, I guess."

"Did you eat anything today yet?"

"I had like three bites of a banana and some juice at breakfast. That was all. It made me queasy."

"Anything for lunch?"

"My mother was over and made me eat some soup. I didn't want it."

"Did you eat it?"

"Yes. A little."

"Anything else today?"

"I had, like, two pretzels. I thought that would help me feel better."

"Good. So it is 2:15 now and you've had part of a banana, some juice, some soup, and a couple of pretzels."

"Right."

"So you are eating something. That is not a lot to eat. But it is not nothing, either. So that is exactly what you should be doing now. Eat what you can. When your appetite is impaired and you are eating so little, it is best for you to make healthy choices, like you are doing, with bananas, soup, and pretzels. That's good. As you start to feel better, you will be able to eat more."

Both of these scenarios illustrate how easily postpartum women in distress get lost in the mountain of symptoms and lose clarity. What's more, your ability to stay focused on a single response and expand it will elucidate the overall clinical picture. Do not undervalue the significance of augmenting her self-care in the aforementioned ways. Attending to all four of these categories – sleep, exercise, laughter, and nutrition – are empirically shown to reduce symptoms in the battle against depression and anxiety and improve feelings of well-being overall.

An act of holding can incorporate all six points at once. In this way, each word you choose, each look of your face or position of your eyebrows, each quality of your voice, each exposed nerve you protect, each bit of confidence that you exude, each stress you endure, and each instruction that you offer combine to contribute to the holding method of engaging a postpartum woman in distress. These are the ingredients that make connecting with you possible, at any point in treatment. These are the skills that make a well-trained perinatal therapist a safe place for a postpartum woman in distress to sit. Connecting with a stranger in the midst of emotional disruption is complicated. It is also essential for healing.

When that connection is made, holding has taken root.

Holding Skill Objectives

Grounding It's. hard being here. I'm hopeful that you will feel better by the time you leave.

1   To reinforce decision to seek support
2   To validate range of feelings
3   To normalize emotional dysregulation
4   To provide initial symptom stabilization
5   To endorse suffering
6   To create environment conducive to safe disclosure

Current state Can you put into words how bad you feel?

1   To elicit self-reported perceived level of distress
2   To assess distress in terms of *frequency* of symptoms
3   To assess distress in terms of *intensity* of symptoms
4   To assess distress in terms of *duration* of symptoms
5   To determine degree of functional impairment
6   Evaluate degree of urgency for child and mother's well-being

Expert What is worrying you the most right now?

1   To reinforce her decision to ask for help
2   To demonstrate precise awareness of her current state
3   To present self as "safe person"
4   To exhibit knowledge and professional competence
5   To prioritize coinciding needs and areas of vulnerability
6   To observe and study both the content and process

Design What were you hoping we might come up with to help you get some relief?

1 To determine most immediate course of action to provide symptom relief
2 To problem-solve in response to her expressed concerns
3 To support her preferences and encourage participation in her treatment plan
4 To provide psychoeducational support and the opportunity to discuss treatment options
5 To deliver options for various levels of intervention, including: social, medical, partnership, biologic, environmental
6 To initiate self-help measures, including: augmenting sleep/rest opportunities, nutritional support, highlighting self-care

Presence Let's talk about how hard it is to get through the day when you feel this bad.

1 To recognize areas of loss as primary means of therapeutic connectivity
2 To understand her narrative as her unique experience with distinct interpretations
3 To remain focused on the nuanced language, expressions, and experiences
4 To remain cognizant of her history and all variables that may be impacting her experience

Safeguarding Are you okay?

1 To protect her at all times, including: her life, her baby's life, her partnership, her level of distress, her physical health, her social network of support, her connection with the therapeutic process
2 To evaluate suicidality at various intervals
3 To monitor emotional state and avoid risky presumptions about her well-being
4 To observe evidence of disconnect or resistance and reset in order to re-engage
5 To take inventory of areas of vulnerability that require ongoing attention

Chapter 7

Authentic Suffering and the Holding Elements

Beyond the holding points, which provide skill-building structure for the holding therapist, let's now take a closer look at the content, as opposed to the process, that each perinatal woman brings into the therapy space – all that she is, all that she does, all that she feels, all that she says – and how this content informs our holding responses. To reiterate, when studying perinatal distress we observe the presence of a common paradoxical theme – the often inexpressible pain that drives her yearning for help and her reluctance to ask for it or follow through with it. This contradiction of desires is crucial to study and is intrinsic to the concept of *authentic suffering*, an overarching construct within the holding framework.

While the suffering of a perinatal woman in distress may be apparent to therapists who work in this area, authentic suffering refers to a more elusive concept, suffering that is eclipsed by pretense. Authentic suffering refers to *that which is obscured by what she wants us to know and what she will let us see.*

- It's the pain she conceals.
- It's the terror that immobilizes her and keeps her up at night.
- It's what drives her anxiety and her fear that she will continue to fall, forever.
- For some women, it's what's in their suicide note when loved ones cry out that *there were no warning signs.*

The reason this concept is so relevant is that authentic suffering influences everything else. It drives her symptoms. It fuels her resistance. It is a steady reminder of how alone she feels. A postpartum woman in distress may or may not be aware of the nature of this suffering and she may or may not be willing or ready to talk about it. So we sit, we listen, we observe. As therapists, we won't always see authentic suffering at first, especially when she doesn't want us to, but our clinical imperative is to access it and connect with it.

DOI: 10.4324/9781003402145-7

She may or may not be aware of the nature of this suffering and she may or may not be willing or ready to talk about it. As therapists, we don't always see authentic suffering at first, especially when she doesn't want us to, but our clinical imperative is to access it and connect with it.

Chapter 4 explored many reasons why postpartum women may be reluctant to disclose and confront the extent of their suffering. We learned how social stigma, fear of judgment, fear of "going crazy," fear of being labeled a bad mom, and fear of having their baby taken away inhibit a new mother's willingness to seek support. These are only a few of the barriers that lead mothers and their support people to an impasse when it comes to authentic suffering. Of course there are mothers who do let us or others know how terrible they feel. For example, a woman may state she has never felt this way before. She may let us know she is afraid she will never feel like herself again. But she may *not* let us know that she cries every morning on the shower floor feeling like she has failed at everything and hoping she doesn't have to be a mother today. She may not let us know that she secretly wishes she had never had her baby. Some women develop thoughts and feelings that their partner and baby would be better off without them. These women suffer from passive suicidal thoughts. They may think, *I'm not suicidal. I don't really want to die. I'm so tired, I just wish I could sleep and not wake up.*

The problem with passive suicidal thoughts – ideation without a specific plan – is that people mistakenly believe that this thinking is not worrisome and it's just part of feeling overwhelmed. Studies of long-term risk of passive suicidal ideation and who may be at risk for suicidal plans of action or behaviors have not produced a clear association between the two (Liu et al., 2020). Thus, passive suicidal ideation should neither be ignored nor disregarded as par for the course. Passive suicidal ideation is thinking that should always be taken seriously and understood as a direct link to authentic suffering. This is precisely why we say that if we are not able to access her authentic suffering, we may come perilously close to missing her true cry for help.

Her authentic suffering is likely what brought her to you. It is why she feels she can no longer function well by doing this on her own or by hoping it gets better by itself. It can be many things or one thing or everything. What is clear is that it is not easy to talk about it and it is fiercely protected. Without awareness of her authentic suffering, we run the risk of letting her leave the session without connecting on a level that helps her feel sufficiently heard. This, in turn, may leave gaping wounds and seriously unmet needs. And while listening to and witnessing her suffering may not feel like "enough" for many therapists who yearn to relieve her of her suffering, helping her feel heard is exactly what she needs most right now. As we repeat in many different ways, our primary holding task at this point is to listen to her symptoms and hear what is not being said, in addition to what she tells. This is when we fire up our senses and learn more about her story and her current state from clues we perceive and from those she presents. As we do so, we pay attention to elements of authentic suffering which provide additional and deeper information.

Loss-Informed Dynamics

One of the markers that distinguish the holding techniques from many popular therapeutic interventions is the extensive attention placed upon the experience of the therapist and how uniquely that experience interfaces with the client and her experience. Well-trained perinatal therapists come equipped with specialized training and a decided passion for treating this population. Moreover, they enter the therapeutic space with astute self-awareness and a burgeoning sense of how their own personal perinatal experiences weigh into this work. This ongoing introspection and recognition of potential consequences is an integral part of the holding approach. Holding therapists must take note of any and all present or past personal involvement with perinatal issues, remain cautious of any possible biases or judgments, and always act on behalf of their client's best interest.

Remember that The Art of Holding Perinatal Women in Distress is a loss-informed approach. We turn toward this intimate feature of her experience and consider all that comes with the agony of loss during a time in her life when she expected to feel endless joy. It is quite possible that the client sitting in front of us has already gone to one or two therapists who have told her that what she is feeling is normal after having a baby. Or, that she will feel better if she finds a hobby. Or, a good night's sleep will take care of everything, with little attention place on the many losses she feels are weighing her down, essentially disregarding the root of her sorrow. One platitude after another fails to touch the anguish sitting in the heart of a new mother wondering what is wrong with her and whether or not she made a terrible mistake.

The holding elements of authentic suffering refer to dynamic forces unique to the perinatal population that influence and can potentially enhance or disrupt our holding efforts and the therapeutic process. We have seen that a perinatal woman is often caught in a push-pull inner conflict of wanting help and not wanting help or not knowing how to ask for help and reveal their suffering. A deeper understanding of these elements will shed light on her inner struggles and, thus, enrich the therapeutic relationship, enlighten our responses, and increase the likelihood that the perinatal woman in distress will experience relief, reduced anxiety, and increased comfort that will enable her to proceed through the treatment process with less resistance and a greater sense of feeling heard.

The holding elements of authentic suffering are:

1 Sitting with Suffering
2 Possessive Longing
3 The Voice of Depression
4 The Paradox of Being
5 Postpartum Stamina
6 Hard-to-Hold

As we review each one, you might find yourself remembering a particular client or a particular interaction that is best understood within the context of these elements. Take note of these thoughts and allow them to bring the holding elements to life. Holding therapists are constantly reflecting as they balance their attention to the client with their attention to the process.

1 Sitting with Suffering
Sitting with suffering refers to:

- The ability to effectively witness, attune to, and tolerate high levels of distress, without any interpretation, by attending to the potential for emotional dysregulation.
- The ability to resist alleviating the suffering, but to help her endure it and eventually seek transformation through it.
- Taking inventory of all holding points concurrently in order to effectively contain and monitor degree of suffering.

Clinician task: To help her find the courage to sit with her own suffering and find meaning in her suffering as she recovers.

Literally sitting with high levels of distress and painful loss does not come easily to many people. Many therapists will, however, confess that they've always been drawn to helping people in this way. Some state that they recognize an innate capacity to tolerate and support others experiencing high degrees of pain. Still, as we are coming to recognize, many of the therapists who do this work have also experienced perinatal depression and anxiety, reproductive loss, or other related struggles which heightens their vulnerability. Some wonder if that makes them more attuned or more qualified in some way because they understand their client's presentation more intimately. I would argue that it is an inherent risk of this profession, and while it can give rise to greater compassion, it can also lead a therapist off course if they are not careful.

Sitting with suffering is hard, whether you have suffered similarly or not. Sitting with suffering requires us to protect ourselves from the invisible daggers that pierce our own hearts while we focus on bearing witness to her pain. This is when we grab onto all holding points at once, take a deep breath, and sit in stillness. How you manage this is largely dependent on your individual and therapeutic style. For me, when I am sitting with unbearable energy, I feel my chest tighten from the weight of her suffering and while I don't feel particularly bad, I do feel as though I am physically trying to steady myself against howling winds. I breathe slowly and deeply to soften my tightening muscles, I plant my feet flat on the floor, and I gaze softly into her eyes. It is powerful. It is magic.

Sometimes, that's all she needs. To be heard by someone who can endure her darkness. To be listened to by someone who will not tell her not to feel this way. To be in the presence of someone who will not judge, will not panic, will not dismiss, and most assuredly will not expect anything from her, other than what she has the courage to share. When we can successfully send the message that she has permission to sit here with us in any way that feels right to her at this moment, and not pressure her to tell us what she might, in fact, need us to know, we paradoxically set the stage to make disclosure feel safer for her, now, or down the road.

As described earlier, our therapeutic goal is not to alleviate suffering. That concept may be counterintuitive for many readers, as it feels like a natural human response to want to stop someone from suffering. Certainly, this would be true in most non-therapeutic settings. Within this context, however, when suffering comes from unexplainable loss, or indescribable depths of depressive thinking, the suffering may serve to a) communicate the level of distress which is clinically essential, and b) ultimately attach meaning to her loss which, somewhat paradoxically, helps us help her. Asking a perinatal woman in distress to find meaning in her suffering is a request likely to be misunderstood and rejected, so we must be careful in the early stages of our work to take this task on ourselves first, as we slowly and deliberately help her see that we may, in fact, find meaning in her suffering. This should be explored later in our work together, but the clinician's task is to help guide the search for meaning as we listen to her stories and her symptoms.

So, we sit with her suffering. While we brace ourselves for the emotional deluge, we understand that this release is only possible by virtue of our messaging that we can withstand the storm. Holding endorses her suffering, which, in turn, validates her and eases the burden of pain, if only slightly. We are reminded that there is extreme uncertainty and senselessness to her suffering, which accounts for her feelings of dread and helplessness. Eventually, as she learns to sit with her own suffering without fear of judgment, finding meaning can manifest as a healing pursuit. There has been much philosophical writing and spiritual contemplation about the mystery of suffering and how striving for purpose can be a profoundly healing endeavor. While this construct is beyond the scope of this book, it does provide substantial food for thought and fuel for our incentive to sit in the suffering alongside her.

2 The Voice of Depression
The voice of depression refers to:

- The language, the non-verbal communication, and the messages she sends us in her symptom presentation and self-expression.
- What she asks for, tells us, aches for, misses, needs, hopes for, grieves for.
- This is manifested in words, in behavior, in silence, in resistance, in desperation, and most impressively through her symptoms.
- A fundamental truism within the context of treating perinatal women in distress: *Symptoms of depression and anxiety do not feel like symptoms to a new mother. They feel like who she is.*

Clinician task: To sit with, to listen to and to assess expression of symptoms and reply with clinically appropriate, holding-attuned language.

The voice of depression model was first introduced in *Therapy and the Postpartum Woman* (Kleiman, 2009). This model will be explored in detail in the following chapter. It is included as a holding element to emphasize the clinical significance of language, hers and ours, within the holding framework. It will only be introduced briefly here, as a detailed discussion appears in the subsequent chapter.

While our goal is to encourage sincere self-expression, the means to guide this process involves observing and connecting with the factors that actually inhibit her self-expression. For example, was she taught to believe that families do not share their private struggles? Or is her instinct to withhold how she really feels an adaptive response to being raised in a home that discouraged open communication? Does she feel unworthy of asking for help? Is she worried she will be judged? And perhaps most important for our purposes here, do her words, posture, and affect accurately reflect what she is feeling in order to inform our holding response?

At all times, we carefully note her language and her presentation, which represent the voice of depression; what she says, what she doesn't say, how she looks, how she speaks, how she sits. Does she look us in the eyes? Does she smile? Is there tension in her face and her words? How she expresses herself reveals clues to hidden sources of distress, such as feelings of loneliness, isolation, and her need and readiness for connection during this vulnerable time.

Our attention to her voice of depression directly instructs our initial response. For example, if she is extremely agitated, we sit still and breathe. If she sits silently, we lean our body in toward her. If she says she has never felt this sad in her life before, we normalize the grief and validate this loss.

These are ways we counter her self-expression with our synchronized holding response. Our unique response to her nuanced self-expression requires critical listening skills and astute observation in order to see past the façade of what she only wants us to see. The voice of depression model is discussed in detail in Chapter 8.

3 Possessive Longing

Possessive longing refers to:

- The instinct to protect and cling to her authentic suffering in response to her pervasive fear of losing her *self*.
- Her desperate desire to preserve what she perceives as her former and "real" self.
- Her response to what she perceives as her inability to cope or a fear of losing control as she digs deep into the very suffering that has propelled her to seek help.
- A core paradox inherent in the understanding and treatment of perinatal distress: The legitimate yet collapsing desire for autonomy and control, in conflict with her very urgent need (and desire?) for help.

Clinician task: To sit with, to honor, and to disarm her commitment to her symptomatic self.

The losses a new mother experiences are extraordinary and often lie at the core of her suffering, whether or not a clinical depression or anxiety is present. When depression invades her transition into motherhood, many women describe an unendurable loss of self. If we recognize this perceived loss of self as the crux of her authentic suffering, we may begin to understand her frantic need to fiercely hold on to it. Some women feel this is all they have left of their former self, or who they were before they had a baby. They miss her. They long for her. Shame permeates their souls as they wonder if having a baby obliterated their previous self, their precious relationship with their partner, and the world as they knew it. They wonder if they will ever feel like themselves again. Some blame their baby. Some blame their partner. Some blame themselves. They wonder if they will be punished for thinking these things or saying them out loud.

What this can translate to is an intense and perhaps ironic desire to hold tight to symptoms and suffer in silence. Quietly, and sometimes quite insistently, she guards her authentic suffering in order to preserve what little she feels she can control right now. This act of resistance is what guides our holding response, as discussed in Chapter 1 and repeated here for emphasis:

Holding within the context of therapeutic work with postpartum women is defined as a loss-informed, strength-based approach that enables the therapist to contain high levels of distress and do so in a way that cultivates the early stages of connectedness. This attempt to contain her symptoms of agitation and despair is accomplished despite the innate pull she feels to repair this herself in order to preserve what she perceives as her dwindling sense of control.

She may or may not be aware of this desire to embrace her lost self. This longing may manifest as a deliberate grip on her former self or it may show up as opposition to the therapeutic process, or reluctance to engage, or any number of other ways that could sidestep the process. Regardless, our ability to interpret this resistance as a *longing to not let go* will enable us to view it as a way in, rather than an impediment. Ultimately, your ability to grasp the nature and passion that drives this dynamic will better equip you to access her authentic suffering. If you perceive it only as resistance, the gap between your ability to hear her and her willingness to disclose will widen. When you interpret this possessive longing not as opposition, but as her desperate attachment to that part of her *self* she wishes she could reclaim, you have joined her process with enough clarity and empathy to help her move through it.

4 **The Paradox of Being**
The paradox of being refers to:

- Her inclination to overidentify with her symptoms.
- How she might feel about herself as she tries to reconcile her transitioning and transforming thoughts and feelings.
- The tendency to express both awareness and confusion at the emergence of her new self.
- An ambiguous self-image: "Is this just what being a new mother feels like?" and "I don't even know who I am anymore."

Clinician task: To normalize this transitional state and to reframe loss.
Many postpartum women wonder if this is just who they are now, if this is what being a mother feels like. They fear that living within this paradoxical sense of self will be their new identity. They are convinced that this is just the way it is, and can stand up against all of our best efforts to help them understand that this is simply not the case. If a new mother's adaptation to their new role is weighed down by an excessive attachment to their heightened anxiety or symptoms of depression, what ensues is a preoccupation with this new self, a disliked self, that can result in a lack of insight into this turbulent dynamic. So, we remind them of what was written earlier in this book:

One of the worst parts about symptoms of postpartum depression and anxiety is that they don't feel like symptoms. They feel like who you are.

We go on to educate them that symptoms may *feel like* who you are, but that, like medical symptoms, when you recover, you will begin to feel like yourself again, a version of yourself without symptoms of depression or anxiety.

If we understand that this paradox of being is largely the result of an intense overidentification with her symptoms and beliefs in her misappraisals, we can understand why our interventions or reframing might fail to resonate with our client. Your responses will be informed by your therapeutic orientation and professional style, but my response in the face of any therapeutic opposition is to process the process. When I process the process, I put words to the impasse or potential misalignment of messaging. I might say, "I imagine it doesn't feel good to hear this right now." Or, "It seems like you're having a hard time believing what I'm saying." Or, "I wonder if you think I don't really understand what you're feeling right now." These are just examples of how we might let her know that while we may very well believe in what we are doing and what we are saying, we also honor her resistance and her disbelief in what we are saying and we might want to sit there for a while with that uncertainty.

5 **Postpartum Stamina**
Postpartum stamina refers to:

- Her physical, psychological, and mental capacity, effort, and determination to manage unyielding distress.
- Her ability to pace herself during the course of recovery.
- Her ability to cope, adapt, and access resources to cultivate resilience.

Clinician task: To identify areas of vulnerability and help her recharge.

Diminishing stamina can lead to feelings of despair and hopelessness. This element signifies the utmost importance of our safeguarding her physical self and reminding all postpartum women – however irrelevant it may feel with a newborn in the picture – that her physical and mental well-being matters. If stamina is defined as the ability to sustain prolonged periods of stress or activity, the postpartum period can feel as though it requires superhuman energy to get through it. Postpartum women are notoriously good at powering through, without asking for help and without paying attention to cues from their bodies or brains that they are overdoing it. Physical depletion can take its toll on our minds and spirit. Likewise, when one is weary of mind, the body weakened. When the very essence of our being feels compromised, it is exhausting on all levels. A woman's ability to recognize when her tank is almost empty is often neglected while she is busy taking care of everyone else. If I detect a diminished capacity, or vulnerability in her ability to function physically and emotionally the way she typically would, I might address it this way:

- *Are you okay?* (Inquires about any pressing physical, mental, medical, emotional, relational, needs.)
- *What do you need?* (Also inquires about any pressing physical, mental, medical, emotional, relational needs.)
- *Are you lonely?* (This is a question I ask to assess the level of isolation and possible detachment from important relationships that may be vital to her well-being. If she perceives she is alone or unsupported, despite the presence of strong relationships in her life, she is more at risk for depressive symptoms to worsen

(Corrigan et al., 2015).

These are a few examples of how to elicit information that might reveal the extent to which she is being worn down by current circumstances and how we help her address this, by advocating for self-care and attention to what she needs on any and every level.

Weakening stamina during the postpartum period can interfere with holding interventions if we are not aware of the direct impact it can have on her overall health and well-being. Women who have not been diagnosed with clinical depression or anxiety may dismiss the importance of taking care of themselves, as they push forward through the exhaustion, sleep deprivation, and ongoing demands of having a baby. While this may feel sustainable to a strong-minded or perfectionist mother who may be quite familiar with relinquishing her own needs, our concern is that if this continues without pausing to take a breath, she can become dysregulated without much notice.

Helping a postpartum woman with weakening stamina recharge will depend on who she is, what she likes, what has worked for her in the past, and what resources she can access. This task is best accomplished by emphasizing the gravity of the situation and how much is at stake if care is not taken to attend to her own needs. Underscoring this too soon can feel intrusive or off track for her since she is focused on the baby, so the objective is to address it with her and help her become aware of the need to restore or fortify her personal resources. If she doesn't feel worthy of what she feels is frivolous attention, our job, however obvious it may be to us, is to assure her that she is.

6 Hard-to-Hold
Hard-to-hold refers to:

- A client, a set of symptoms, or a therapeutic moment which strains the connection, confronts our professional sensibilities, and challenges our holding response.

- Any therapeutic circumstance which triggers a forceful emotional response in the therapist. This may or not be in response to a personal and identifiable shared experience.
- The therapist's belief that the alliance has been compromised by variables which necessitate further attention.
- When activated, any hard-to-hold experience requires immediate self-reflection.

Clinician task: To identify personal triggers and initiate emotional regulation.

As with the voice of depression, the hard-to-hold concept was initially described in the first edition of this book and is included as an element here due to its significant impact on the therapeutic relationship. Because this particular element can be so challenging and therapeutically distracting, Chapter 10 discusses the concept of hard-to-hold in greater depth, considering some of the nuances and complexities.

To simplify this construct, consider the following questions when thinking about a client who may activate you in some way which prompts you to wonder *what is happening to the process right now?*

- What do you *feel* when you first notice you are uncomfortable?
- What do you do in response to that feeling?
- What is happening that is making you feel that way?
- What client-centered issues are in play?
- What therapist-centered issues are in play?
- Are there any issues about her or about her situation that trigger you?
- Are there any issues about your current situation that are contributing to how you feel about the session or the client?
- Have you noticed any pattern in how you respond to certain clients?
- Is there a particular diagnosis or personality type or symptom that you consistently find hard-to-hold?
- Are you aware of your own personal vulnerabilities that may be contributing to this response?
- Do you find yourself leaning in or leaning out when someone is hard-to-hold?
  - What does that depend on?
  - Does your response tend to make it better or worse?

Sometimes, these hard-to-hold experiences are expressed as unpleasant commentaries of the therapist's misperceptions of the relationship, such as, *why does it feel like this client doesn't like what I am saying?* Or, *why is this client not complying with our plan?* Or, *what is this resistance I am feeling?* Or, *I wonder why this client keeps cancelling appointments? What is this strong emotion I feel when I meet with this client?* and so forth. These are questions which may be uncomfortable for a therapist to acknowledge and are red flags that signal a potential disconnect that should be addressed through personal reflection, clinical consultation, or supervision. What distinguishes the hard-to-hold element from the others is a strongly subjective component which renders it more difficult to discern objectively and elicits extensive personal scrutiny. After all, when our reflexive experience to a client's distress denotes anything other than unconditional support and empathy, it behooves us to examine our sensibilities and take a closer look at what's going on. We owe that to her and to ourselves. Chapter 10 explores some variables that can result in hard-to-hold scenarios.

Accessing Authentic Suffering

Understanding the elements of authentic suffering enables us to take a close look at how these dynamics inspire our holding interventions and how paying attention to her suffering through this lens can equip us to better align with what she came hoping to find. The elements of authentic suffering provide the backdrop within which the precise holding skills are engaged. This prepares us to consider how best to use each holding point as we synthesize the information we are collecting. In sum, accessing her authentic suffering may be the key to facilitating the requisite therapeutic space in which reliable self-disclosure can take place. While each therapist will rely on their individual training, personal style, and skill set, it will help to elucidate some tips to gain entry into this well-defended territory.

How to Access Authentic Suffering

Therapists with specialized training in perinatal mental health are obliged to consider the best way to access authentic suffering. How do we unlock the door guarding the deepest emotions, fears, and insecurities of a new mother in distress? Imagine, for example, why a client might deny access to her authentic suffering. She may not want to put words to the thoughts and images she deems monstrous. She may not want us, or anyone else, to hear her inner thoughts or know how bad she really feels. *She* doesn't want to know, either. She may believe that if she puts her suffering into words, it becomes more real. It becomes more a part of who she is now. She cannot pretend that it will go away by itself. Shrouded by layers of shame and personal disgrace, she works hard to keep loved ones and professionals from digging in too deeply. The shame and stigma attached to such profound grief and sorrow rests just beneath her well-rehearsed pretense that she is "fine." When this authentic suffering is missed, by well-meaning therapists and healthcare professionals who may not be trained to address the nuances that characterize perinatal suffering, women are likely to leave the providers' office feeling unheard and more hopeless. The unintended conundrum ends up sounding something like this: *I will do everything in my power to make sure you do not know how bad I really feel. And if you, as a professional, can't figure that out on your own, then I will leave and there is no hope of me ever getting better.*

The general framework of our holding task to access authentic suffering looks like this:

First and Foremost We:

- *Ground* her by helping her feel comfortable, and
- Assess her *current state* and ability to function, and
- Present your best therapeutic *expert* self, and
- Stay *present* with her suffering, and
- *Design* a plan of intervention, and
- Make sure she has the resources, insight, and support to protect/*safeguard* herself.

We Must Also:

- Fortify our capacity to sit with her suffering and acknowledge that her suffering is deeply embedded and paradoxically disguised by her search for relief
- Honor her possessive longing and her desire to cling to her perceived lost self
- Recognize and embrace her misguided inclination to resist help and remain attached to her symptoms
- Take close note of and monitor all aspects of her well-being and resources and how this may be impacting her ability to function
- Pay close attention to how she is making us feel and what, if anything, is getting in the way of our ability to apply all holding points.

The "how-to" portion of accessing authentic suffering depends on your professional style and comfort level. What works for me may not work for you. It may help, however, to have an idea of how I do it, as a template to start from. Let's start with this reference from the book *Therapy and the Postpartum Woman* (Kleiman, 2022):

> "How bad are you feeling right now?" This is a question can work well to penetrate resistance, in spite of, or perhaps because of its simplicity, though it may need to be repeated. When women have new babies, they

are used to people asking them if this is the best time of their lives. They are used to others asking them if they are tired. They are even used to strangers who ask them how many other children they hope to have. But most are not asked, even by their healthcare providers, are they feeling bad? Or how bad are they feeling?

(Kleiman, 2022, p. 9)

When we ask a postpartum woman in distress how bad she is feeling, we immediately bypass the expectation, imposed upon her by others, that she present and express the culturally reinforced prospect of pure blissfulness. Instead, it presumes a certain level of sadness, which endorses her suffering and reassures her that we are listening, we hear her, and she is safe here.

So when a client comes in and I suspect she has not expressed the true extent of her suffering, or at least her understanding of that, I assume the expert posture by doing the following:

- I sit still and tall.
- I take a deep breath.
- I look her in the eyes.
- I lean my body in her direction.
- I say her name softly and firmly.
- I pause.
- I make sure I have her attention, awaiting some response to her name, such as, "yes?" or "what?"
- I say her name again, slowly and softly, with intention, to ground her and make sure she is listening and to let her know there is nothing on my mind other than her.
- Then I ask her, "How bad are you feeling?"
- Then, if I believe she is only scratching the surface of her suffering, I will repeat the question with a new emphasis on the word "bad." As in, how *bad* (pause) are you feeling?
- If/when she says something like, "bad," I probe calmly by asking, "how bad?"
- Remaining still and focused will send the message that I am not proceeding beyond this point until *you tell me how bad you are feeling*. This is not the case, of course, and it is certainly not spoken, but her perception of my determined stance emphasizes my presence and concentration on her pain.
- Some expressions of authentic suffering sound like this:
  - I have never felt this bad in my life.
  - I don't think I can endure one more day of this.
  - I can't take this anymore.

- I told my partner that I don't think I can do this.
- Tell me I will not always feel this way.
- Please tell me I'm going to be okay.

The immediate response to any expression of authentic suffering should be unwavering comfort and endorsement that you have heard how bad she feels and that you will now, together, take steps toward helping her feel better. Between revealing her suffering and inserting a design for intervention, it is important to re-clarify what suicidal thoughts are, how her thoughts may or may not indicate clinical worry, but her level of suffering does necessitate a swift and purposeful response.

Be mindful that our access to her authentic suffering may feel terrible to her. While it will lead to intimacy and empathy, it may feel excruciatingly vulnerable for her and this can manifest as an insufferable burden, or sometimes it can feel like an incredible relief. Sitting with this open-hearted vulnerability further cements our presence and, again, models that the intensity of her disclosure is endurable and does not clinically alarm or intimidate us. Once this delicate yet powerful interaction takes place, she is in a better position to accept your help and you are in a better position to help her.

Chapter 8

The Postpartum Voice
of Depression

If you do a search on Google for the words *the voice of depression*, you will find a list of links referring to the negative chatter invading the mind of a depressed person. I found "The Critical Inner Voice that Causes Depression" and "Turning Off the Inner Voice of Depression." And then there was "Depressed? We Can Tell by Your Voice, Academics Say." Most often, references to any voice of depression is likely to conjure up related discussions on the pervasive negative voice that lingers long after any negative experience, if there even was one in the first place. It is a voice that bellows back and forth between how someone perceives the world around her and how bad she feels. The voice is often loud and relentless.

When referring to The Postpartum Voice of Depression Response Model, it means something different. The Voice of Depression paradigm depicts the function of depressive symptoms as messengers on behalf of one's inner self. Symptoms are viewed as representations of what she cannot say or do right now. They are her ticket back to her *self*, when she finds the right place to express them and learns what they mean. This chapter examines The Postpartum Voice of Depression and the Response Model in its revised form, first introduced as a theory of intervention in *Therapy and the Postpartum Woman* (Kleiman, 2009). In this review of the intervention, scripts are presented to elucidate how specific holding techniques apply.

The Voice of the Elements

Whereas earlier references to a depressive "voice" refer to the exasperating inner talk, the obsessive chatter, the intrusive and pervasive negativity, in this context, the Voice of Depression describes how depressive symptoms can, at times, serve as an agent to protect and advocate for the individual. Although this may be a time in a woman's life when she feels most out of control and powerless, it may also be a time when she is in the best position to get the help she needs, possibly help she needed before her

DOI: 10.4324/9781003402145-8

postpartum depression set in. In this way, the voice of depression is her language, her words, her non-verbal communication of her authentic suffering and what she believes she needs right now. It is the way she manifests her suffering.

Imagine a woman who has spent a lifetime taking care of others or has disregarded her own well-being in support of others. Regardless of her particular set of historical circumstances, psychological predispositions, or relational tendencies – personal vulnerabilities suddenly collide after the birth of a baby. Despite increasing awareness, experts acknowledge we do not entirely understand why one woman with few risk factors may experience postpartum depression and another woman with a long list of risk factors might not. We can express a bona fide opinion on the origins of that discrepancy, but we do not always know why this occurs. The Postpartum Voice of Depression puts forth the notion that regardless of her personal or family history or what led to the depression, she has shut down to some extent. Variables from her past and present experience, both external and internal, directly affect whether or not she perceives aspects of her pregnancy and postpartum experience as losses that are inconsistent with her expectations.

Her body has shut down; her mind and her spirit have shut down. In this way, the depression serves to speak on her behalf, saying ostensibly, "That's it. I'm done. I cannot do this anymore. I'm tired. I'm weak. I'm completely done. I need to sleep. I cannot do this by myself, not for one more day" (Kleiman, 2009, p. 56). Thus, depression serves as a mediator for the self, an effort to protect her raw and exposed essence. One way to interpret this is to understand that when incapacitating stress is present and a woman feels forced by life circumstances to maintain control of her emotions, the depression acts as a provisional state of shelter. It eases the dissonance. In this way, depression is an illness with a purpose. It is the only way she knows how to get help when nothing makes sense and she cannot function. Depression becomes a vehicle to find her way home, as per Connelly's title, *All Sickness Is Home Sickness* (Connelly, 1993). When we attune to this voice of depression, we can zero in on the elements, e.g., Is she overidentifying with her symptoms? (paradox of being) Are we able to tolerate what she is saying or not saying? (sitting with suffering) Is her distress feeling difficult for you to contain? (hard-to-hold) Is the way she is expressing herself pulling us in or pushing us out? (possessive longing; voice of depression) in order to gain insight into her resistance, her suffering, and her readiness for therapeutic engagement.

One group of women who appear to be at risk for depression includes those who repeatedly engage in mutually dependent relationships where they assume more than their share of responsibility for the well-being of others (Kaplan, 2023). Women who tend to turn outward and pay more attention to the needs of others over their own may do so out of compassion or necessity, but may also, in fact, be acting to protect a fragile or underdeveloped sense of self. Her ability to establish and maintain boundaries may be weak. Self-esteem may be low. The need to please or be approved by others may be high. The desire to engage in caretaking relationships may be strong. Fear of rejection may be present. The ability to express her own needs may be limited.

Although these characteristics do not always lead to depression, they predispose her. When women at risk often do not guard themselves by reaching out for help preventively or by communicating their need for help if symptoms emerge, feelings may be suppressed. We know what happens when powerful feelings are suppressed. Often they transmute into something else, something undesirable: depression. anxiety, and distress (Nelson et al., 2024).

An adaptive, strength-based interpretation of this model of depression – admittedly small comfort to the suffering woman – is that symptoms represent a distressed woman's best effort to seek support and obtain relief. It is her way of letting us know that we should look harder for her authentic suffering and her possessive longing to enable us to guide her toward the best course of action. Although there is no upside to suffering, we have all seen countless women transform in response to their painful experience with depression, developing self-awareness and personal insight. If you, as a catalyst for healing, can steer her in the direction of hope and reframe her symptoms as evidence of her strength and capacity to reach out for help, you have set recovery in motion.

Many online and social media outlets focus on the crusade for increased openness about vulnerability and needs experienced by women with postpartum depression. *Do not hide from your symptoms. Do not be afraid to ask for help. Talk about your postpartum depression.* These statements, which emanate from the hearts of women who have recovered from a variety of postpartum mood and anxiety disorders, have remarkable influence to ease the suffering of women who currently struggle. A mission is to defy the stigma. *Speak up on your own behalf. Do not be ashamed of your symptoms. Do not let shame interfere with your right to feel better.*

Depression is agonizing and undeserved. Still, understanding that one function of depression may be to act as a mechanism for self-expression can be a useful frame of reference. Our goal with this shift of perspective is to help her differentiate symptoms from her *self*, and recognize how these symptoms might help her to express – *and help us understand* – what she needs. This viewpoint can begin to reframe her feeling cheated by her symptoms into a more thoughtful understanding of what her symptoms might be revealing.

Model Revisited

The Postpartum Voice of Depression Response Model, developed though clinical observation, comprises four primary emotional domains, which have been observed to take precedence over others. These four sets of domains are A) powerlessness/confusion, B) sorrow/grief, C) fear/anxiety, and D) shame/dependence. When first presented, the Response Model had three emotional domains. Since that time, the model has been expanded to include a fourth domain, sorrow and grief, to reflect the predominance of loss.

In order for the postpartum woman to feel held and cared for, she needs to believe that feeling powerless/confused, sad, fearful, anxious, and/or guilty or dependent is acceptable and that these are not necessarily pathological states. She needs to know these emotional states are expected, are normal within the context of her postpartum experience, and will subside as treatment progresses. Early validation of these disturbing states through holding can significantly reduce her distress from the outset. As a clinician aligned to protect and guide her, your fundamental task is to respond to these early states of intense vulnerability with holding techniques specific to each one. In this way, you establish initial parameters of the therapeutic alliance, which is one of the most consistent predictors of therapeutic success (Buchholz & Abramowitz, 2020).

As you consider the voice of depression response model, it is helpful to be mindful of the holding elements as they are believed to engender her language and expression of symptoms. The domains described in the response model are noteworthy within the postpartum setting due to their inner-directed nature. Self-absorbed states present with sharp contrast to the insistent demands of the infant. Complicated by social and personal expectations and obscured by self-generating symptomatology (e.g., *I am ashamed of my shame. I am anxious about my anxiety. I am depressed that I feel so down*), these emotional states directly influence a woman's sense of self-esteem and self-identity. Consequently, she may perceive herself as worthless and undeserving of support, reinforcing her desire to vanish into thin air. The preference for invisibility can manifest as withdrawal and isolation, or it can appear as scorn, contempt, or disgust directed at herself or at others, including you. Her perception that she is deeply flawed and incapable is totally unacceptable to her and without proper holding or therapeutic intervention can mutate into a chronic and sustained negative belief.

To repeat, the holding intervention is implemented as a loss-informed, resiliency-based approach. This model builds upon the concept of loss of self introduced in Chapter 4 and on the reframe explored further in Chapter 7, loss of self as a driver for the prevailing collection of postpartum symptoms including grief, helplessness, anger, ambivalence, self-blame, and distress (depression and anxiety). The Voice of Depression adds that these symptoms may be understood within the context of domains of peri-natal emotional states. Some symptoms can be interpreted as belonging to more than one domain, such as anger, which could be understood as belonging to any one or all of the domains, depending on the woman and her circumstances. The domains are not mutually exclusive. They are relevant with respect to our holding responses in order to ensure we are in sync with the associated emotional state. Understanding whether a particular symptom emanates from shame versus anxiety can guide our response. Remember that symptoms can shout for attention, misdirecting our focus. Remaining attuned to the domain keeps us focused on the primary emotional state to which we respond.

The diagram (see Figure 8.1) illustrates the symptoms of postpartum depression and anxiety as defined by the four domains of emotional states. Listed below the domains (powerlessness, sorrow, fear, shame) are corresponding means in which holding may be introduced to her through a) reassurance, b) hope, c) control, and d) nurturing.

When symptoms are attended to with the suitable holding responses and your client directly or indirectly accepts your intervention, *engaged empathy* emerges. You might observe this acceptance through her nod, her smile, her tears, her sigh, her words, her gratitude, her silence, her questions, her curiosity, her surrender, or her eyes. Therapists may note there is

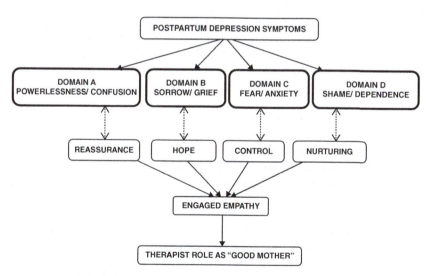

Figure 8.1. Voice of Depression Response Model Revised

© The Postpartum Stress Center, LLC.

a dynamic exchange of energy taking place. At first, emotions are high. Focus is intense. Deprivation is striking. Urgency is conspicuous. Although your presence and skills exude empathy from the beginning, this action and reaction, which takes place between her emotional states and your holding responses, is what identifies the engaged part of the empathy. Your skills are indispensable, but without her readiness to accept this process, without her willingness to participate on some level, there is more work to be done.

You can proceed regardless of her resistance to the process. Even so, at some point, you will likely discern some word or some gesture, whether restrained or demonstrative, which indicates her permission to press on. Engaged empathy is essential for the advancement of the therapeutic partnership beyond the initial connection. Without it, the energy dissipates, and she may or may not be able to sustain the desire for connection. Consider the following scripts when holding a postpartum woman in distress. Each begins with a statement from a client followed by sample holding response options.

Domain A Powerlessness|Confusion

Feelings of powerlessness, whether perceived or actual, can incapacitate a new mother. Confusion will aggravate a sense of powerlessness leading to greater anguish. Postpartum women report that feeling out of control and defenseless exacerbates their current state of distress.

What is an example of a grounding response as a means of calming this current state? A therapist's optimal response to powerlessness is the expert expression of steady encouragement and *reassurance*. Reassurance within a therapeutic environment does not refer to words of optimism she might hear from loved ones or healthcare providers who hope to help her feel better. Our expert words of reassurance indicate that we know how to help her feel better and that by seeking support she has already begun to reclaim her power.

Imagine you are supporting her through her feelings of powerlessness. Others might tell her, "C'mon you can do it, you are strong, let's go, you'll feel better if you get up, don't cry, let's go." What you convey, in essence, is:

I know you feel bad, of course you feel bad, look what you have lost. Let me help you slowly get up, I know it's hard, I know it feels easier not to move, but let's start with a tiny step. After a while you will feel better. Right now I will guide, but soon you will feel powerful enough to go on without me.

Consider the following dialogues. Keep in mind that holding points over-lap. Any therapeutic statement can encompass two or more holding points at once. Each point in parentheses has been teased out for emphasis, but others also apply.

Client Statement of Powerlessness or Confusion

I'm afraid I will never feel like myself again. I don't know what is happening.

Therapist Holding Statements of *Reassurance*

Option #1 I know it doesn't feel like you will ever feel like yourself again, but you will (Grounding). You will not always feel the way you feel now (Current state).

#2 This feels terrible now for you, I can see that. I can hear it in your voice (Grounding). We will come up with a plan (Design) to help you feel better.

#3 You will feel better again. It may be hard to hear that right now or believe it, but you will feel like yourself again. Right now, all you can feel are your symptoms. Your symptoms feel like who you are (Current state). But that's not who you are. You are not your symptoms (Expert).

#4 I am sorry you feel so bad right now (Current state, Presence). Can you tell me more about what worries you so I can be sure we take the best steps toward getting you feeling better (Safeguarding)?

#5 I can see that things feel overwhelming right now (Current state). Let's start with one thing at a time (Grounding, Design) so I can help you cope better with things that are overwhelming you and ease some of your stress (Safeguarding). Why don't you describe what yesterday was like for you, starting from when you first woke up (Current state)?

Holding her in response to feelings of powerlessness fosters the earliest stage of engaged empathy. That is, as we hold, we position ourselves alongside her in her suffering. In doing so, we invite her to lean toward this process and participate with us, bringing her closer to the heart of the therapeutic alliance.

Domain B Sorrow|Grief

Chapter 4 discussed the overriding loss in terms of a postpartum woman's sense of self. Although grief reactions are commonly associated with preg-nancy loss or infant loss, bereavement is not the only perinatal circumstance that leads to grief. As discussed, loss pervades the postpartum milieu. When sadness and grief are experienced within the context of a miscarriage or infant loss, it is expected to some extent. When grief is experienced by a woman who gives birth to a healthy baby, it is often met with denial, disbelief, discontent, or judgment.

It will not surprise any postpartum woman to learn that feelings of loss complicate and compromise emotions after the birth of a baby. Confirmation that grief is a natural emotion that results from any sense of loss related to this time period can be comforting to a mom who is stunned by such a seemingly random emotion. It can mitigate guilt over her perception of unfounded grief. It can infuse a sense of hopefulness which may be the first hint that healing and recovery are possible.

Client Statement of Sorrow and Grief

I don't feel like myself. This is not who I am. I have never felt so sad in my life.

Therapist Holding Statements of *Hope*

Option #1 I know you didn't expect to feel this way or think some of the thoughts you are having. It's hard to imagine now, but when you feel better, you will no longer think this way (Grounding, Current state).

#2 You have shown courage in your ability to advocate for yourself; by calling, by coming in, by sharing your story, by exposing your pain (Grounding). What that shows me is that you know how to take care of yourself. And even though you don't feel like you are doing a good job with that right now (Current state), I can see the qualities that make you resilient (Expert). When you begin to feel better, you will see what I see (Design, Presence).

#3 Of course you feel sad. So many things have changed for you. This sorrow is a natural response to what you have been through (Grounding, Expert). It is okay to feel sad right now (Current state, Safeguarding). Yes, I have seen women be this sad and they get better. Really this is not about being a mother. This is how depression feels. Once we treat the depression (Design), you will no longer feel this way (Expert).

#4 As we go forward, you will find renewed strength. You are tired now (Current state). You are tired from taking care of everyone else, aren't you (Presence)? For now, how 'bout we take a look at ways you can take care of *you* so you can have a break and your body, mind, and spirit can begin to rest and recover (Design, Safeguarding).

#5 I know it feels hard to move when every feeling weighs you down so much (Current state). It's hard to imagine it ever not feeling like this.

But the darkness will lift. Not as quickly as you would like. You will feel bad for a while longer. But you don't have to do this by yourself anymore (Safeguarding). I will keep my eye on you and make sure you stay on track (Grounding, Presence). If you have any concerns after you leave my office, you know how to contact me, right (Safeguarding)?

Domain C Fear|Anxiety

Anxiety is a hallmark symptom of postpartum depression, distinguishing it from other depressions unrelated to childbirth. It is worth noting that a full-blown anxiety-related diagnosis is not always applicable and many women experience feelings of anxiety that are distressing but may not meet criteria for one diagnosis or comorbid diagnoses. Women describe feelings of acute anxiety as if they will lose total control, or that they are losing their mind, or that they must, in fact, be going crazy. They cannot stand the way they feel, physically and mentally. *I want to crawl out of my own skin. I cannot think. I cannot breathe. I will never be okay again.* As with any pervasive and distressing somatic feeling during this period, it is important to have all concerns be assessed by a healthcare provider to determine whether or not the symptoms need to be treated.

Client Statement of Fear|Anxiety

I've never felt so out of control. I'm so scared every second that something bad is going to happen. I keep thinking awful thoughts.

Therapist Holding Statements of Control

Option #1 I know this is scary for you (Presence). You might feel better if we talk about some of the thoughts you are having that scare you (Grounding). Did you know how common it is for new moms to have scary thoughts? It is. It is extremely common (Expert). I am not worried that you are having thoughts that are scaring you (Safeguarding). However, I don't like that you are feeling so bad (Current state) so let's see what we can do to help reduce some of your anxiety (Design).

#2 You have told me that you are *not* having thoughts of hurting *yourself* (Grounding). Do you want to tell me about the thoughts you are having about your baby that scare you? Some women feel better if they talk about it and get it out (Presence, Current state).

#3 Did you know that 91% of *all new moms* report negative, intrusive, scary thoughts of harm coming to their baby? (Expert) 91% of all new moms! That is almost every single mother who gives birth saying that she has these scary thoughts (Grounding). That's how common this is. I know this statistic doesn't make it feel better (Presence, Current state), but it might help you worry less about it, right? (Safeguarding)

#4 I can see how anxious this makes you (Current state, Presence), and you know what? That's a good sign (Grounding). You feeling so bad actually tells me these thoughts are anxiety driven. We know what this is (Expert). We know how to treat this (Design). I know you feel terrible (Presence), but you will not always feel this way (Safeguarding).

#5 It's okay that you are anxious right now (Current state). Even though it feels terrible, nothing terrible is going to happen. You can sustain high levels of anxiety and nothing bad will occur (Expert). As you continue to heal, your anxiety will lessen. In the meantime, I will be watching this with you and I will not let anything bad happen (Safeguarding). Our work together will help you learn to cope with your anxiety so you are not so afraid of it (Design).

Our best response to her endless anxiety is to use your expertise and knowledge to increase her sense of *control* over the commotion in her head right now. This is where what you know specifically about perinatal mood and anxiety symptoms is useful. For example, sharing your knowledge that the majority of new mothers experience unwanted intrusive thoughts and that you have the clinical tools to treat this symptom communicates the clear message that there is a tried and true path you can follow to contain a situation that feels unpredictable to her. Our composed response to her anxiety will send the message that we accept her unsettling symptoms, we can manage the situation, we are not alarmed by her crippling anxiety, and that she is in a place where things do not feel so uncertain.

Domain D Dependency|Shame

Postpartum women do not often expect to feel so reliant on others, which can quickly transform into an uncomfortable feeling of neediness and guilt. This is a state of being that contrasts fiercely with their anticipation of how this all would unfold. For many postpartum women, feeling dependent is unfamiliar territory, as they find themselves in the disagreeable position to need, ask for, and accept help. The discomfort this dependent role gives rise to can be so disquieting that it prevents postpartum women from seeking the help they need.

Shame, which can result from constant misappraisals related to the self as undesirable or bad (Mills, 2005), is closely related to this discomfort with being dependent on others. Shame-related cognitive states and behaviors surround a new mother who is immersed in depressive ruminations. It is understandable that shame would interfere with relationship-building behaviors because it is associated with the fear of negative evaluation from others (Lewis, 1986), reinforced by stigma and misperceptions. The presence of shame hinders the collaborative rapport between the therapist and the postpartum woman and can potentially contribute to her failure to disclose when asked, regardless of holding methods. Shame will eventually reveal itself, but if deeply entrenched, it can hinder the holding process.

The holding response to this state of dependency and shame is grounding in the form of *nurturance*. It may be the last thing she wants, but it is exactly what she needs. Think about it from a basic need perspective. When we are sick, it can feel good to have someone take care of us. If we are stuck in bed with a fever, it feels nice to have someone bring us some cold juice with a straw that bends so it reaches our mouth with little effort, doesn't it? When we are in any weakened state, it feels good, *if we let it in*, to have someone who cares help us attend to our most basic needs. If it doesn't feel good, it is possible that it is the result of a defensive rebuff. When we offer nurturance to her dependent self, and if she accepts that, her shame will ease and she will begin to feel better.

What does it mean to nurture within the constraints of a therapeutic alliance?

It means we encourage her; we educate and gently guide her. We help her develop greater tolerance for her hard-to-tolerate symptoms; we assess her self-help management and we help foster healthy relationships that will provide much-needed support during this time of transition. When we provide emotional support and monitor her physical well-being, we nourish her soul. Nurturing implies worthiness.

Nurturance with respect to shame is a bit more complex, but briefly, it should be understood within the context of compassion and quintessential holding. Sitting with someone shrouded by shame compels us to learn how to sit and hold in silence. Sometimes, we have to hold her without saying anything or doing anything. She just has to know we are doing it. She does not have to believe she is worthy of it, not yet. She just has to allow it to take place.

How does that work? Imagine yourself with your 8-year-old daughter who is sick with a virus and frightened that she is going to throw up. You go into her room and check with her and when as she sits up in bed, she vomits. In her bed, on the floor, all over her pajamas. She immediately cries. You tell her that *everything is going to be okay*, as you guide her to the bathroom. How does she know everything will be okay? How does she know you will clean up her bed? How does she know she is in safe hands? How does she know you will take control of the chaos? How does she know she will not be condemned for messing up the house? How does she know she can trust you without you saying a thing?

She just knows.

She knows because of who you are and what your relationship has been. She knows because of how you make her feel and what you have said prior to this moment. She knows because she believes in you and when she is scared, you are there. When we are comforted by the essence of relationship, it is because we have connected with the core authenticity of that bond. Your job is to make this possible within the therapeutic framework.

Client Statement of Dependency and Shame

I am so embarrassed. I cannot believe I am thinking these things. I am mortified.

Therapist Holding Statements of Nurturance

Option #1 I know this is uncomfortable for you (Current state, Presence). You might be surprised to hear that in a short time, you will be grateful that you came here, once you realize you feel better. Have you ever been to a therapist before (Grounding)?

#2 I know it feels like you are the only one who has ever felt this way, but when depression descends after a baby is born, it can feel this bad, this dark, this overpowering (Grounding, Current state). It's hard to envision yourself laughing or enjoying yourself again, but it will happen (Presence, Expert).

#3 It's hard to take care of yourself when you feel this bad (Current state). Are you able to eat? Are you able to get out and take a walk? Are you able to rest when you cannot sleep? Are you avoiding alcohol and caffeine? Are you drinking enough fluids to stay hydrated? Are you setting limits with friends and family so you can avoid feeling overwhelmed (Design, Safeguarding)?

#4 Are you able to allow me to help you with this (Expert)? I know you don't feel like doing anything right now, but if we can take baby steps, you might discover that it is not as impossible as it feels right at this moment (Grounding). Can you tell me what you have relied on in the past for relief, for relaxation, for escape from stress, to replenish your spirit? Is there anything that gives you even the tiniest bit of pleasure now that we can draw upon (Design)?

The exchange of energy that takes place when your client relinquishes some of her power over to you temporarily can be one of the most loving and most rewarding gifts of the early therapy experience. This surrender, which may not always feel like it was in her control or a deliberate choice of hers, can emerge either from a place of trust or from sheer despair.

This event marked by engaged empathy puts you are in position to listen closely to her symptoms and determine what can be gained from her specific voice of depression, her words, her presentation, her story, and her pain. Therefore:

- You offer solid *reassurance* to a woman feeling helpless and confused.
- You offer *hope* to the woman who cannot see beyond the darkness.
- You create an environment of safety and *control* for the woman experiencing irrepressible anxiety.
- You provide therapeutic *nurturing* to the woman who feels weakened and shamed by her unsettling reliance on others.

When you properly acknowledge your clients' emotional states, accept them without judgment, and respond with points of holding, you convey empathy. When she accepts this from you and remains connected to the process, engaged empathy is achieved.

Treatment Conundrum

The therapist is prepared to intervene when it comes to making sense out of a postpartum client's contradicting emotions and potential treatment options. A postpartum woman may not, on her own, think she needs to see a therapist. She just needs to get better. What she may not realize is that getting better involves more than just taking a pill or admitting you don't feel good. Getting better may mean finding support and explanations for crushing symptoms so she can stop blaming herself. It may mean understanding that she is not going crazy so she can stop beating herself up and worrying herself sick about what might be happening. It may mean having her anger validated so she can settle down and stop hating everyone around her. Therapy can help with that.

She may think or hope that if she runs this by her healthcare provider, she will get the magic pill or the quick fix and be done with it. It can, of course, be as simple as taking the right medication for some people, but for most, it doesn't work that way. Not for the long run. One might also think or hope that once the postpartum woman finds the courage to reveal how she is really feeling to her healthcare provider, she would immediately be guided on track toward relief and a favorable outcome. Unfortunately, we know it doesn't always work that way, either.

It is astonishing that the shocking tragedies of women hanging themselves or driving their cars into the ocean with their babies have failed to catapult healthcare providers into action. Too many providers remain cavalier about the presence of postpartum depression and anxiety. Regrettably, an uncomfortably large number of women continue to report that their health practitioners are patronizing and misinformed.

- Let's see how things go. Call us in a few weeks.
- Oh, it's just the blues. You'll enjoy it in no time.
- Every new mother feels this way. You'll be fine.
- It's normal to be weepy for months. You've just had a baby!
- Just try to get some sleep. Everything will be better if you get some sleep.
- Have a glass of wine to help you relax.
- You'll feel better when she's older. This is the hardest part.

These words of empty consolation mean little to the woman who is not sure how she will get through the day. They are glaringly condescending to the woman who thinks her baby would be better off without her. If women do not take it upon themselves to be clear about how bad they are feeling, and if healthcare providers do not take the responsibility of screening for prenatal and postpartum depression and anxiety seriously, all of our advocacy work and push for greater awareness will continue to fall upon deaf ears.

So the conundrum is that therapy implores postpartum women to talk about their postpartum depression, tell someone how they are feeling, do not suffer in silence, let someone you trust know how you feel, and so forth. This perspective, although driven by an ambitious – if not idealistic – expectation that healthcare providers are sufficiently informed, often pushes women further into the direction of misguided responses. It can result in a blatant underreaction to severe symptoms.

Or an overreaction to uncomplicated symptoms. Many experts expect that the surge in attention to maternal mental health awareness will bring rapid and abiding changes in responsiveness and protocols. But it's complicated and much continues to be unknown. Suffering can be subjective and symptoms can bewilder even well-informed family, friends, and healthcare professionals. There is no way to standardize symptoms or quantify shades of distress. Nor can we operationally define the heartrending descriptions of any one woman's pain.

Thus, we are left with this:

If we tell postpartum women to let us know how they are feeling, we must know how to respond. If we tell healthcare providers they are obliged to be on the lookout for postpartum depression and anxiety, they need to know what they are looking for and where to refer for treatment. This is why the task of the therapist extends beyond the therapy office and into the territory of psychoeducation, marketing tactics, screening protocols, and teaching opportunities for those who are inclined to follow that path.

Another problem is that there is not one tried and true treatment option for postpartum distress. There are a number of opportunities for recovery, each requiring a careful risk–benefit review from a very personal and individualized perspective. Without a detailed discussion of these options, women and their families may be left uninformed or confused. Another part of our job is to be aware of the treatment possibilities so we can help guide her through the maze of choices. Whether it involves ongoing psychotherapy, alternative therapies, medication, hospitalization, psychiatric evaluation, or a day program, we make sure we have information, resources, and referrals at our fingertips. Postpartum women need information. Hopefully, their physician, midwife, nurse, or other medical professional will lead them in the right direction.

Our job is to reinforce their lead or, when necessary, initiate or augment it. Postpartum women also deserve a conversation about these options. Much of the time, they ask for ongoing conversations about the options. Their feelings of helplessness, sorrow, fear, and shame will cloud their view back to their former selves, obscuring any vision of recovery. We are often in the best position to clear the way by exploring options and sharing control of these choices until she feels stronger.

And finally, although the encouraging shift of attention from the government and advocacy groups is welcome, we caution against premature expectations of compliance and positive outcomes. Unquestionably, the current emphasis on screening protocols and recently approved oral medication for postpartum depression are encouraging. But if we lose focus on the stigma that inhibits women from disclosing how they feel, or if we rely on unskilled screeners to elicit shocking secrets, or if we do not have access to the new treatment options, we risk conflating our advocacy efforts. We have much more to do.

As her therapist, you are poised to help her navigate this network of contradictory emotions and messages. As her symptoms surface with varying degrees of impact, each of them seeks separate but equal responses in line with her impending recovery. As you securely hold these burning emotions with her and on behalf of her, she begins to engage in this process, dial back her fear, and let go of her resistance.

This is how holding provides access to treatment.

Chapter 9

Hands On
How to Hold Better

When we hold a postpartum woman in distress, we do so with a combination of precision, purpose, and our best self. This combination provides the ingredients our client needs to begin to engage in the process of therapy and recovery. Therapeutic styles are as varied as the temperament of each therapist, and although evidenced-based skill building for psychotherapists is ideal in many ways, it is simply unattainable due to the role human interaction and personality play in this work. The study of an intuitive therapy with postpartum women therefore warrants careful consideration of the skills involved in order to work toward the development of reliable training and treatment standards.

Skill Training for Holding Points

When we consider the six components of holding, we begin to see how the significance of each point is weighted toward the initial or early session(s). As sessions proceed, holding continues. Throughout your work with each postpartum client, you should regularly consider the influence the holding elements have on your work and monitor use of the six holding points: your efforts to ground, to convey your expertise and confidence in the therapeutic process, to assess her current state, to design a plan for her relief, to be present, and to safeguard her.

The role of the expert has been singled out for this chapter because it is the holding point that many therapists struggle with from the outset, which can have a direct effect on the success of other holding points. Our aim is not to point out that what you know renders you an expert; rather, we will discuss how increasing your confidence can help to develop a client's trust in the process of therapy and in the therapeutic relationship. Although increasing your knowledge and training throughout your career is certainly an important objective, your confidence in yourself matters. Postpartum women in distress need to trust that you know what you are doing. Remember, a postpartum woman is in a hurry to feel better. She is in a race

DOI: 10.4324/9781003402145-9

to return to her baby and her previous level of functioning. If you appear hesitant or lacking confidence in your ability to help her, she may wonder if she is in the right place. This is not to say you need to have all the answers to her questions. Nor should you mislead her into believing you have the answer when you are unsure. Of course not. It means you should assume the role of the expert, the role of someone who communicates clearly, *I can help you.*

Beginning practitioners might rely on external validation for feelings of expertise, either from a supervisor, a colleague, a mentor, or professor or positive outcomes, for example. More seasoned therapists, who enjoy a fuller sense of competence, learn to rely on an internal register of their expertise (although external validation may always be appreciated, and supervision or consultation is always important at any career stage). This internal mastery of our craft enables us to put forth an air of confidence and competency, which makes an important impression to clients in acute distress.

The first stage of becoming an expert is *belief in yourself as a therapist.* Self-assurance is an attribute that you should aspire to achieve, particularly if it does not come naturally to you. You can also cultivate self-assurance over time. Your conviction that self-assurance will develop, therefore, is enough to start. How does one look, sound, and behave like an expert? The following descriptions will illustrate how assuming the role of the expert interrelates with the other five holding points. Remember, there is no discernible endpoint or timeline for these components, as they are all germane to successful holding.

What follows is a close look at how one might convey confidence while *grounding* the client, attending to her *current state*, embodying the *expert*, *designing* a plan, remaining *present*, and *safeguarding* her, all at once. The following tips are what work best for me. This is my style. My comfort zone. It is a blend of my personality, my nature, and my experience. Again, it may or may not represent what feels best to you, but it can serve as a template for you to build upon.

1 | Sit Up Tall

My posture is not great by default. I have to remind myself to hold my stomach in and keep my shoulders back on a moment-by-moment basis. Sitting at the computer for hours on non-clinical days does not help, so when I am in session, I have to fight the urge to curl up in my comfy therapist chair or slouch into spinal misalignment. I remind myself on a regular basis how important it is for her, and for my own well-being, that I sit up tall.

How you sit and how you present yourself makes a difference to someone meeting you for the first time, particularly to a client who feels out of control. When anxiety is heightened and a client comes to us feeling out of control, one of the best ways for us to ground her is to model our most confident and comfortable self. Our non-verbal body language is a powerful way to convey self-assurance and competence which can ease her anxiety.

2 I Maintain Eye Contact

Eye contact is a funny thing. Just because you are looking at someone's eyes does not necessarily mean you have good eye contact. There can be too much eye contact, too little eye contact; there can be aggressive eye contact. We have all felt when someone makes eye contact that feels uneasy or disingenuous. Have you ever been to a party and looked someone straight in the eyes while they were blathering on about something that did not interest you? While you were looking into their eyes, you were either nodding to counteract your disengagement or you decided to plan your grocery list at that precise moment in time. Either way, understand that it is possible to look at someone's eyes without actually caring very much. You need to be alert to this phenomenon as it relates to the experience shared by both of you in the therapy space. Peculiarities of her eye contact or lack thereof may indicate something that is hidden from her words. She may glance up or away from you if she is anxious, uncomfortable, upset, or any number of reasons that prevent her from connecting. Factors such as anxiety, social awkwardness, and psychological impairment may also interfere with eye contact (Akinci et al., 2022). Keep an eye on her eyes, and on yours. Your eye-to-eye contact should be relaxed and natural, warm, and welcoming. Of course, many client-oriented factors could interfere with eye contact, such as anxiety, social awkwardness, and severe psychological impairment, to name a few.

Research has noted that sad people tend to avoid eye contact, which reinforces their feelings of isolation (Hills & Lewis, 2011). This presents an incentive to do your best to engage your client with her eyes. If you watch carefully, and are good at it, you might actually help her get better at looking at you by creating an expectation that this is a part of therapy. Looking someone in the eyes when they are talking is largely an instinctive response as well as a precondition for secure attachment (Corwin, 2012). While it can be difficult at times, eye contact is a relatively effortless way to connect with your client and communicate that you are entering an alliance with a common goal. If this feels awkward or especially difficult for you, practice with a partner or someone close to you. Start by sitting together and looking into each other's eyes and see what it makes you feel. Take note of any discomfort or tension you feel so that you can address these feelings and sensations using your coping strategies, supervision, and supports as tools.

Also worth mentioning is this warning: be aware of your facial expressions. I have curiously expressive eyebrows. I have been told this my entire life. One of them seems to arch up without provocation and I have no idea why or when it happens. People tell me this. I am not at all sure what it means or how I look when it happens, for that matter. Apparently, I appear chronically worried. People randomly ask me, "What's wrong?" I reply, "Nothing, why?" "Oh, you look worried." So, whether this is a facial manifestation of a persistent emotional state or whether I have been blessed and cursed with expressive eyes that do not always accurately reflect what I believe to be my current emotional state, I am not sure. Either way, I know it is necessary for me to monitor my eyes and facial expressions so as not to convey the wrong message, both in therapy and out of therapy. This is not easy because although it may be too obvious to mention, it is not just the eyes and the eyebrows. I am an emotional and reactive person by nature. Although that predisposition contributes to my ability to empathize, connect, and hold, I counterbalance reactions on a regular basis in order to remain neutral. It is a tough balance that many readers are familiar with, staying true to your own and your client's genuine emotional state while presenting yourself as in control and unbiased.

3 I State My Confidence Aloud

Postpartum women do not need to read your resume. Nor will they be impressed with your diplomas from prestigious universities. They do not care if you went to 20 trainings on how to treat postpartum depression. They will be fairly unenthusiastic about your personal passion for this work.

They just need to know you can help them feel better.

Asserting one's expertise should not be a declaration of your years of preparation or your success in treating perinatal mental health disorders. It should not be a recitation of your knowledge or education in this field of study. Although these are decidedly attributes that may enhance your ability to help her, they remain in the background when trying to display your confidence. Expressing your confidence and your belief in your ability to help her is another way to bring your best self into that session. An example of how you can say this is:

I know this feels terrible for you. I am sorry you are struggling right now. I can help. Let's start by making a plan that will guide you to feel better.

This is not said with arrogance or empty guarantees. Clearly, we have no idea what direction her recovery will take. For that reason, we need to be cautious about promises, quick fixes, or any sense that we can predict or influence the course of her treatment and, ultimately, the outcome. At an early stage, we do not have enough information about her diagnosis or the clinical challenges that lie ahead. We can only work with what we know, and right now, we only know that she is uncomfortable with her symptoms, and she has come to us for relief. Relief which begins with that first handshake, or first eye contact, or first soothing words.

You have come to the right place. You will not always feel this way. It will take time. You will find your way back to your former self.

4 I Speak Softly, Slowly, and Purposefully

Voice tone is considered an important channel of communication. How we sound to someone who is agitated and perhaps skeptical of our first meeting can make a difference in how holding proceeds. Here, we witness another paradox unfold as we use an easy soft-spoken quality in order to signify grounding and control. Various qualities of our voice, such as pitch, volume, rhythm, speed, and intensity, are influential from the beginning of all early relationships (Papousek, 2007). Moderating our voices requires attention and control to inhibit our automatic response. Although this eventually becomes second nature to experienced therapists, controlling involuntary functions such as voice quality is a diligent effort.

Becoming a parent is the time when many of us learned first-hand how much power and authority our voice could carry. There is much evidence that infants respond differently to different voice qualities (Tobin, 2020). Interestingly, it has also been shown that individuals who perceive the voice of their healthcare provider to be more supportive report higher satisfaction, perception of control, and medication adherence (Orena et al., 2022).

Your voice should sound kind and gentle. Strong and focused. It should sync with your eye contact and posture. It should sound exactly like what you would want to hear if you were feeling so bad.

5 I Am Explicit

The words you choose can impact the holding relationship significantly. I use plain language, which is relatable and down to earth, to show that I am an ally who will collaborate with her in a way that she will understand and find meaningful. To some, going to a "doctor" or medical authority can feel intimidating. I try to work through these dynamics early in treatment and reduce her anxiety by acknowledging it. I remind her that I am here to help her find her way back to herself. Be careful and thoughtful about the words you choose, as they cannot be unheard. Anxiety has a sneaky way of embedding your words into her swirling thought process and while you may not remember saying something, she might remind you that something you said impacted her tremendously, either positively or negatively.

Remember when you first heard that your own anxiety could make your children anxious? Many people know this to be true only too well and continue to wrestle with the transference of their own mental health challenges onto their children and the inescapable guilt. However, in session with your client, there is no place for ambiguity. Whether her symptoms make you anxious or whether you have never treated anyone with a specific manifestation that troubles her, your ability to speak clearly about what you can do to help her feel better is imperative.

Your ability and readiness to guide her toward healing is unequivocal. This may mean you refer her to someone else. This may mean you need to consult with a colleague. This may mean you need to connect her to resources with which you are unfamiliar. Regardless of the paths that follow, the clear and direct expression of your willingness and capacity to help her get the help she needs should be firm and resolute.

6 I Acknowledge What I Am Not Clear About

After being thrown into the frenzied world of media sensationalism years ago, an important trick of the trade was revealed to me: when you are unsure how to answer, emphasize what you do know. Headline-grabbing postpartum catastrophes send a ripple of anxiety throughout communities trying to make sense of the tragedy. Well-meaning journalists bombard experts with troubling questions which reflect widespread anxiety. *Why did she kill her baby? Why did she jump? Why did she do something so horrific?* Clearly, I could not know the answers to these questions and if this mother had been my client, I could not give any explicit or specific response. Therefore, you learn to say what you can and what you know. Similarly, when someone, a journalist, an interviewer, or a client asks you something you do not know the answer to, you answer with what you do know, alongside of any explanation of why you don't know. In other words, it's okay that you do not know the answer, but the emphasis of your response should be on what you do know. And in some circumstances, what you can do to find the answer if there is one.

Some questions might have a straightforward answer that you do not know, such as,

Is okay for me to breastfeed if I take such-and-such medication?

You would defer this question to her prescribing doctor, while reassuring her that many women can successfully breastfeed while taking various antidepressants.

Or, she might ask something more ambiguous such as,

Why do women get postpartum depression?

You might offer a supportive yet imprecise reply such as: There are so many variables that contribute to the emergence of depression. Let's take a closer look at what specifically impacted you and your experience.

If she asks,

How long will I have to feel this bad?

You might say something like:

Symptoms can last anywhere from weeks to months if they are untreated. That is why it's so good you are here. That is why it's so important that we begin to take steps to help you feel better. There are things we can start doing today that will help you feel more in control of your life again. Let's begin by...

Postpartum women in distress want answers. Unfortunately, there are not always clear-cut answers to their many questions, and this can momentarily leave us feeling unqualified or inadequate. Remember when asked a question we do not know the answer to, *we say what we do know* and we offer to find additional information. Stand strong in your conviction so that even if we do not know she has the chance to feel cared for and grounded. Sometimes, her question is in search of an answer. And sometimes her question is a more undefined hope for someone she can trust during this unsettling time.

Say what you know.

7 I Am in the Moment

Regardless of your best intentions, your years of skilled listening, and your dedication to the practice of excellent clinical care, sometimes everyone succumbs to the temptation to drift off course. It is not something any of us like to admit, but it happens. You might find yourself thinking about other things – most often, it is about your own life, your own pressures, or your own intrusive thoughts squawking for attention. This is why we need a *thing*, some kind of reminder that will bring us back into the therapy space with focus.

My thing is a tiny, round, white sticker I put on the wall behind the spot that most clients sit on the couch in my office, or on my computer screen, off to the side near eye level. My brain is trained to respond to the sight of that sticker with immediate scrutiny of my focus to the task at hand. Literally. If I glance at the sticker, I instantly assess whether or not I am entirely in the moment with my client. If not, there is on-the-spot refocus.

Being present with our clients encompasses all that we have previously described regarding eye contact, voice, and posture. It also compels us to monitor our gestures or any facial expressions that might unintentionally give off messages that could be open to misinterpretation. We cannot overlook how our client's vulnerability makes her susceptible to feeling judged, on many levels. Even raising an eyebrow in response to her mention of scary thoughts could send her into silent and permanent retreat.

What does it mean to be fully present? This is a huge topic worthy of a lengthy discussion by experts in fields such as mindfulness, but for our purposes, being present refers to that act of being fully engaged with our client at the expense of everything else. Every one of us has experienced that dreadful void when the client spends a good portion of the session venting or hyperfocusing on the details of an event, and suddenly we find we are out of time and we've done nothing! *We've made absolutely no difference at all. She could have been talking to her friend or muttering her thoughts to herself.* Or so it seems. Promptly we fall back into line and zero in on what needs to be done. Allowing a client to unload has its place and can provide relief. But calling attention to the nuances of her unbridled vent and using that information to guide her toward a more purposeful end should be our objective with any rant in a counseling session. Otherwise, the dialogue can run circles around any good therapeutic intention; in some cases, allowing clients to draw attention away from vulnerable issues.

And my mother-in-law doesn't listen. She absolutely does not consider my feelings when she bolts into my house unannounced. Uninvited. Unwelcomed! I mean, I know you had four children and I know you love your son more than I love him, but give me a break. Anyway, she comes in and starts warming up a bottle and I'm like, "I need to put the baby down for a nap," and she's like, "oh, it's no problem, I'll just be a few minutes" and I just turn away. Don't you think she's wrong? I mean, am I supposed to just give up my routine and my baby's routine because she is in the neighborhood?

This is when we might steer her slightly off of the contextual details and move toward the process itself, curious about how she experiences the context: "You don't like it when your mother-in-law behaves this way? What does that feel like for you?"

Or, say she is talking about a difficult subject then changes topics. I might ask, "What just happened there?" in an effort to help her see how she avoids talking about her feelings.

This is "processing the process." In both instances, we stay present with her and with the process while she navigates the content, then, we review it together. Our ability to remain present with her can enable her to remain present with her own experiences and feelings. Although she may not think she wants to be there in the present moment, since it feels so bad sometimes, you increase the likelihood for insight and change if you can bring awareness of her actions and reactions into the present moment.

8 | Tune In

Content refers to what is said, what words are used, what topics are being addressed. Process refers to a complex dimension of our work, one that is less concrete, more relational, and more focused on underlying issues. We listen to the words that are spoken and unspoken, we stay attuned to the non-verbal cues, and we consider therapeutic interaction at all times.

We recognize that a significant complication inherent in working with the postpartum population is the overlap of symptoms that are normal reactions to postpartum adjustment with those that are clinically and diagnostically relevant. For example, the context, details, and issues at hand, which feel so pressing and so distracting, exist as challenging aspects of any normal postpartum period, and yet may also be the object of an obsession. *How can I think when I can't sleep? What if the baby dies in her crib? I had to stop breastfeeding. I feel like such a failure.* It's hard, if not impossible, to tease out which questions, concerns, and anxieties are normal to new mothering from those which are symptoms of a mood or anxiety disorder.

Listening with the "third ear" is an enduring concept first introduced by psychoanalyst Theodor Reik (1948), which refers to the practice of listening for deeper meaning in order to glean what is not being said. It means taking into account the emotional underpinnings associated with words being spoken. We must at all times listen to what is not being said, particularly when it comes to secrets, hidden fears, or unwanted intrusive, scary thoughts. I refer to this as *listening to her symptoms*. The emergence of fruitful material is often found in the silence or in distracted discourse. Wandering narratives can be rich with information that will help you help her.

9 | Am Proactive

As a therapist, I prioritize active listening to validate and reinforce that my clients' preferences for her treatment are important. However, I recognize that she needs my clinical judgment in order to guide her on the most efficient pathway to recovery. Typically, I strike a balance, encouraging her to lead the course of treatment that feels best to her while she accepts my recommendations when necessary. Proactive, in this setting, refers to my tendency to take a stance and express myself if I feel strongly about something on her behalf. This reflects a personality trait and a professional style and may not be comfortable for everyone.

As postpartum specialists, we are required to ask hard questions: *Are you having thoughts that are scaring you? Are you having thoughts of hurting yourself? Do you have weapons in your house? When was the last time you had a drink? Have you ever been abused, emotionally, physically, mentally, sexually, by a stranger or by someone you knew? Do you ever wish you could leave this situation? Do you feel your family would be better off without you?* These are some of the questions that need to be asked of every single postpartum woman who comes through your door, even before you have a relationship with her and, most likely, before she is comfortable with you asking the questions. She needs to know you are asking them as a matter of protocol, but also because you understand the association between her scary intrusive thoughts, her history of trauma, her alcohol or drug use, or her suicidal thoughts and her current set of symptoms, and that your response to her disclosure will be supportive, helpful, and in the best interest of her and her baby.

Although there are numerous schools of thought and many personal styles of therapeutic intervention, postpartum women repeatedly express irritation with traditional styles of therapy: *I do not have time to talk about my childhood, nor am I interested. It has no relevance to why I'm here or what I need.* Instead, they may be calmed when they discover your primary objective is to provide symptom relief.

As quickly as possible.

I am devoted to psychodynamics and have respect for many of the principles of psychoanalytic theory, yet I recognize there is not time for this process with postpartum women. Not at first. In-depth therapy can take place after there has been significant resolution of the symptoms that brought her into treatment in the first place. Postpartum women are very clear about their desire for a therapist who, in addition to listening and caring, will speak to them, advise them, and walk them through the unknown territory. Operating from a proactive stance is more comfortable for some therapists than for others. This may be a function of a therapist's training, level of experience, personal preferences/style, history, and personality. It is not a prerequisite for good postpartum treatment; it is a style that has shown to be beneficial.

10 / Disarm with Psychoeducation

One of the most efficient and effective ways to counterbalance distress in this setting, especially distress that is anchored in misinformation, is to provide good, reliable information on postpartum depression and anxiety. Turning to social media or online resources for guidance and advice is increasingly commonplace. These outlets can be invaluable sources of strength, connecting like-minded women who seek companionship and support. Unfortunately, inaccurate information can spread like wildfire via these means, misleading and confusing postpartum women, including extremely anxious or symptomatic women. Women can be bombarded with words that sound like facts or assistance that appears consoling at first glance, only to be left swirling around the drain ruminating, comparing themselves to others, and wondering why no one is feeling as bad as they do. This can be confusing at best, leaving postpartum women overwhelmed with information and seeking clarity. Suddenly, everyone within reach knows more than she does and everyone has an opinion that turns them into self-proclaimed experts.

You may be one in a line of several people telling her what to do about her moods and what they indicate. Keep things simple. Be clear. Straightforward sound bites carry much weight in our work. Uncomplicated, concise words expressed with authority and compassion can provide much needed support:

You are not your symptoms.

Postpartum women can become extraordinarily attached to their symptoms. They are inclined to overidentify with them and view themselves and the world around them through a lens of fear, helplessness, and dependency. When I reframe her guilt, her pain, and her fear that she is a bad mother as symptoms, reinforce that these symptoms will resolve with treatment, and reflect that these symptoms are not proof that she is a bad mother, she may, for the first time, believe she will feel better one day. I explain further that one of the worst parts about the symptoms of postpartum depression and anxiety is that they don't feel like symptoms. *They feel like who you are.* A notion worth repeating: we recognize postpartum emotions that interfere with our client's positive adjustment as *symptoms*, but they are experienced by our clients as *self*. To a postpartum woman, it does not feel possible or productive to separate her feelings of guilt and shame from who she fundamentally is, which is part of what puts her at high risk for suicide. It is essential that you explain this phenomenon of symptoms and self in a way that makes sense to her, even if she rejects it outright. You might need to restate it a couple of different ways. The same is true about many things you say; she may not need to believe you yet, but she needs to hear you say it.

Additional information about postpartum depression and anxiety will not only ease her discomfort, it will also instill confidence that she is in the right place. This aspect of holding is a significant component of safeguarding. Your expertise and motivation to help her recover serves to protect her from anyone and everyone who has previously disregarded her concerns.

11 I Validate Her Experience

I trust a postpartum woman's instincts when she tells me she doesn't feel right. I realize that she may exaggerate or underestimate her symptoms, but if a postpartum woman tells me this is not who she is or this is not how she usually acts or feels, I believe her. She will know from the outset that I am not a healthcare provider who is going to patronize her by telling her everything will be fine. I tell her, instead, that I am sorry if she has felt dismissed by other healthcare providers or people in her life and I am onboard to ensure that she feels on track.

- I tell her she doesn't have to go through this by herself anymore.
- I tell her if she doesn't feel good, it will not help to hear that everything is fine.
- I tell her we will do this together.
- I tell her it is not okay for her to suffer, and we will take the necessary steps to give her a break from her symptoms, providing a glimmer of hope that things do not have to continue to feel this bad.

My objective is to join her journey in a way that inspires her to take care of herself and trust the process. It will not help her if I withhold my interpretations of what I think may be contributing to her current state. Always keeping in mind her level of functioning and how severe her symptoms are, I do my best to include her wishes and preferences as we move forward with treatment planning. If I feel strongly that a particular preference will be counterproductive or not in her best interest, I will make my viewpoint known. I worry about postpartum women who are either overprotected or under protected. I tell them what I am thinking so we can collaborate and agree on a plan together.

A word of caution here is that efforts can spiral off course and unsettle her if you expose too much uncertainty in the wrong manner. You can articulate a lack of knowledge with the strength of your conviction (*I can get that information for you*), or you can express it with a tentative voice and lack of belief in your abilities (*Hmmm, I'm not sure... maybe, um, we can try to...*). Working on your confidence in your ability to hold space for her regardless of what you may not know will enable you to address many unknown variables from a position of strength.

Faking It

Researchers interested in the origins and outcomes of how we perceive ourselves and how we judge others have studied the role non-verbal behaviors play. In our training classes, when we talk about "acting like an expert" or "fake it 'til you make it," we explore the notion that not only are you likely to be perceived as more competent, you will actually feel and become more competent.

Amy Cuddy and her colleagues (2015) investigated the relationship between acting "as if," which she calls "power posing" (Carney et al., 2010), and physiological changes that take place, affecting how one feels. The researchers begin by defining a power pose, a posture that is expansive, such as arms up and open, with chin up. When people feel powerful, they tend to posture themselves in ways that extend or expand their limbs and stretch out their body. This is true across the animal kingdom. The interesting result of their research is that this goes both ways: when you pretend to be powerful, when you act as if you are powerful, when you adopt a power pose, you are more likely to actually feel powerful.

Though this research has been debated due to weak replication of her findings, critics of Cuddy's work do agree that there's a connection between our posture and how we feel (Elkjær et al., 2022). I love the way her work calls attention to the control we can exert over how we present ourselves and steps we can take to prepare our minds and our bodies for challenging moments in our clinical work.

It is important to practice cultivating resilience, particularly in our difficult line of work. Take the time to discover what works for you – whether it's a power pose, or breathing, or a grounding exercise – finding ways to prepare yourself for the day's work or a difficult client will fortify your holding resources and establish you as a primary source of support.

You have seen how important it is to present ourselves as someone who is in a position to help. Who you are, how you sit, how you feel about yourself, and how you present yourself make a difference in your work. Below is a review of some salient points for you to incorporate into clinical practice.

Beyond the Words: Holding Language and Posture

Holding Language

Remember it is not only what we say, but how we say it. Do not underestimate the power of the *how*. To summarize, the how is what you look like when you are speaking, how you are sitting, how the words are coming out of your mouth. What your facial expression is, the tone and cadence of your voice. All of these factors combine to determine whether or not your client will be influenced by what you are saying. Keep in mind that your client may be coming to you with presumptions and misbeliefs that predispose her to disengage (*No one can help me; This is a waste of time; I don't even think anything is wrong with me; Something is really wrong with me,* and so forth.) While your job is not to convince her to stay, your job is certainly to do your best to make her want to and believe that it is in her best interest to do so. Our language, the words we choose, the way we say them, can directly influence level of comfort with you from the outset.

Remember that all of the holding points work simultaneously as the therapist navigates high levels of distress. Perinatal women in distress are presenting with a nervous system on fire. They are apt to overreact or feel hyperaroused by any slight deviation from what they hope or expect to hear. All perinatal therapists should pay close attention to the words they use and the manner in which they express themselves.

The following questions and statements are a few examples of prompts that have been shown anecdotally to elicit authentic responses from a woman in distress, when presented with a soft, controlled, gentle, confident tone:

- Are you okay?
- What do you need right now?
- Is there anything you haven't told me that you might feel better if I knew?
- Does anyone know how bad you really feel?
- I can see how hard you are trying and how tired you are.
- Do you feel comfortable here with me? (If not, is there something I can do to help you feel more comfortable?)
- You are such a good mother.

Holding Posture

Holding posture refers to the disposition you set forth – what she sees, what she hears, what she feels, and what she overall experiences when she sits with you. This is a fundamental part of feeling confident and reflecting that confidence.

The following list will serve as reminders that how you are perceived by a perinatal woman in distress will directly impact the influence you have on her and her willingness to engage in the therapeutic process.

- Sit up tall and open – This suggests confidence, readiness, strength, and steadfast attention.
- Maintain genuine eye contact – While challenging in a virtual setting, this is nonetheless one of the most significant ways you can demonstrate and reinforce connection and empathy.

- Remain focused – Again, virtual therapy can make this challenging, still, any distraction will instantly convey lack of attention and lack of caring, and feel dismissive.
- Regulate breathing – It is believed that when we model the behavior we hope to elicit, there is the potential for mirror neurons to become activated, motivating the receiver to literally mirror this behavior (Aragón et al., 2014). This potential encourages us to make sure we, ourselves, are regulated and calm. Breathing exercises are one of the most efficient (and easiest to conceal) ways of calming oneself in the moment.
- Harness the power of stillness – There is great power in one's ability to sit and sustain the posture of holding distress. When one sits with intentional relational awareness, the energy that is transmitted easily translates into empathy and compassion.
- Modulate voice and word choice – As mentioned, how you express yourself can have a huge impact on how she hears and feels what you are saying. This is particularly true if she is acutely agitated. Aim for a slow, gentle, self-assured tone alongside unwavering eye contact.
- Be explicit – When we sit with a highly anxious new mother, we are not always aware of the extent to which our words and our demeanor may affect her. Any ambiguity on your part may be interpreted as a lack of confidence or more uncertainty in her very uncertain world. Be clear. Let her know what you know. Access your inner expert and speak with the authority of someone who can help her.
- Be real – Saying what you know is half of the authenticity equation. The other half is saying what you don't know. When we say something from strength, instead of weakness, it is perfectly fine to let her know that you need more information or clarity and you will get back to her. You don't have to have all the answers. You just need to let her know that you can get the information she is seeking and reduce the uncertainty as best you can.
- Monitor facial expressions and gestures – Never lose sight of the fact that her anxious self is clinging to you for hope and, more likely than not, reading between your lines. She is hungry for reassurance and guidance but also ripe for misinterpretations and distorted thoughts. Again, pay attention to the messages you are communicating to her, verbally and non-verbally, as you do your best to strike the balance between being neutral while still being engaged and compassionate.

In summary, it should be clear that each holding point complements the others, but that the expert point for the holding therapist is ever-present. The earliest stages of holding begin with the first phone call or the first session with words, gestures, tones, behaviors, looks, and the belief in what we do. These forces at work become codes for communicating and engaging with the postpartum woman on a level that connects to her petrified core. How is this different from the way any non-postpartum therapist would behave? I cannot say with certainty; I can only say that for over 36 years postpartum women have been telling me what they need. Now they tell me that many of the therapists they seek help from "do not get it." Postpartum women in distress are being missed because they do not look sick enough. They continue to fall through the cracks after seeing one too many therapists who misread or failed to understand the signals. If therapists do not engage her properly, know what to look for and how to respond, she is less likely to divulge that she is having thoughts that are scaring her and less prone to reveal the extent to which she is suffering.

Holding skills will increase the likelihood that she will open up to you.

Chapter 10

Hard-to-Hold

What makes any particular postpartum woman *hard-to-hold*?

When a postpartum woman is hard-to-hold, it is challenging, confounding, and always elicits a strong emotional response in the therapist. It is as if your well-planned words bounce back with little or no impact on her. You take note of this feeling, this lack of connection. *What is wrong here? Why does this feel off track? Why isn't she responding the way I presumed she might? Why are my words not helping? Why are we not connecting? What is getting in the way? What is not working? Why am I feeling what I am feeling? Is it me? Is it her?*

It can feel oversimplistic and disrespectful to her suffering if we rush to construe a client's disconnect with the process as resistance, especially when we consider the magnitude of existing disruption in her life. Our previous discussion of the holding elements can shed light on this misalignment, encouraging us to lean in and learn more, rather than perceive it as a therapeutic impasse. Even so, patterns of hard-to-hold scenarios offer some conceptualization of how this opposition to the process emerges and how you might respond in order to facilitate an early connection.

Even a hint of misgiving in the mind of a postpartum therapist can indicate that something is getting in the way of holding. As we've seen, there are countless explanations for early disconnects in psychotherapy, but with respect to the needs of postpartum women, holding is often hampered by one of two sources. Ruling out, for now, contributing factors attributed to the therapist, a woman who is hard-to-hold is exhibiting a) hard-to-hold symptoms, and/or b) a hard-to-hold personality. They are not easy to distinguish, and they are not mutually exclusive. Moreover, that which presents as hard-to-hold for one therapist may not be experienced the same way by another. Therapists have their own sets of idiosyncrasies and personality characteristics which contribute to any hard-to-hold dynamic. For the moment, let's focus on that which is emanating from the client. If you

DOI: 10.4324/9781003402145-10

find yourself scrutinizing the holding process with some of the previous questions, it is an attempt to tease out the distinction between how much of this is symptomatology and how much is who she is, how she has been raised, what her expectations are, what socioeconomic and cultural factors are influencing her, how her marriage is, and so forth. In other words, the question, *what's going on here?* reflects a single-minded quest for clarity: Are you experiencing the fallout from her symptoms or are you experiencing pushback from who she fundamentally is? Or, of course, is it a little bit of both?

Severe symptoms of mood and anxiety disorders may also impede holding. Unstable psychiatric symptoms of depression, anxiety, PTSD, OCD, panic, bipolar illness, and psychosis can abruptly dislodge your most sincere therapeutic endeavors. The pursuit of holding is challenged by the force of these symptoms. You can, at times, move through the symptoms and grab a glimpse of who she is, who she was before she was inundated with symptoms. There will be times when a woman's personality, history of trauma or environmental stressors, personal narrative, and family-of-origin dynamics combine to predispose her to resist holding. You might see this in women with whom you immediately connect – you like her, she seems to like you, it feels right, you proceed. Then, you are waylaid by an unexpected response. Perhaps you have made an empathic comment to join with her and she fails to accept that. Or even picks up on it. She doesn't seem to care that you care. Still, you like her. You feel connected. This juxtaposition of energy can feel like you are doing something wrong.

She rejects your attempt to hold her.

Perhaps she takes it a step further. She minimizes your effort to hold her. She denies it or rejects your words. It may feel personal, though your professional self tries to remind yourself that it is not. You readjust your inner dialogue. *Is it too much? Am I coming on too strong? Am I misreading her cues? Are we not a good fit?* Perhaps.

It could also be about her.

Imagine she has a history of trauma and feels overwhelmed by your words of comfort. Imagine she has spent considerable time shielding herself from relationships so she can avoid further suffering. Imagine she perceives any shred of intimacy as an uncomfortable threat. She is hard to read, despite your resolute intention and efforts. She wants it that way. Now what? You must learn to honor her defensive posture and continue to lean into the holding process.

What about a woman whose affect and attitude causes you discomfort? A woman who thinks you don't understand, nor ever will. She is only here because someone else thinks she should be. She is agreeable but insists on doing this her way. She may ask for your help but has no intention of making use of your suggestions or your expertise. She is irritatingly self-absorbed, quite the know-it-all, condescending, and a bit of a phony. There may be helplessness, but if it's there, it is shrouded by her strong-minded and dogged convictions, which she points out are not up for discussion.

Or, what about a woman who is so riddled with anxiety that she presents as disinterested in your interventions or supportive introjections. Each suggestion for relief hits a nerve and flickers into space as if she did not hear or does not care. But she does, it is just that her symptoms may not leave space for her to convey her caring or perhaps accept yours.

If you find yourself sitting with a postpartum woman who feels hard for you to hold, ask yourself *why*. Use this question of why as a compass to find your way to her. Sit back. Reconfigure your strategy. Pay less attention to random feelings of ineffectiveness and more attention to her and what she is experiencing. All holding points need to be adjusted to accommodate who she is and what she needs. How do I **ground** high levels of agitation? Do I have sufficient information about her **current state** right now? Does she acknowledge that I have the **expertise** to help her? Am I demonstrating my capacity to remain **present** in spite of her opposition? Can she sense that I am here for her, in control of the session, **designing** our next step? Does she know I am thinking about her best interests, **safeguarding** her, despite knowing that she may be silently composing an exit strategy during our session?

When Symptoms Distract

Keep in mind that a postpartum woman in distress may be unable to distinguish between her symptoms and *who she is*. She may believe her distorted thoughts. She may believe she is a bad mother. She may believe that you are not in a position to change that. She may feel desperate and dispirited, and she fundamentally does not believe that you or this process can help change the way she feels. For your client, her lack of trust in the process might feel worrisome, or it may embed itself into her irrational belief system, reinforcing her belief that no one can help her. For you, your client's lack of trust in the process obliges you to embody the very control she seeks.

Unruly symptoms can unhinge any session. If symptoms distract the session, pay attention to what is happening. What is it about what you are observing or experiencing that is tugging at your ability to concentrate? What is it about the way her symptoms are expressed that is hindering your focus? Or her focus? Keep in mind that a couple of things may be happening here. Symptoms can *feel* bad, or they can *be* bad. The former is scary for *her*. The latter is clinically significant for *you*.

A Surge of Anxiety

Whether it is a case of nervous energy or full-blown panic attack, anxiety can be immensely disconcerting. It is pervasive. It can be harsh, breathless, agonizing, provocative, loud, intrusive, and alarming. It can startle a novice recipient. It can worry an inexperienced therapist. Severe anxiety can invade a therapy session with such force that any and all agendas are left in the dust. It may be the only thing she is able to attend to and the only thing you observe. Anxiety can also privately persuade her that her irrational thoughts carry way more weight than your words. The force of an anxious mind is crafted to defend her from perceived dangers. She is not quite sure whether you are a safe person for her. If you are not careful, you will find yourself joining her fixation.

This is when your own inner voice should repeat: *This is anxiety. This is okay. No matter how bad this feels to her, or to me, I can tolerate this. I can help her.* Anxiety has contagious qualities and can provoke intense emotions in uncontrollable proportions for both the mother in distress and the therapist. When anxiety rages and all holding points instantly fuse, your instinct to ground to achieve mental focus should pull rank over the other points at the outset.

Good grounding techniques often include sensory awareness tips to help her engage with her present surrounding environment.

- Everything is okay.
- You are in the right place.
- Nothing bad is happening.
- Look at me. Look me in the eyes. It is okay.
- Can you feel your feet on the floor?
- Can you hear the birds outside the window?
- Can you smell the coffee brewing?
- Breathe.

Each therapist is comfortable with their own strategies for helping others, and helping themselves, cope with anxiety. The take-home point here is to acknowledge that high states of arousal can disrupt your agenda. The best response is to identify this, name it for her, ground her, and move through it. Resting in place with her distracting symptoms for too long, without a plan, is likely to reinforce them.

The Black Haze of Depression

When depressive symptoms are severe, they can misconstrue our most sincere intentions. A postpartum woman with profound depressive symptoms feels hopeless yet longs for help. She is tired beyond description and may have little to offer in terms of history taking, participation in assessment protocols, or the expression of how she feels or what she needs. She is lost. It can make you feel as if you are doing all the work.

When symptoms of despair inundate the air you both breathe, you may feel as though you, too, might choke from the thickness. If this happens, pull back, breathe, and ground yourself first, but remain focused on your distressed client. Keep your eyes on her even if she is unable to meet your gaze. Stay there with her. You may notice that she warily peeks toward you every so often to see if you are there. Your eye contact is vital when she feels lost. Grounding her with your gaze is an effective holding tactic. You demonstrate to her that you have her back. You remind her you know what you are doing. You reassure her that you are not troubled by the extent to which she is suffering. You do this with your eyes.

In the meantime, be mindful of any added weight carried in your eyes and brows. You may need to check and literally refocus or reposition your eyes and how you look at her. *Do you appear worried? Can she read uncertainty in your eyes?* Soften your eyes. Relax your brows. Breathe. Stay with her.

In the following vignettes, we see that despite women's efforts to disguise or deny their symptoms we must never lose sight of the fact that their symptoms remain just below the surface.

Lindsay and Her Obsessiveness

Lindsay, mother of a 2-month-old, called our office and reported she had too much anxiety. She could not stand it. She said she was unable to get through the day. I had a cancelation and was able to see her for an initial assessment that afternoon. She was asked to arrive 10 minutes early to fill out some forms; she came 20 minutes late.

I was struck by how "healthy" she looked and sounded. I always am, despite how accustomed I am to seeing that pretense. The paradoxical presentation of looking good and feeling bad is a constant reminder of the energy a woman puts forth to look good despite her suffering. Lindsay was a bit chatty and seemed comfortable enough to engage in an ice-breaking casual exchange.

"Was traffic bad?" I asked following our standard meet-and-greet introductions, as we found our way to my office.

"No. Not really," She replied nonchalantly. "Do you want me to fill out these forms?"

"I do, but let's wait. We lost some time, so let's talk a bit first."

The reference to traffic and lost time was my attempt to ascertain any early connection with the process. She didn't appear to notice she was significantly late, which is rarely overlooked by clients who realize that they have to pay for a full session, even when the session is shortened because they arrived late. Lindsay didn't appear to notice much around her; it was as if I accidentally walked into the middle of her conversation she was having with herself. Sometimes, you can almost see the internal thoughts buzzing around. You can feel it. Lindsay was smart, friendly, articulate, and scrupulously in sync with the rhythm of her fixations. There was little room for me, or for anything else.

She talked a lot about her symptoms of distress but didn't appear particularly distressed. When asked about her ability to "hide" her symptoms, she said she's really fine, it's just that everyone around her is tired of hearing her "worry and whine."

"Why do you think they are tired of hearing you worry and whine? Have they said that to you?"

"Yes. My mother, my father, my husband, and my brother. They all keep telling me I am worrying too much and looking things up on the internet too much." She giggled nervously. "I am on the internet all day."

"What do you do when you are on the internet?"

"Well, I'm reading about inflammation and how that can cause some of the symptoms I'm having, you know, like that pain I have in my stomach. And then I took those stupid antacids and I'm sure that made everything worse. Now I have diarrhea and I'm sure it's my body protesting. I blame myself for making everything worse and I'm trying to figure out how to counteract the antacids. I knew I shouldn't have taken them. I took them for a couple of weeks; I don't know why I did that. I never take pills. I hate putting things in my body. See what happens when I do? I probably would be fine now if I hadn't added antacids to the mix. I don't know why I did that. I read that antacids can cause acute hypermagnesemia. It's a rare complication in people who have underlying causes. I'm sure I have underlying causes. It is especially a problem with antacids that have magnesium in them. Mine had magnesium in it. I looked it up."

Holding is difficult when the early stage of relationship building is prevented by the onslaught of relentless and acute anxiety symptoms. It feels as though wheels are turning but no one is getting anywhere. You ground with psychoeducation; you reassure with your present attention to her distress; you assess and validate her worry; then, you repeat. Nothing seems to stick.

Your rational response to an irrational symptom does not attach to her sensibilities as easily as her own distorted explanation. Though you continue on track, her gravitational pull keeps her spinning. It feels as though holding is not taking place, especially early on.

I asked her if she understood what I was saying. She said, "Yes, but..."

I asked her if she understood that her anxiety was taking the form of obsessive thinking and that was making it hard for her to understand what I was saying. She said, "I know, but what about..."

I asked her to stop talking for a minute and look at me. She did. I smiled and told her I know how hard this is and that it feels like I'm not listening to her. She said, "I know you're listening, but I just think if..."

I discovered, after subsequent sessions, a few phone calls, and an anti-depressant in response to her strong family and personal history of anxiety, that Lindsay did hear what I was saying. She described how my words would knock at her head but it was as if her brain locked them out. We talked about how acute anxiety symptoms can do that and how easy it is to be fooled by the brain. We talked about the fact that we need to address and treat the obsessive nature of her anxiety and not necessarily the object of her obsession. We also talked about how much she appreciated having someone to talk to about this and how comforting that felt, even when she was frustrated because I declined her request to focus on her obsession. We discussed how counterproductive it was for her to seek information and justification for her obsession and how hard she worked to convince herself and others that her illogical worry was logical. We talked about the value of staying off the internet.

Our sessions brought us to a comfortable balance between her world of worry and ways she can learn to accept and reinterpret the content of her thinking. Eventually, she was able to apply and incorporate cognitive interventions.

Early stages of holding don't always create warm and fuzzy connections.

When the holding therapist imparts healing properties and perspective into the heart and soul of an anxious mind, holding finds its early foothold.

Annie and Her Petulance

When I first met Annie, she was oozing with rage. She hated everyone around her. It didn't seem to matter who they were or what they meant to her. Everyone pissed her off. She walked in with an attitude and made sure I knew that. Annie was the mother of twin toddlers and a new baby and had her hands full. She sarcastically remarked that her husband conveniently works late on her most tiring days. He is majorly pissing her off. Everything enrages her. The kids are in the way of everything else she wants to do. Her doctor is an ass because he said she should find a hobby. Her best friend is a bitch because she doesn't have any children and cannot stand spending time with whiny kids. It is stupid to go to therapy because no one can really help. She just shouldn't have had this baby, whom she loves very much, but she is not going to win any Super Mommy pageant. Her brother is a jerk because he said he would come over last week but ended up canceling at the last minute because he had something more important to do. Her mother is useless and if she could get her own shit together, maybe then she could be a help to Annie but until then, who has time for her mother's nonsense?

I knew I was next in her line of fire.

"It's ridiculous for me to sit here and grumble on. What good can that possibly do? I've been to therapy. I know the drill. Honestly, I don't even know why I am here; it's a stupid waste of my time and money. I'm sure you know what you are doing, and I don't mean to be rude, but I already know what's going on. There's nothing you can say that's gonna make any difference whatsoever."

She spoke with far too much bitterness in her voice befitting our first moment together. Like a soldier in line, we put on our bulletproof vest and do not to take these comments personally. Nonetheless, if a client's anger raises issues for you, be aware of this and tune in promptly so you can stay on track with her. If this is a point that requires further attention or supervision, never hesitate to take notice and action on behalf of your emotional responses during this work.

Raging irritability is a common symptom of postpartum depression. Although we should not be surprised to see it when it emerges, it is a fierce emotion that manages to surprise many of us.

"Annie, how did you get to us, did someone refer you?"

"My friend Caroline told me to come. She thought it would be helpful. She's a pain in my ass. She has this better-than-thou attitude going on and just because she thinks therapy is a good idea, she thinks everyone should go to therapy. She's like this entitled rich girl who's crazy if you know what I mean. And I do mean crazy. I'm not crazy. I'm tired."

"I imagine you *are* tired, my goodness, with three little kids? Two of them twins? A new baby? That can make you very tired."

"Oh thank you for that bit of wisdom. Glad I came in for that. That is certainly worth my money," she sneered as she shook her head, fiddled with her phone, and let out a loud breath.

My eyebrows raised in time with her snarkiness, I am quite sure. "Glad you came in for what? What just happened here?"

She can be angry. She can be symptomatic. But when her symptoms provoke rudeness or offend others around her, you can presume that her relationships outside of this office are strained and need to be addressed. Even without knowing the extent to which her history or predispositions may influence the current behavior and suffering, it is helpful to address it from a present-moment perspective.

Annie frowned; her foot started tapping, "What do you mean, *what just happened*? You just told me something I already knew. I mean, it's obvious. Yeah, I'm tired. Thanks for telling me." She rolled her eyes and bounced her crossed leg back and forth, imagining a way out.

We sat in that awkward awesomeness known as psychotherapeutic silence, where magic can happen. Or not.

"Why are you looking at me?" she continued her rant. "Oh now we're just going to sit here. That'll be worth it."

I waited. About 15 seconds. A psychotherapy nanosecond which feels like an eternity to someone who isn't comfortable with it.

"This *does* feel like a waste of time, doesn't it?" I smiled a crooked smile to join her disapproval and offer a slight mockery of her premature interpretation while also not wanting to increase her anxiety. "What should we do about this? We have 40 minutes left. Can you come up with something you want to talk about during this time? I mean, you're here... we might as well see how this works..."

"No, not really."

I waited.

"This is stupid," she chimed in.

"Want me to come up with something?" I asked.

"I don't care."

"Okay," I agreeably responded with a voice way too perky for my own comfort. "How about we talk about how bad this feels for you right now."

"Oh great. Why would we do that?"

"I'm not sure." I paused. "I guess I'm wondering if some of the people close to you make you feel as bad as I'm making you feel right now. I wonder if you might be pushing away people who are in a position to help you."

"Are you freakin' serious?"

"I am." I smiled again.

"Jesus. I knew this would be asinine. You sound like my husband."

"I do? Does he say that? What does he say, Annie?"

"He says I have a bad attitude. He says having this baby has turned me into a mean-spirited, ungrateful, angry, tired lady."

"How do you feel about what he says? Is he way off base or is he right?"

"Oh. Great. This is just great," she said with waning defiance.

We wait.

Her eyes averted mine, rolled up into the top of her head, and rested behind her closed lids.

Her leg continued to tap in unison with her impatience.

She looked up, "Do me a favor? Can we just pretend I didn't come in here?"

"Not really," I tilted my head and replied with the most loving whisper I could muster.

She sighed deeply, taking in the words.

"I wonder if there is some truth to your husband's description," I repeated softly, trying to access her pain, her loss. "Are you angry and tired, like he said?" I teased out the two words from her description that I felt would be the least antagonistic and most readily identifiable for her.

She nodded affirmatively.

We wait again.

"Well," I took the lead, "if you are walking around angry and tired, and perhaps, a bit mean-spirited and ungrateful, as your husband claims, then it is possible, that it is not so 'stupid' that you are here and maybe, just maybe, we can find a way to help you feel less angry, and, perhaps, more grateful, and, hopefully, less tired. What if that were possible? Perhaps being here could help you feel better? Maybe a little? What if I know what I am doing and you might not have to continue to feel so bad?"

She sat with her hand covering her mouth as she gazed down at her tapping foot.

She took in a breath.

"Okay." She looked straight at me for the first time since walking in.

"Okay?" I repeated for reassurance and for permission to proceed.

"Okay."

"Good."

How Do You Distinguish between Symptoms That Scare Her and Those that Are Clinically Significant?

As much as I hesitate to respond to this huge concern with a cliché sound bite, I rely on my confidence in the intuition that good therapists in this field possess when I say, *trust your instincts*. Often maternal mental health therapists refer to this truism when guiding a postpartum woman toward help. *Trust your instincts*, we say, *if you think something is wrong, it probably is. That doesn't mean anything terrible is happening, but if you do not like the way it feels, let someone know.*

The same is true when you sit in a session with a postpartum woman in distress. How can you tell the difference between a symptom that requires immediate intervention and one that is non-threatening to the safety of a mom and her baby? Often, you will know, but this can be difficult to discern at times, especially when you are a new therapist in this specialty. If you are not sure, err on the side of overprotecting her, safeguarding at all costs. You cannot afford to misinterpret a symptom that is screaming out for help as a disruptive nuisance. You cannot afford to misconstrue her despairing withdrawal as introversion. You cannot afford to misread her manic expression as anxious rambling. Holding requires an ongoing inventory of current state by maintaining your (and her) grounding and presence. When symptoms roar for attention, the design is put on the back burner.

When in doubt, ask more questions. In addition to standardized screening tools as a guide, you should address the particular symptom that concerns you and ask her about it. Speak softly, lovingly, directly, and with confidence.

- Can you talk to me about your tears? What is happening now? Can you tell me?
- Have you ever felt this bad before? Did it look like this then? How is this different?
- I can see how bad you feel. What is worrying you the most right now? What are you afraid will happen?
- Is anyone else worried about you? What are they saying?
- I know it's hard to be here. Can you help me understand how bad this feels?
- Can you put words to your pain?
- I know it's hard to talk about this. Can you help me understand what is scaring you the most about the way you feel right now?
- When you sit there quietly, I wonder if you don't trust that I will understand this. Are you okay in here right now? Is there anything I can do to help you feel more at ease?
- I'm wondering if you might take a breath, for a moment, and answer some questions I have so I can better understand what you are experiencing. Would that be okay?
- Who am I seeing right now? Is this who you usually are? Do you feel like yourself right now? Can you describe what you are usually like and how this is different?
- The way you are expressing yourself right now, is this the way you usually express yourself? Do you typically talk this fast or is it because you are feeling anxious right now?
- Is there anything you are worried about that you are not telling me?
- Is there anything you are thinking about that is scaring you? Or you feel too embarrassed to share with me?

When all is said and done, do not hesitate to tell her if you believe another opinion would help or if a psychiatric evaluation is indicated. Remember you are safeguarding her when you express your uncertainty with authority. If you need help determining the best course of action for her, offer to collaborate and give referrals to appropriate resources. Avoid sending her out the door without sufficiently addressing your concern. Talk to her. Tell her what you are concerned about. Discuss the option of reaching out to her family. Trust your gut, then reach out to your colleague, supervisor, or mentor for further validation or support. Although it may initially unsettle her, we are trying to convey the degree to which we are concerned and devoted to making sure she is okay. Above all, your most pressing determination is your assessment of the presence of suicidal ideation or psychotic symptoms. Either of these situations is an emergency. Although passive suicidal thoughts may not call for urgent intervention it can be very difficult to predict future behaviors of someone experiencing suicidal ideation (Ross et al., 2023). Therefore *any* thoughts of suicide, whether active or passive, must be taken seriously.

Uncommon "Magic"

Postpartum women who come to see me soon learn that if they believe in magic, they will feel better, sooner. If they hang on to the hope that traces of joy are within reach, they increase their ability to let in a shred of goodness rather than inhabit the hardship of the moment. Magic opens up possibilities. It introduces hope. It helps women defer negativity. It makes them smile. I sprinkle in magic throughout my attempt to hold whenever and wherever possible.

Even at the risk of exasperating her. I think it is that important.

The unexplainable events and transformations that transpire throughout a therapeutic relationship can be understood through evidence-based studies that measure the reported feelings and changes, or they can be understood through something less tangible. Less measurable. Less reliable.

Magic in the face of symptoms that are impossible to bear and hard-to-hold can sound like an oxymoron at best. Still, the primary objective is to introduce hope and the belief that good things can happen. Our ever-present, implicit message is:

You will not always feel this way.

The principles behind magic in this context originate from listening to the voice of depression. Excluding the use of supernatural powers, there can surely be something enigmatic about the therapeutic process, especially to a client who is unfamiliar with the practice. Bringing the concept of magic into the space can lighten the weight. It represents an unknown power that can be harnessed through our relationship to influence her ability to control that which seems to lie beyond her control at the moment. It helps loosen her resistance. It helps her suspend disbelief. It helps her believe the unbelievable.

I always ask a client if she believes in magic.

I have toys and trinkets laced with magic, such as the hand-crafted worry dolls from Guatemala. According to the Mayan legend, when worry keeps a person awake, a person can express this worry to one of the tiny dolls and place it under her pillow. The dolls then take over the worry, thus allowing the person to sleep peacefully. In the morning, the person awakes without the worry! Women appreciate the illogicality of such myths, but many can relate to the promise of a miracle when desperation sets in.

Another is the "magic bracelet" (Kleiman, 2009) that comes with a guarantee that it only works if she believes in magic. I have a magic wand and fairy dust in my office. The practice of magic in this context demonstrates the use of hope as a legitimate intervention in combination with her readiness for change.

When therapy is done exceptionally well, there is magic in holding.

The Upside to Being a Witch

Magic in psychotherapy resides in responsibly, mindfully, and creatively honoring the transformative power available within each client. We listen to her narrative, we cherish her words that define her pain, and we rely on our sincere belief that we can make a difference. Asking her if she believes in magic as the prelude to offering my gift of the magic bracelet endorses the process. *It will not work if you do not believe*, I tell her, with a sincere voice and a wink of sarcasm. Usually each woman responds with a smile, or a smirk, or a roll of her eyes as she mocks my silliness. Then she notices I am serious about this. *It will not work unless you believe in magic*, I repeat, with an unyielding look of an earnest belief in what I am saying. "Okay. I believe in magic." She always acquiesces, often shaking her head in opposition at the same time. When I introduce this and other magic, I am acutely aware of how badly she wants to feel better. When she opens herself up to an intervention that rests solely on her willingness to suspend disbelief, we share in a critical holding moment. Despite any misgivings, if she concedes and leans into the magic, she is allowing us to engage her playfulness, creativity, and imagination. For an instant, she sits with the possibility that something good might transpire. If we sit quietly with this, we can catch a glimpse of her belief that she won't always feel this way.

The use of magic in the postpartum milieu implies that one surrenders, to an extent, and succumbs to the forces that be, whatever that means to her. It is defined in the spirit of letting go, acceptance, and hope. Most students of psychotherapy feel more comfortable with things we can see and measure. Research and validated studies have tremendous value in our field. But just as a woman can score low on the Edinburgh Postnatal Depression Scale (EPDS) (Cox et al., 1987) and still experience clinical depression, some things are not measurable.

Magic happens somewhere between the conscious and the unconscious, in the relational space between you and your client.

Introducing the concept of magic to a postpartum woman needs to be done with precise timing and careful consideration of her current state. If symptoms are acute, whimsical tools are set aside until symptoms are more stable, allowing her to be more open to various solutions, options, and magic. The reference to magic in therapy transcends a woman's religious beliefs or any personal views on mysterious supernatural phenomena. It represents a mechanism by which she can momentarily postpone her fear and turn her attention to a force greater than herself and the host of possibilities that lie ahead.

In the interest of full disclosure, I believe I have "witchy" qualities. As a super empath, I am intensely tuned in to how other people are feeling – sometimes, I have been told, before they are even aware of how they are feeling. My husband jokes that I would know he was having an affair before he would, which would be funny, except it's more true than not. He is better at living in the present moment than I am. I take any present moment and madly process what is going on, why is it going on, what else is happening, and what should I be doing about it? I am thinking, feeling, experiencing, wondering, worrying, processing, and considering the moment while he is, well, he just is.

Being witchy has its obvious drawbacks. But in a therapy session with a woman who may or may not be good at expressing her innermost reality at the moment, being witchy enables me to help her put a name to what she is feeling. You will discover that some of the tools and tricks of our trade that you are already using will work better if you attribute magic to them. The use of metaphors, guided imagery, or creative language has proven to be a useful tactic in psychotherapy for some time. This approach helps by reducing the anxiety that comes from focusing on the issue itself. Identifying this as magic empowers the strategy of intervention and can distract her from the anxiety.

Meg and the Russian Dolls

Meg came for treatment when she was 7 months postpartum after her second son was born. Her very short hair red framed her petite facial features. When she smiled, which was not often, she would light up, but most of the time, her eyes and mouth sulked downward framing her mood. Meg was tired. Tired from not sleeping, tired from trying to make sense out of her unfulfilled expectations, tired from taking care of everyone else. She has never been good at taking care of herself. All the way back to when she was a child when her mother died at a young age from cancer, Meg learned the hard way that she would feel better if she focused on taking care of everyone else. Compartmentalizing her feelings worked for a long while, until her first son was born. The birth was a rude awakening that thrust her into a deep depression, missing her mother and retreating into the eerie comfort of darkness.

By the time she came to see me, she was familiar with her tendency to stuff her emotions and rarely did she reveal her more vulnerable side. Over and over again, she would cling to the shield of her grown-up self and push through her weariness until she felt she could no longer move. As I listened to her story, I could hear how hard she worked at looking good, being good, doing good. I could see the exhaustion that dated far back and long before her first pregnancy, to the years around her mother's premature death. The energy that emanated from the tales being told was tired and tattered from years of worry and caretaking. With each postpartum period, Meg became increasingly more drained, expressing words of hopelessness at the thought of caring for one more person. Her life had been a series of complicated relationships since losing her mother, and becoming a mom herself continued to raise questions about her own ability to take this on.

I turned behind me and reached into my treasure box of magic and selected a small Russian nesting doll set. It's a miniature plastic version of the traditionally larger wooden variety; I like it because it has eight pieces of nesting dolls, rather than the more common five, taking us to a minuscule and quite precious-looking figurine.

I take the entire doll, with all layers intact, in my hand between my thumb and first finger (it's that small). I say:

"Meg, look at her for a moment. Let's pretend this is you." She plays along because she is tired. And because she believes in magic. I place the doll on the table between us.

"This is you. Working hard. Strong and capable. Put together. She looks good, doesn't she?" Meg nods.

Playing along with magic is evidence of a desire to engage with a hint of hopefulness.

"You know how we all have outer layers, the part that others see? When we perform, when we produce, when we pretend we are grown-ups, when we act a certain way? These are very real parts of ourselves, to be sure, and they serve an important purpose," I say as I lift the outer doll off the stack. "Underneath this layer of what we present to the world is a deeper level of ourselves, one that we share with close friends, or our partner. One with a bit less protection, a bit more vulnerable. Can you feel her?"

Meg listens intently. I remove the next layer, exposing a smaller doll, and then a smaller one.

"Each doll takes us closer and closer to our deepest, private childself, so to speak, our core child, or deepest fears, our most vulnerable self." As I remove each single doll, I comment about that particular "self" customized by the history of our work together. "This is Meg when she goes to work and manages her staff and has the answers to everyone's questions." She grimaces in discord. Revealing the next doll, "This is Meg coming home, being her best mommy self with your 4-year-old, easing her pain when she tumbles on the sidewalk, feeling some anxiety but having full access to your resources to take care of her." Another doll, "This is Meg with your close friends, or husband when you try so hard to only let them see your strong self but sometimes uncomfortable emotions break through, expressing themselves as sadness or fear." And so forth until we expose the teeniest of them all. I softly place this wee little painted doll no bigger than my pinky fingernail into the palm of my hand. I then bring her closer to my chest while I cradle it with my second hand. I sit quietly with the smallest of the dolls and I breathe. I look at Meg.

"Do you see her? Do you see little Meg? Can you feel her sweetness? Can you feel her vulnerability? Look at her," I say as I extend my arm to share the cradled doll with Meg.

She cries as she speaks:

"I miss her. I worry about her."

"I know you do."

We sit together in that revered quiet space.

"We need to take care of her," I tell Meg. She sighs in harmony with my words. "We need to make sure she knows it is okay to feel sad and scared and she doesn't have to work so hard all of the time pretending she is okay when she feels so bad sometimes. No wonder you're exhausted." I return the baby doll inside the stacking cups, gently placing one doll on top of the other.

"See? Here she is, right at the center of everything, nicely covered up by your grownup defenses and fabulousnesses. Do not forget she is there. Do not forget to take care of her, always. Do not forget to let her express herself." I hold the stacked set between my fingers again as I did when we started, "This is you. Remember, little Meg is in there. She needs you to remember that for now. She is crying out, you know. You discover that you won't be as tired when we find a better way to take care of her. Does that make sense to you?"

She closed her eyes and nodded.

Meg was relieved to find a safe place for her sad self to rest. It's hard to be a mother when you have unfinished pain from the past or present that doesn't know where to go. Externalizing the pain enabled Meg to see that she could do both; she could do a better job addressing her sadness and honoring her younger self, and at the same time, she could admit that she has spent way too much time worrying about everyone else and it was time to focus on her own needs right now. It was a way to reorient her focus. To embrace her perseverance. To pay tribute to her strengths.

Horton Hatches the Egg

I love Dr. Seuss. His brilliance crosses the boundary between the enchantment of childhood and those tender teaching moments we might miss as adults if we do not pay attention. On occasion, I will read a children's book with a client, when appropriate. This is a stylistic preference and quite personal; in fact, I've been surprised to discover that many therapists are not comfortable with the notion of reading a children's book to a client. I am, but only when the timing is right. That's an important distinction. Falling flat with an intervention that doesn't hit the mark as you intend is, beyond the obvious, a therapeutic misstep, a waste of precious time, at best, and an insulting, condescending intrusion, at worst.

Therefore, if you are not comfortable with it or are unsure, do not do it.

If you are, on the other hand, interested in dabbling in the magic of reading the right book to a client at the right time, consider the example of using Dr. Seuss's *Horton Hatches* the *Egg* with an adoptive mom who expresses feelings of inadequacy or feeling anything short of being her baby's mama. When we talk about the "right time" to bring an interactive, dynamic intervention such as reading a children's book, complete with animated inflections and silly voices, we need to be sure our mom is symptomatically stable, interested, and, perhaps most important, sufficiently engaged in the process and our relationship to trust this far-fetched but meaningful life lesson.

Reading together can be a playful and powerful interaction that allows her to smile through her suffering. Make sure to check that she stays engaged in the process. Do your best to differentiate between her being a compliant client and her genuinely agreeing to take the time to listen to the story. If you get the sense that she loses interest, stop reading. Lean in toward her and put the book away.

If you do share this journey with an adoptive mom struggling for confidence with her new identity and get to the part at the end that reads, "and it should be, it should be, it SHOULD be like that," you will know exactly why you read that book to her.

So will she.

If this style of intervention appeals to you, there are countless books from your own childhood that might resonate for any particular client. I can't say that I do this often, but just like so many other things, it seems that something whispers in my therapeutic ear when the opportune time presents itself.

Finding the Right Words

Magic is useful when particular symptoms pronounce themselves with heightened ferocity. There is great healing power in the belief that something will work. Research has shown physiologic changes take place in the brain of someone who believes that the treatment will be helpful. At its most extreme, this notion can be dangerous and potentially misguide someone in a medically critical situation who might, for example, choose an alternative treatment over a medical treatment because it feels "safer" or "natural." But in scenarios that are not life or death, belief that a treatment works holds substantial merit. There is evidence that placebo interventions have important clinical effects (Kirsch, 2019), which, when applied to our work, lend credibility to our soft reference to the use of magical thinking to augment belief in the therapeutic process. *You will begin to feel better if you believe that good things will happen. If you believe I can help you.*

In the face of unstable symptoms, it can be the symptom itself, or it can be a woman's perception of the symptom, or her tolerance/intolerance of a symptom, or sheer panic that leads her to believe she will never feel better. Regardless of the starting point, symptoms that gush forth leaving you little room to process compel you to respond. One response is to utilize the magic of a sound bite. The virtue of any sound bite is found in the clarity of its message and the earnestness with which it is presented. If she is exceedingly anxious, it needs to be repeated. And then repeated again.

"I can't stand the way I am feeling. I am such a horrible mother. A good mother would not have these thoughts."

"I know it feels that way to you right now. But, *you are not your thoughts*. The thoughts you have are symptoms of your depression and anxiety. When these thoughts are treated, as we have started to do, you won't think this way."

"Yeah, but I cannot be a good mother with these thoughts. It's not okay."

"These thoughts are not who you are, I know that. These negative thoughts are symptoms. There is *you*, a core *you*, your essence. And there are your symptoms. Like a terrible cough. Or a fever. These are symptoms that respond well to treatment. I know it doesn't feel that way now, but you will feel better. These thoughts are awful symptoms. But they are not you. You are not your thoughts."

Sound bites are effective because they give your client something to take home with her. They are concise expressions of holding that she can grab on to. She can practice cognitive reframing; she can repeat the words; she can train her brain; she can hear your voice. She can log it; she can record it and listen to it. She can use this to transition from your office to her life at home. And she can effectively substitute her current ruminative expressions with words that hold more healing power. Many therapists have their own sound bites that work with various scenarios. Each of you will develop your own style and toolbox of magic. What works for me will not work for others, or others may be uncomfortable with my words. Find what works for you.

The following are some phrases that can work with specific symptoms to temporarily reassure:

OCD: You are not your thoughts.

Scary thoughts: Did you know that 91% of all new mothers report scary, unwanted, negative thoughts about harm coming to their baby? That's almost every single one. And that's all new moms, not just moms with depression. Having a scary thought is not associated with anything scary happening or acting on these thoughts. They are symptoms of anxiety.

Psychosis: You are not okay right now, are you? (After further assessment you might say…) I don't like the way you are talking right now. I'm concerned that you are not thinking clearly. We need to call [partner] and make plans to get you help right now. Do you understand?

Excessive worry: No, this is not how being a mother always feels. What you are feeling are symptoms. When you get treatment and feel better, you will no longer think or feel this way.

Anxiety: I know there is a lot going on right now. It's okay for you to be anxious. But you can learn to be anxious better, and we can work together to reduce the level of distress your anxiety causes you.

Postpartum posttraumatic stress disorder: You need time to cope. If you feel guilty for feeling so bad because your baby is beautiful and healthy and you are not feeling grateful, take a pause. Being grateful will not resolve your trauma. You can love your baby and you can honor your pain.

Bipolar illness: Even though you feel good some of the time, I'm worried that you are not sleeping and that your words and thoughts are racing. You might be wondering why things feel so out of control. You are in the right place. You will feel better again.

Postpartum stress syndrome: This is a new normal, but you can expect to feel more like yourself again with the right information and support.

Attachment concerns: I am not worried about you bonding with your baby right now. As long as your baby is being cared for by wonderful and reliable substitute caretakers, you need to focus on getting better. In the meantime, spend small amounts of time with your baby, skin to skin. If you begin to feel anxious, let someone else hold the baby for now. That's fine.

Suicidal thoughts: There are not a lot of absolutes in this work, but one thing is certain. If you think that you not being here is the best thing you can do for your children, you are very wrong. This is indisputable and undeniable.

Using concise phrases of comfort or clarity have their place, but they cannot stand alone. They must be delivered and followed up with use of good holding techniques and comprehensive therapeutic treatment.

There will be women whose symptoms, personalities, or circumstances make holding difficult and challenging. Sometimes, it is unfeasible, bad timing, or a bad fit, and they will find someplace else to go, or they will decline help altogether. As we've seen, this may or may not have anything to do with you or your therapeutic competence. Most often, it does not. Your expertise in this field and your attention to the nuances that characterize postpartum women in distress will arm you with insight and the tools you need to connect with her under the most demanding conditions. Remember this:

• You cannot fix her problems.
• You cannot make her pain go away.
• You are not responsible for her grief.
• You *can* ease her suffering.
• Hold her.
• Let her feel.

How do you know you are helping her? You are.
How do you really know? Ask her.
How do we know when holding takes place?

There is usually a turning point in the session. There is a shift of energy. A sigh. A look. A moment. A recognition. A connection. You will see it. You will hear it. Or you will feel it. That is when you know. When you unreservedly endure the anger, the rage, the pain, the total shit show that can present in your offices, paradoxically, you initiate the process of holding. When you transform her fear into hope and her panic into a belief that this is not a permanent state of being and that she can expect to find her way back to herself, when you can see that in her eyes and you can feel it from her heart, you are holding her.

Chapter 11

The Anatomy of Holding

Psychotherapists never stop learning. We learn something each time we see a new client, or even a client we have seen many times. Observing our clients objectively while we engage in holding practices and good clinical techniques can feel second nature to experienced psychotherapists.

Regardless of how proficient our holding instincts and skills are, we are always learning. How to do our work better. How to do our work differently. How to enhance our holding skills so we can best support our clients and protect ourselves. And so we open our hearts to the possibility that we can always do our work a bit better. Or a bit differently. This is what we often hear from our advanced training participants at the end of our course: *I think I was always holding my clients. Now, I believe I will do it better.*

On-the-Job Training

Although I aspire to one day achieve spiritual enlightenment and eternal peace, I confess it is difficult for me to sustain the practice of relating to my inner state of consciousness. So much so that it makes my head ache to read too much on the subject. I am not sure if this is my brain protesting such an intrusive demand on my preference to ruminate or if it injures my brain to attempt such a radical modification. In any case, I avoid it and I yearn for it. I am able, nonetheless, to teach it to others.

After many failed trials and tons of books, YouTube videos, and podcasts, Eckhart Tolle, a German-born spiritual leader and author of *The Power of Now* (2004) is the spiritual teacher who resonates for me and inspires me to work as hard as I can toward achieving whatever this is that I find myself seeking. There is something about the way he writes, but for me, it is also the way he speaks. Most likely, his appealing German accent is comforting and reminds me of my mother's loving family. I learned that strawberries (or anything yummy) taste better when you don't just *eat* them – you must *savor* them, *Das muss mann ja genießen!* That must be

DOI: 10.4324/9781003402145-11

why I listen to Tolle rather than read his books. Regardless, I love to hear to him speak, and when he does, I listen. Painstakingly so.

It really does hurt my head to hear him instruct me to stop paying attention to my thoughts. Even though this is precisely what we instruct our anxious clients to do, I find it infuriatingly impossible. He says not to take our thoughts too seriously and that we are often imprisoned by our minds. Thoughts confine us and restrict our experience. Our presence, our attention, our awareness is the experience, not what we think of it. He claims that discovering this dimension frees one from suffering. Suffering, he says, is something we impose upon ourselves with our thoughts.

I do not comprehend his heartfelt lesson. Surely, I am misinterpreting what he is saying. After all, much of my professional and personal success has been a direct function of paying very close attention to my thoughts. So his coaching to free myself from my thinking mind is both maddening and invigorating.

Of course it is. That is the point.

This is an example of why I am so attracted to and exasperated by Tolle's work:

> One day you may catch yourself smiling at the voice in your head, as you would smile at the antics of a child. This means that you no longer take the content of your mind all that seriously, as your sense of self does not depend on it.
>
> (Tolle, 2004, p. 21)

I take the content of my mind extremely seriously, as most overthinkers do. Therefore, this is a most exasperating challenge. But I remain enthused about the possibility that one day I will achieve this elusive gold nugget of enduring inner peace.

One of Tolle's inspirational notions is his reference to "watching the thinker" (Tolle, 2004, p. 14). This lesson guides us to pay attention to the noise, thoughts, and voices in your head, but do so without judgment. Pay attention to the complaints, the speculations, the worries, the protests, but *just notice it*, without identifying with it in any way or attaching any relevance to it.

> When you listen to that voice, listen to it impartially. That is to say, do not judge. Do not judge or condemn what you hear, for doing so would mean that the same voice has come in again through the back door. You'll soon realize: *there* is the voice, and here *I am* listening to it, watching it. This *I am* realization, this sense of your own presence, is not a thought. It arises from beyond the mind.
>
> (Tolle, 2004, p. 18)

Tolle teaches us that there are ostensibly two parts to ourselves. There is the thinking, acting, talking, and doing self. And there is the observing self, the healthy dissociating part, the part that watches, witnesses, and takes note of the thoughts and behaviors but does so with stillness and control. Tolle says that the most significant thing that can happen to each of us is the shift from thinking to aware presence as we become more comfortable with the state of "not knowing." He says that suffering begins when we label a situation as bad, which creates what he calls an emotional contraction. Releasing that response by letting go of the negative appraisal and letting things be what they are without our evaluation makes more positive energy available. The act of witnessing without judgment is not easy to do. It is a mindful practice that can be learned.

This is a concept that I teach my postpartum clients to help them pull back from the quicksand of their negative internal chatter. Together, we practice mindfulness techniques to help them begin to let go of the power these intrusive thoughts can hold. *Watch them. Notice them. Let them go.* This is not easy. Still, it is an important lesson and one that can immediately offer a sparkle of hope, the possibility of freedom from unwanted thoughts.

Likewise, this is a concept that you should embrace as you hold each client. When you pull yourself back from yourself, so to speak, monitor your own emotional state, and stay present with the unknown, you hold yourself while you hold her. You teach yourself as you teach your clients. You practice what you teach. This parallel process is paramount to the art of holding.

Disclaimer on Behalf of Good Therapy

Therapy is not for everyone. It is never your job to talk anyone into engaging in a therapeutic process if that is not what she wants to do.

Or, is it?

Respect for a client's decision not to enter a therapeutic relationship takes precedence. Postpartum women are burdened with ambivalence toward seeking help during this vulnerable time. No matter how much they want the help. It just doesn't sit right for many women to associate new motherhood with "needing therapy." As mentioned, this ambivalence can set up an initial challenge for both the therapist and the client, but early resistance to therapy does not appear to be associated with treatment failure, premature discontinuation, or non-compliance in my experience with postpartum women. Rather, it appears to come with the territory of heightened emotional reactiveness and possessive longing, as mentioned earlier. Postpartum women tend to be either decidedly eager to get to the first appointment in search of relief or they are disinclined to come and are anxious about the experience. Or, a little bit of both.

Our Clients as Mirrors

How do you know if holding is working?

This is a question we ask throughout this book. It's a question that bears repeating and entails continual introspection. Your clients reflect your work. They represent your finest mirror. Depending on the factors that contribute to each individual's response, such as her history, her symptoms, her diagnosis, and her personality, as well as other variables, each woman is in a position to respond to your holding attempts uniquely. Holding doesn't always play out the way you presume it will, which leaves space some therapists might fill with doubting their effectiveness.

Therapists are constantly monitoring what is being said and done and try not to lose sight of the impact their words and choices have on each client. We check in with our clients as they work in sessions, aware that our clients, particularly our postpartum clients, are susceptible to misinterpretation, misleading impressions, and distorted thinking. We are mindful to respect that current state when we present the information she needs in order to feel better.

This is where your witchy senses come in again. Most of the time, you will know when it is working and when it is not because you work hard to remain attuned to her and her responses. This continuous process enables you to monitor the holding experience, indicating whether or not it is moving in the right direction. Focus on your observing self and while you are talking, listening, or otherwise engaging with your client take notice of how she looks, feel how she feels, listen to her tone, her breath, her energy.

- Is she connecting with you?
- Is she able to make eye contact?
- Is she resisting?
- Is she getting more agitated?
- Is she relaxing a bit?
- What is she saying?
- Is she able to distract herself from her symptoms for an instant with a laugh or a smile?
- Does it seem to feel okay for her to be there?
- How is she responding to what you say?
- Can you feel that you are connecting?
- Do you need to recalibrate?
- Do you need to slow down? Or look her in the eyes, or find a better way to reach her?

Carefully, mindfully, and adaptively, you align yourself with the process of the moment, rather than focusing solely on the content. The art of holding depends on your ability to stay present with the process at all times, regardless of what she may be saying at that moment. Even if she is excruciatingly agitated, or if she is sobbing, or if she is angry or withdrawn, even if her words wildly insist that you take immediate notice, staying present with her suffering will enable you to contain the holding experience as well as monitor it from the outside in.

Getting in Your Own Way

Mentoring therapists allows me to enter that unique space between their work as a professional and the use of self in their work. Lauren, a young mother herself, recently immersed herself in full-time clinical practice. During our mentoring session, Lauren presented a case where her client was besieged by guilt over some choices she made on behalf of her own mental health. Both Lauren and I agreed that the choices themselves were reasonable, but her guilt was noteworthy. Later in our session, Lauren asked:

"Do you see a lot of this? Guilt. I see it as such a big problem in my practice."
"What do you mean you see it as a problem?"
"I see guilt all the time as a huge problem. Don't you?"
"No, actually. I mean, guilt is present much of the time, as a symptom of the depression, but I don't see it as a huge problem."

It dawned on me at that moment we were stymied by a semantic hiccup. Was Lauren telling me that the symptom of guilt was pervasive and interfering with the functioning of a high number of clients, or was she telling me that she is challenged by that particular symptom?

"What does the guilt mean to you? Is guilt an issue you have difficulty with in your own life, Lauren?" I probed.
"Yeah. I guess it is," she seemed to scoff at her own humanness.
"Tell me what that means."

This is when the connection between who we are and how we work is elucidated and why, at times, it is difficult but imperative that we disentangle our own issues from those belonging to our client.

"I guess, guilt is big for me in my own life. You know, balancing work with a houseful of kids, asking myself if I am making the right choices on a day-to-day basis, and so forth. I am forever monitoring my life to make sure things line up in a way that best meets the needs of my family as well as my passion for my work. So, yeah, guilt is a big one for me. This is interesting. So, do you think I am more sensitive to the guilt of my client because it triggers me in some way? Or, hmmm... what if I am actually making guilt a bigger problem for her, because it's a problem for me?"

"Good question." I love learning from the therapists I mentor. They are wise and so thoughtful. "What if you are?"

"Maybe that's why you don't see guilt as a big problem in your practice," Lauren correctly surmised.

"Probably," I gently confirmed. "I don't see guilt as a huge problem in my own life. I mean, I make some of the same choices you do on a regular basis, or I did when I was at that stage of life, with small children. I do not, however, remember feeling guilty about most of them. That isn't to say I did any of it better than you do it. I just didn't feel guilty."

"Wow. That's so interesting. So what *do* you see a lot of in your practice? What symptom is the most difficult for you?" Lauren loves to turn the conversation back to me. She learns a great deal about who she is by digging into my experiences – especially those experiences in which I am most vulnerable. "I don't mean to pry, but I'm curious."

"I have the most trouble with relentless, piercing anxiety that manifests as constant unanswerable queries, with repetitive OCD momentum. When anxiety symptoms are a 6 or 7 on a 10-point scale, some women can find a pause button. If the anxiety presents as a 9 or 10, with cyclic statements or questions that inhibit her from responding to or from listening to any explanation, it is challenging for me, for a couple of reasons. First, I know if she could actually hear my response, she would get some relief, but she can't hear, because her symptoms are deafening. Insight is limited, even with the most intelligent women, because her brain will not let the information in. Her distorted thoughts trump any rational assertion. Second, it makes me anxious. I can feel my tension rise when, regardless of what I say or how I say it, nothing seems to penetrate her highly agitated emotional state. I regroup and try another tactic. Still, the ruminating persists. Because, well, that's how it works, right? But when my repeated efforts to grab hold of this symptom fail to provide relief for her, I feel frustrated. The nature and expression of this symptom set are so fierce, it can feel as though it transcends any intervention. This is when I rely on tools to help refocus my attention away from my own emotional response and back to her. Make sense?"

"Yes. It makes perfect sense. Thank you. And it makes me understand that this is why guilt always feels so big to me and so present in so many women. It's almost like I'm looking for it, or focusing on its presence, or it smacks me in the face because I'm vulnerable to it myself."

"Yes. Being aware of this will be helpful. We should also discuss ways for you to work on this with your client so you can minimize the impact of it for her, rather than have her constantly focus on it, which may indirectly reinforce the guilt."

"Ah... that is true. So how do I respond? Can you give me an example of a response that helps minimize the guilt without dismissing her?"

"Of course, I can." We share a silent smile. "Can you?" I quipped back, returning to my best therapist self.

"Um. I'm not sure," she hesitated. "Maybe by validating her guilt? I'm not sure how to say that."

We wait together.

"I don't know, Karen. This is where I get stuck."

"How do you validate her guilt?"

"Hmmmm. I'm not sure how to say that."

"How do we validate any emotion?"

"By naming it?"

"Yes. Exactly. So we say something like: 'It's hard, isn't it? To feel these feelings? To feel so bad and so sad, and now, to feel guilty on top of that. It is really hard.'"

"Yeah, I like that."

"And remind her that guilt is a common symptom (Current state, Grounding), she won't always feel this way (Safeguard), and perhaps refocus to a discussion about how she can better manage this symptom when it feels overwhelming (Design). By discussing coping options you validate that you are clinically unconcerned about her guilt and that there are actions she can take to help decrease it. Such as, accept it, not beat herself up, understand that it is common, and distract her brain with tasks that you and she come up with together which have meaning to her."

"This is so helpful. I can tell by talking about this with you that much of the emphasis on guilt has actually come from me, and not as much from her. That's so interesting and important for me to recognize."

"Good," I confirm, as she reminds me how gratifying it is to hold excellent therapists.

"It feels so right to redirect this onto her and help her feel better by acknowledging and dealing with the emotion instead of feeling afraid of it, in a way, like I tend to do in my own life."

"Yes. Good. And you can work on managing and reducing your own guilt another time."

"Definitely."

An Unforeseen Hold

Recently, while joining forces with a colleague, I experienced what it felt like to be held, unaware of what was happening until it happened.

I do not consider myself an avid music fan. I love music in the background, as long as it remains in the background. It seems I have been blessed with senses that are instantaneously overcrowded by stimuli, and too much of anything doesn't feel good. The wrong music turns into noise. The wrong smell turns into an allergic reaction. And so forth.

When I met with Meredith in our staff meeting to discuss her music therapy and how that might be an asset to our treatment model at The Postpartum Stress Center, I was curious, interested, and skeptical.

"Tell me how it works. I don't know much about music therapy, although I'm intrigued by it. I wonder if our clients will find it helpful." I have no idea why I began with a negative slant, but it turned into an opportunity for her to advocate for her life passion and promote her work as we explored the possibility of collaborative services.

"I appreciate music, but honestly, it doesn't hold a huge place in my life, it often feels distracting to me," I continued to confess.

She sat and listened, nodding her approval of my apparent search for meaning.

"I wish I could enjoy it more. I'm easily distracted, so I often prefer quiet. Especially when I'm relaxing, which is counterintuitive, I suppose. Oh, well lately, I have serendipitously discovered the pleasure of listening to music while I write. It's a first for me. I have been listening to classical guitar music, not sure why, but now, I have it on in the background while I'm writing at the computer."

Meredith loved this. She nodded and appeared slightly amused by my introspection.

"What's really interesting is that I notice it when it's not there and I love having it on now. It keeps other noises out and helps me focus."

"What do you like most about the music in the background?"

"I don't know. I don't actually think I hear it. If I heard it, I wouldn't like that. It's as if it blends well with my crazy sensibilities and it gets neutralized somehow, and my brain is able to synthesize it without effort. It's nice."

"Where do you feel it in your body?"

That question always rubs me the wrong way. I'm not sure why. It feels trite and contrived. I feel slightly put on the spot, similar to how a yoga class full of limber deep-breathers makes me feel when everyone is relaxing except me. Perhaps it makes me aware of how out of touch I am with my mind–body connection or how undeveloped my mindfulness practice is.

"I don't know where I feel it."

My response was too cerebral; my wish to comply fell short of any good response.

"I don't feel it anywhere."

At that moment, I brought my mind home to my computer and imagined the guitar melody strumming in my head. Meredith could see I was thinking, imagining, feeling.

"Where do you feel the music in your body?" She repeated. "I think I know, but I'd like you to tell me... Try not to think so hard. Try to feel it."

Pushing past my reactive temptation to think way too much and reject her suggestion that the music meant more to me than I claimed, I brought my hands closer to my face, palms up. I looked at my hands. "It's weird," I remarked, looking at my fingers as if they held the answer. "I hear the music, so first I guess I feel it in my ears. Then it goes straight to my heart (clearly bypassing my brain, or I wouldn't like it), from my heart..."

I closed my palms and turned them downward, slowly stretching my fingers open as if typing.

"From my heart, it moves down my arms, into my fingers. Like the music comes out my fingers and turns into words."

I felt unexpectedly calm.

I continued, "It inspires me. Hmm... It helps me think and write. I love it."

Meredith smiled, "When you feel the music and can notice what happens in your body, you have connected with the music. You are more aware. More mindful. The more nuanced your awareness becomes, the more you are likely to bring about a deeper state of consciousness."

It felt amazingly good. When I stopped thinking and let myself feel, I felt the connection.

Ah, Eckhart Tolle would be so proud.

Sitting there with Meredith enabled me to appreciate both the value of the music while I work and the importance of the work she did to promote a serene birth experience for her clients. Most importantly, I experienced what it felt like to be held.

A dubious mind can come in handy as long as it remains open enough to allow convincing or a change of heart. Just when I think I'm getting too old to change my mind, someone teaches me that this is not even close to being true. Remember that your clients are skeptical, too. They are doubtful that anything can help. They may mistrust your suggestions or scoff at your belief in magic. They may feel doomed by an insufferable black cloud. They may interpret your sweet music as a clamoring nuisance.

If you stay with them, if you remain present and ground them with words of reassurance and expertise, it is possible for holding to take place whether they fully invest in that process or not.

Is It Working?

You have seen that holding can manifest as a smooth transition from sheer panic to palpable hopefulness. Or, it can unfold circuitously in spite of her resistance, her wish to escape, or her belief that no relief is possible. Either way, you hold. That is your overriding assignment when you meet a post-partum woman. Whether it is your first meeting or your last. Whether you are engaged in a playful repartee as she leaves your office or entangled in a troublesome exchange of reemerging symptoms. Holding takes precedence. Implicit in this directive is your steady assessment of the process, which includes both her well-being and yours. Consider hers, first and foremost. Scanning her face, her body, her reactions, her emotions, her expressions, her words, and her energy should occur within each moment you share. You should never lose sight of how she is doing at any given time.

Take Inventory

Somewhere between random free association and acute perceptiveness lies your ability to assess the current state of how you are holding.

Check In with Her

A primary and most efficient method to assess holding is to ask direct questions to identify how she is doing. This is especially relevant if you sense she is uneasy.

- Are you okay right now?
- Does being here with me feel okay for you?
- I know it's hard to talk to a stranger about all of this. Is this okay for you?

Notice the use of the word "okay," which I rely on throughout therapy with postpartum women. It is a word that safely bridges the medical/pathology aspect of your work with the nurturing/good-mother aspect of your role. The word references her physical well-being (*Are your symptoms taking over too much right now? Too much anxiety? Can you sit here?*) in addition to her emotional well-being (*Do you feel comfortable with me? Do you feel you can trust this situation at this early stage?*)

Appraise

Below are prompts to help you review your use of the holding points; to facilitate greater awareness and close monitoring of the process.

- Are you using words and exhibiting behaviors that serve to **ground** her? Remember that what might work for one woman may not work for another. Stay attuned to the manner in which she responds to what you are saying or how you are saying it. Do you observe a decrease in agitation and better focus?
- Are you addressing, assessing, and acknowledging her **current state**? Out loud to her? Do you think she feels validated and safe to disclose? Are you discussing her symptoms and the problems they continue to cause for her? Are you reviewing the small increments of progress she may be making? Does that seem to offer a bit of relief to her?
- Are you sitting up tall with confidence? Are you embodying the confidence of an **expert** in the room? Can you feel that she trusts that you know what you are talking about? Are you using words that are both substantive and supportive?
- Does she agree with your treatment plan? Do you believe she feels cared for by the actions you want her to take? Do you believe she feels able to comply with the plan you have **designed** with her? Is there more for you to do to help facilitate that?
- Are you **present**? Are you sure? Does she feel heard? Are you sure?
- Can you determine whether or not your words and presence are absorbed in a positive light? Does she nod with approval? Does she sigh with relief? Does she smile with affection? Does she express her appreciation? Does she exhibit a decrease in distress? Does she acknowledge her agreement? Do her questions demonstrate a willingness to proceed with caution and trust? These are all signs that early efforts of **safeguarding** are making a difference.

Biological Basis?

As we continue to learn more about the process of neuroplasticity, we are now able to use brain imaging technologies such as MRI (magnetic resonance imaging) to view the inner workings of the brain to study changes that take place during psychotherapy. In fact, neuroimages have shown that psychotherapy can affect brain structure the same way that biological mechanisms do. In one study, when comparing images, the brain activity after CBT intervention was similar to the changes noted with the use of selected SSRI (serotonin reuptake inhibitor) antidepressants (Gorka et al., 2019).

This notion of being able to change brain structure and function through psychotherapy is promising for our field. While a discussion of neuroscience and brain development is unrelated to this book, we have learned that some fundamental principles of psychotherapy have shown to create structural and functional changes in the brain (Malhotra & Sahoo, 2017). Imagine a postpartum woman in crisis who is functioning in survival mode. To be sure, it's hard to retrain one's brain while gasping for air, but one of the things we strive for in psychotherapy is that the client learns how to think and feel differently. Anxious, toxic thinking patterns tend to self-perpetuate, creating a vicious cycle of entrenched pathways in the brain. Psychotherapy can be viewed as a tool for learning and a catalyst for changing brain chemistry.

If a woman enters therapy with her amygdala on hyperdrive, one of our objectives is to reduce this hyperactivity, regulate her "fight, flight, freeze" response and move her into a state more conducive to learning. It has been reported that the relationship between therapist and client aspects of therapeutic engagement, such as empathy and trust, can help regulate this state of arousal (Good & Beitman, 2006). When you ground and assess with expertise and a plan, and with your most authentic presence and safeguarding measures, you contain her emotions and mirror the early stages of a secure attachment. When clients feel safe, they are more capable of self-observation, according to Beitman, which relies on the healthy function of the prefrontal cortex. When learning takes place, new pathways are created and new options for responding differently, more effectively, become available. It creates the space for therapeutic changes to occur. This coincides with our understanding of the brain's stress response. If we activate the parasympathetic nervous symptom through grounding and relaxing techniques, we can help move the client from "fight or flight" into "rest and digest", promoting calming responses and thus stabilizing the nervous system.

Holding will take root if you know who you are and you believe in your ability to do this well. Your determined and sustained presence will counterpoise her unpredictability. The moment you question your ability to accomplish this is the moment the connection weakens.

The Seeds of Progress

In psychotherapy, our objective is to provide healing and the alleviation of suffering through the management of symptoms. Whether postpartum women initiate this therapeutic relationship willingly, whether they are coming in response to their unbearable distress, or whether this action is requested by their provider or partner, ultimately, you need to check in and monitor how the process is going for them. Many postpartum clients move through the process of therapy in a predictable pattern marked by an up and down course. Often, if you ask them to explore the intersection of their parenting stressors and the ebb and flow of their symptoms, they will realize that this pattern is consistent with the demands of new motherhood, sleep deprivation, exhaustion, hormonal influences, and the emotional roller coaster built in to this life transition.

Monitoring Progress: What Criteria Do We Use?

As your clients progress, consider assessing the following four variables to determine whether holding is having an impact. Although these factors may seem obvious, they are noteworthy determinants when continuing to assess her current state and ability to get through the day. You assess her general functioning, her level of autonomy, her ability to internalize, and the degree to which her daily life improves.

1 **Functioning.** Look for improvements, however slight they may be, which include a decrease in the symptoms of anxiety and depression that brought her to you initially. Remember that some symptoms might have preceded her crisis and it is important to tease that out in history taking. Moreover, certain symptoms, such as intrusive thoughts, may persist beyond the point where others begin to resolve. Clients who are successfully held in therapy should have a clearer understanding of these lingering symptoms and feel better able to cope, even when certain symptoms last longer than they had anticipated. Her symptoms and areas of poor functioning can represent an inventory that the two of you can review together by asking her what she believes is a little bit better, what, if anything, feels worse, and what feels the same.

2 **Autonomy.** Within the context of treating postpartum women, autonomy refers to the decreased dependence on external support, including the therapeutic relationship. As holding gains traction, dependence lessens, and the client moves toward autonomy. We learned from Winnicott that the infant's journey toward independence moves from absolute dependence to relative dependence and ultimately toward independence (Winnicott, 1965). Likewise, holding, which embodies empathy, enables the client to feel more secure as she moves from dependence to autonomy.

3 **Internalization.** This refers to the client's ability to assimilate and apply what is being discussed and experienced in a way that enhances her current level of functioning and helps project the possibility of ongoing healing. Checking in to endorse her understanding is essential because her ability to think clearly is likely impinged by symptoms. If her level of insight is good, it is reasonable to expect a client to make changes that increase her ability to cope.

4 **Improvement in Quality-of-Life Experiences and Relationships.** When holding is progressing, the client should be able to report incremental progress both in the way she is feeling about the therapy process and how she is experiencing her life outside of therapy. You may also notice that her connection with you feels more steady and comfortable. The parallel between the lessening of symptoms and her feeling more

engaged in the therapeutic relationship is not a coincidence. The reciprocal nature of this makes it hard to say for sure which affects which. Whether the symptoms are, in fact, remitting has less of an impact than her a) belief that they are, and/or b) appraisal of them as less invasive, and/or c) perceived ability to cope with them better.

5 **Gridlock.** Sometimes, effective holding slides off course and the therapeutic relationship can feel at an impasse. This is *idle holding*, which can occur well after holding techniques have been established as successful. It can be the result of many factors, belonging to the client or the therapist, or it can be the product of the interaction between the two.

Idle holding can result from:

- **New content brought into session** (e.g., medication) may cause a distraction to the holding process.
- **New environmental stressors** enter her life and the session.
- **Change in her diagnosis**, experience, symptomatology, or her attitude or perception of her current state.
- **Emotional fatigue**, which may arise if expectations of the process disappoint her and she becomes frustrated or impatient.

Whatever the origin of this intermittent standoff, it is again something you can *feel*. In the previous chapters, you saw how a therapist's style can contribute to ineffective holding. You also learned that some postpartum women are repelled by holding techniques and would do better with a different style altogether. In addition to reviewing the suggestions in the previous chapter, each therapist should consider the following points of clarification when idle holding presents itself:

- Is this stalemate a consequence of her current state, your approach to her, or something in the middle?
- Do you feel capable of shifting gears and confronting the situation in order to assess this block? Remember, it may be something that only *you* feel. Take care not to misappraise her experience in therapy. Remain open to the possibility that the process might be progressing just fine from your client's perspective. If that is the case, what is it, then, that you are responding to with such scrutiny?
- Perform a rapid self-inventory: *Am I focused? Am I listening? Am I paying attention? Am I okay? Am I holding? Is something distracting me?*
- If/when a client resists with such force that holding points prove unsuccessful, it may be pathologically driven. That is not to charge the client for all holding failure. It is simply to say that if a woman walks into a therapist's office with any glimmer of hope for symptom relief and she

stonewalls any/all attempts to engage, often her guard may be diagnostic, so study it carefully.

- Gridlock, like any dynamic within the therapeutic relationship, can be processed directly with the client. The difficulty here is that we are talking about an early dynamic within the short time span imposed by the postpartum urgency. Fundamentally, it may come down to whether or not you feel you can work through this with her.

- Ultimately, if holding points do not work, even after modifying, and you feel you will not be helpful to her, process this with her to make sure there isn't a schism in the relationship and determine whether or not a referral to another therapist would be in her best interest. Idle holding can ensue during the most cohesive therapeutic relationships and always warrants diligent attention.

Missing the Mark

We all slide off course once in a while. Sometimes, we fail to ask the right question and only realize this after the client has left. Because postpartum women are so adept at presenting themselves as well put together and healthier than they feel, it is likely that you might miss something. This is why you always employ the holding points, fine tuning them in response to each assessment question in your attempt to remain aligned with her. The truth however is that you need to be emotionally prepared for the possibility that you might still miss something.

Remember, *she is not telling you everything*.

Healthcare providers are similarly in a position to miss signs. If postpartum women visit healthcare practitioners with the façade of being in control and doing well, they run the risk of reinforcing widespread misconceptions. If not trained to see through this, healthcare providers are led off course. It has been reported that general practitioners feel confident in their clinical intuition, which would alert them to signs of postpartum depression, as opposed to using a formal screening instrument or even actively making an effort to assess or ask questions specifically about depressive symptoms (Chew-Graham et al., 2009). However, some of these same doctors who report that they are intuitive enough to spot depressive symptoms within a five-minute window of opportunity are missing the mark. That discrepancy is unsettling.

Bethany and the System Fail

We received a phone message from Bethany, who was 2 weeks postpartum and extremely agitated. Her voicemail message said she had her baby 2 weeks ago and experienced a trauma related to her birth. She wanted to come in that day and could not stand the way she was feeling anymore. I called her back promptly:

"Hi, Bethany, this is Karen Kleiman from The Postpartum Stress Center returning your call. Are you able to talk for a few minutes?"

"Yes. Hi. I feel terrible. I can't stand this. Thanks for calling so quickly." Her voice sounded frantic and sweetly apologetic.

"Sure, Bethany. I'm sorry you're feeling so bad. Let me see what I can do to help you. Your baby is 2 weeks old?" I usually start by referencing something I know from the referral source or from her message on the phone.

"Yes. She just came out of the NICU yesterday. Everything is fine, now. She's okay. But she stopped breathing right after she was born." She paused to catch her breath and another deep inhale, "I watched everyone scramble and run around freaking and giving her CPR and yell things like 'she's not breathing.' Oh God. But she's okay now. I'm not. I am not at all okay."

"My goodness, Bethany, how scary for you. I'm not surprised you feel bad. I'm glad to hear that your baby is okay. What is her name?"

"Alicia."

"What a pretty name, *Alicia*. And what a relief for you that Alicia is doing well now. Good. Then let's talk about you. Have you ever felt anything like this way before? Do you have a history of any depression or anxiety?"

"No. Nothing. I did go see a counselor this week, though. Someone I was referred to from the hospital when I had the baby."

"Okay. You had one appointment? Did that go okay for you?"

"It was awful, really awful. It was terrible, actually. I felt so much worse after I left there."

"Oh, I am sorry to hear this. What happened? Why was it so 'awful'?"

"Oh my God. The therapist kept asking me questions. I mean I can't even breathe. She gave me like a nine-page questionnaire thing. Like I can sit there and fill that out?! I couldn't even sit! I couldn't think. I couldn't focus. My head was pounding. Then she kept asking me questions about my family and my past and shit like that – I'm sorry, I'm just upset – I told her I felt traumatized or something like that. I told her I couldn't function," she cried as she spoke. "I mean, she could see I was shaking. Like this wasn't me. It isn't me at all."

"Bethany, I'm sorry you had to go through that and felt so misunderstood. Did you tell her that? Was she aware of how you were feeling?"

"YES! I said, *why are you asking me so many questions? Why can't you help me feel better?* She said she needed to ask me those questions so she could get to know me. Really? After what seemed like forever, I finally got up and walked out."

"You walked out before the session was over?" (I think that's when I started scowling to myself, to the tune of, *I can't believe she had to go through this...*)

"I did. And I'm not going back. No way."

"What did she do when you left? Did she come out after you? Or call you back in, or call you later on the phone?"

"Nope. She did not."

Bethany was then scheduled for a session with our clinical director the next morning and I reassured her that she would be in good hands. We spoke a few more minutes about what she could to do get some short-term relief between now and then, and we ended the conversation with her saying, "I feel so much better already. Just talking to you on the phone makes me feel better."

That is a golden nugget.

Bethany had been sent to a program that specialized in treating women's issues so she was right to expect good care. In this particular instance, however, she left feeling uncared for and angry. "Like I wasn't feeling bad enough when I got there!" she exclaimed with righteous indignation. Her annoyance seemed justified and matched by my own frustration with healthcare providers who still do not get it. It is not that the therapist did anything wrong, per se. It is that she failed to reconfigure her assessment protocol when it became clear that interference from the client's symptoms made compliance impossible. This is when a therapist should put down her pen and paper and look the client in her eyes to determine what the best next step should be. Assessment questions and interview procedures mean nothing if the client is not listening or attending or able to answer the questions. This is when all best efforts break down and should be redirected in response to what she needs.

This is about the connection between her and you.

Bethany was told to call us that night if anything scared her and we would see her in the morning and help her start to feel better. When her appointment time arrived, she sat in our office with her mother. As I passed through the waiting room, I noticed her curled up in the chair, with arms crossed, each hand grabbing the opposite elbow securely wrapped inside both sleeves. She was gently rocking back and forth, with legs bouncing from nervous energy. She caught me glancing her way.

"Are you Karen?" She asked with wide-eyed curiosity.

"I am. Are you Bethany?" I smiled.

"Yes." I heard both the anxiety and the relief in her voice.

I sat down in the chair next to her, introduced myself to her mother, and turned back to Bethany, "I am so glad I was able to meet you before you went in to see Marcie. You doing okay for now?"

"I dunno. I hope so."

"Well you are in the right place. Marcie is our clinical director. She knows exactly what to do to help you feel better. I am glad you came." She made great eye contact with me through her tender tears and told me again how good it felt to be there. Her mother also expressed gratitude. I sat with them for a minute or two until Marcie came out to greet her.

After her first session, Marcie and I met to discuss what had occurred. She reported that Bethany was easy to connect with and that most of the session was spent reassuring her, assessing her degree of trauma, evaluating her access to support and resources, and evaluating her coping potential. Marcie also called her obstetrician before Bethany left to discuss the option of her taking a small dose of benzodiazepines for her acute anxiety until the antidepressant they started her on kicked in. Everyone agreed.

A week later, Marcie stopped into my office to report how well Bethany was doing after her second session. Her anxiety had markedly reduced, and she was able to enjoy her baby. Both Marcie and Bethany were surprised and pleased with her rapid return to her previous level of functioning. Although she was feeling significantly better, they made an appointment to follow up because she was early postpartum and it is helpful to hold for a bit longer than they might think is necessary. While hormones are recalibrating and sleep deprivation is at an all-time high, we err on the side of caution and monitor moods and symptoms a bit longer, even when we witness an early return to improved functioning. There are times when postpartum women can go from feeling that bad to that much better that quickly.

This example of an initial therapeutic misstep is what we hope to avoid. Let's see where things veered off track for Bethany.

Take-home points to minimize holding failures:

1 **Do not let paperwork undermine your clinical interview.** Anyone who has worked for a mental health agency or organization, especially one that accepts insurance, is well aware that they require massive amounts of paperwork, which for the most part is now electronic. Still, therapists often require clients to fill out assessment forms prior to their intake session, which is fine, as long as symptoms do not interfere with that process. If they do, therapists should be tuned in to this and follow the course that is most comfortable for the client in distress. Consider the holding points. How can we be expected to ground according to her current state, remain present as an expert, make a plan, and keep her safe if we are more interested in adhering to

protocol than we are to her words and the voice of depression? In fact, how can we possibly hold at all if we prefer that she follow a formal structure despite the added stress it may create for her? For women who are able to complete the paperwork without incident, there is no downside to doing it in any way that best meets the needs of your individual clinical practice. For those who are unable, consider establishing a protocol for your practice that allows her some grace and you some flexibility.

2 **Do not ignore her cries for help.** Although this may seem like an obvious directive, it is alarming how often cries are missed. It does not matter if she is crying aloud in pain or if she is trembling with excessive adrenaline. It does not matter if she knows how to answer your questions or if she wonders why she's there in the first place. If her symptoms get in the way of your early agenda, be sure to sit with what she needs and spend more time grounding her and being present. Our job at this early stage is to meet her where she is and find out how we can help ease her distress.

3 **Do not presume you know more about how she is feeling than she does.** Emphasizing the importance of maintaining the expert role does not mean you undermine her priorities or what she thinks she needs right now. Her self-report overrides what you think is going on at the outset until you have more information to draw upon. Her story and her perception of its impact need to be told and heard. Be careful not to make assumptions as these can take you off course just enough to misalign the therapeutic endeavor. Clear your mind of what might or might not be in front of you and allow her to express herself. Remember to listen to what she is not saying as well. The gap between her thoughts and her words is significant.

4 **Trust your instincts.** Always. Even though this may appear to contradict point three, you must always balance her self-report with your intuitive reflection. If you think she is too upset to follow your line of assessment, shift gears. Or ask her. If you think you might be pushing her, check it out. If you think she might feel too uncomfortable to proceed, confirm that she is okay to go on. Intermittent emotional check-ins are excellent holding techniques that maintain the connection while you scan for interruptions.

5 **Follow up.** Do not let a client storm out of your office, visibly agitated, without following up with her. If she cannot tolerate the experience and abruptly leaves the session, are you not professionally, morally, and ethically obligated to make sure she is okay? Act in a way that is appropriate for the moment. The end of any session should round off all holding points, leaving her feeling valued and respected.

Although there is little you can do to modify the errors in judgment of other professionals, educating those in a position to help may be part of your comprehensive professional strategy. Hopefully, excellent holding opportunities and practices will eventually find their way into all healthcare offices. In the meantime, do damage control.

With so many unpredictable variables at play, there will be times when therapists either miss the mark or second-guess their judgment. This is standard practice for a conscientious therapist who is self-aware and open to growing as a professional. It is highly probable that readers of this book are devoted to this work with superb credentials and deep passion. Still, we must always remain vigilant. That's because postpartum distress is not what it looks like. Postpartum women can fool the best of us. They are good at that. They have to be. They have tons of family and social expectations and stigmas to contend with and challenge. As one client expressed so powerfully, "I wish I felt as good as I look like I feel." Your job is to recognize that and, above all, make them feel comfortable enough to loosen the facade.

Rigorous Holding

There will be times when holding doesn't seem to work. Either from your perspective or hers. There are a million reasons why; some we can decipher; others are lost forever in the mysterious abyss of psychotherapeutic unknowns.

Typically, women who may not initially respond well to holding techniques are:

1 Women who experience acute, excruciating (either real or perceived) symptoms that obstruct interacting on any meaningful level (including psychotic symptoms).
2 Women who are self-absorbed by their symptoms and unable to fathom any experience outside of their current state right now.
3 Women who experience sensory overload as a result of their symptoms. Intense symptoms can inhibit her ability to hear what others are saying, see things from another's perspective, or feel things in a different way than how they are currently experiencing things. These women might feel suffocated or intruded upon by well-meaning holding attempts.
4 Women who may have significantly impaired primary relationships with their own mother or father and attribute negative transference to the therapist, which thwarts their attempt to connect.
5 Women who misperceive the intent of the therapist either because they misread it or the therapist is off track.

190 The Anatomy of Holding

6   Women who have been raised to believe that it is better not to let others know how they feel or who resist the therapeutic process and are present solely in compliance with a doctor's suggestion.
7   Women who are predisposed to overintellectualize, overanalyze, overscrutinize, who are logical thinkers and whose personalities prompt them to be emotionally unavailable or constricted.
8   Women who have low self-esteem that prevents them from letting others in. This may be accompanied by a deep fear that if others saw who they really are, they would judge or reject them.
9   Women who respond to being cared for by others with disdain, mistrust, or contempt. This prickly response can be managed well by a skilled therapist, but holding attempts need to be modified to accommodate the potential for hostility and detachment.
10 Women who come in with their own agenda, whether it is characterologically driven or symptom propelled, with a single-minded or provocative objective, which may or may not leave them open to your style or intention.
11 Women who may or may not be clinically depressed but who may have been overindulged and overprotected, which might generate feelings of entitlement, privilege, or a prerogative that discredits or rejects holding gestures.
12 Women with a vulnerable and variable clinical profile whose personality predispositions or disorders create a wedge between the two of you.

None of these states are incompatible with holding, but they are apt to inflame the process and challenge the holding points and subsequent course of treatment.

Intuition and Revision

Regardless of the reason, if you sense that your client is repelling your efforts, you readjust and revise without delay.

Holding revision requires that you promptly:

- Assess what you said and how you said it. Review what you did and how you did it.
- Assess how she is feeling and reacting in order to determine whether or not it is a direct reaction to what you said or did.
- Check your intuition and ask her directly how she is feeling right now.
- Consider the possibility that this may be a critique of you and your style or it may be a reflection of who she is and have nothing to do with you. Either way, you need to ensure that she is okay to proceed.

- Determine whether there is something you need to do to modify your words, your behavior, or your thought process.
- Give her permission to let you know if something is not working for her and be prepared to accommodate your skills to align with her appraisal and her needs.

If a client responds in any way that feels unfamiliar or unexpected, your best response is to gently and honestly confront it and ask her how she is feeling. Your ability to readjust in support of what she needs will be enhanced by your genuineness and willingness to accommodate. This also holds her accountable for her responses that may benefit from a closer look. We know that expertise does not mean you have all the answers. Nor does it mean that your client's personality will naturally mesh with your therapeutic style. Being an expert means you are confident in who you are, what you do, and how you do it to surrender some of that on behalf of what she needs and are brave enough to ask her what that might be. Always be prepared to ask for help from a colleague or refer for further evaluation. Having a relationship with a trustworthy psychiatrist will be useful in numerous ways, particularly when working with difficult or complicated cases. In the ideal world, every perinatal therapist would have an ongoing relationship with a psychiatrist who shares a special interest in this field.

Holding in Crisis

When symptoms are extreme, dangerous, potentially life threatening, or out of control, holding techniques morph into something else. Suddenly, the moment urgently requires even more of your undivided attention. Take into account that what feels like a crisis to her may not, in clinical terms, be a crisis. When it feels like a crisis to her but does not actually represent an emergency situation, the response model in Chapter 8 is appropriate, relying on tools of reassurance, hope, control, and nurturance. If, on the other hand, you deem the situation to be critical in terms of suicidal intent and her safety, you command the moment and respond with immediate management of the situation. All holding points merge instantaneously as you shift into high gear to protect her. Once you determine that immediate intervention is required, depending on the circumstances, you:

- Explain your specific concerns to her.
- Describe your plan. (Contact primary support person? Call hospital? Activate support network? Take steps to remove weapons from home? Initiate safety contract? Contact psychiatrist?)

- Contact her partner. Speak to her partner in her presence. Ideally, have her partner join the two of you, if feasible; if not, let her hear your phone conversation.
- Make arrangements for your client to stay with you until her partner arrives. If not practical, contact another support person to assist you.
- Contact her healthcare provider when appropriate, with the client's permission.

In crisis, holding points converge. Her current state of crisis means that in order to ground her, you must remain present in response to her serious predicament and activate the design to keep her safe.

Transformation Through Suffering

The suffering that can accompany a woman's transition to motherhood is profoundly grievous and heartbreaking. Both to witness as well as to experience. It's hard to find an upside to suffering, but one of the therapeutic endeavors we must sanction is our belief that a postpartum woman can grow personally and develop a new level of resilience out this anguish. It's a notion that doesn't come without protest if spoken aloud to a woman in distress, but it is something most of us have gleaned from our work.

The Postpartum Stress Center's *Model of Transformation Through Holding* illustrates a trajectory postpartum women may take as they move from the suffering that brings them to therapy through stages of empowerment and, ultimately, toward healing. The belief that transformation through suffering is attainable is best understood as a process involving a series of seven stages, (see Figure 11.1 The Postpartum Stress Center Model of Transformation Through Holding).

While not applicable to every postpartum woman, this outline of stages provides insight into the trajectory that many postpartum women in distress will follow. We see here that when holding is introduced to the suffering she can learn to accept her current state, hope that she will return to her previous self, begin to tolerate periods of uncertainty, cultivate resilience, and thus begin to heal. If we believe in her capacity to heal through and beyond her suffering, she can begin to believe that, too.

Just Knowing...

In this chapter we have taken a look into the mechanics of holding. Sometimes, successful holding can transpire when you least expect it. Other times it can elude you, despite your sound intentions and efforts. You have seen that holding attempts can be substantive whether you are

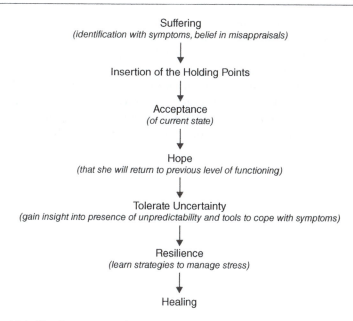

Suffering
(identification with symptoms, belief in misappraisals)

↓

Insertion of the Holding Points

↓

Acceptance
(of current state)

↓

Hope
(that she will return to previous level of functioning)

↓

Tolerate Uncertainty
(gain insight into presence of unpredictability and tools to cope with symptoms)

↓

Resilience
(learn strategies to manage stress)

↓

Healing

Figure 11.1 The Postpartum Stress Center Model of Transformation.

introducing yourself in the waiting room or convincing her you need to keep her safe from symptoms.

I am a huge fan of intuitive work in psychotherapy. Emergent awareness can inform our responses and interventions with gifts of honesty and humanity. Although your vast body of knowledge and endless pursuit of continuing education credits can inspire you, never underestimate the power of who you are and how to use your clinical intuition. In the classroom and in the academic literature, there is not a lot of attention placed on clinical intuition. In practice, however, it can be a vital component to healing. This is perfectly expressed by Terry Marks-Tarlow (2012) in her book, *Clinical Intuition in Psychotherapy: The Neurobiology of Embodied Response*:

> Clinical intuition is defined from a neurobiological perspective as a right-brain, fully embodied mode of perceiving, relating and responding to the ongoing flows and changing dynamics of psychotherapy.
>
> (Marks-Tarlow, 2012, p. 3)

Your gut reactions, your sense of humor, your playfulness, your hunches, your good instinctive responses all contribute to the client's connection with you and, ultimately, her ability to move toward lasting positive changes and growth, if she is not in crisis. There can be great power in intuitive thinking, which is the guiding force behind my assertion that you will *just know* when holding takes place. My hope and presumption is that you have entered this field of clinical work as a result of your innate talents and creative processes. If you do not allow your good intuition to fill that gap between clinical theory and practice, you risk interpersonal misalignment and may fail to notice significant moments and opportunities.

The convergence of knowledge and intuition is what constitutes holding.

Chapter 12

Your Professional Identity

During our professional training classes, I have the privilege of gathering with clinicians who are dedicated to this field and wish to enhance their practice by delving deeply both into the process of providing therapy for new mothers and the impact of this work on themselves. It has become one of the most cherished aspects of my work, and it provides a unique opportunity for me to get to know many motivated and devoted therapists up close and personally.

This intimate exchange between the clinicians and me is enlightening on so many levels. Of particular interest is how the group dynamics unfold as unfamiliar guests from around the world assemble with one common goal; each hopes to leave being a better, more informed, more effective maternal mental health specialist than when they came in. It doesn't take long for the atmosphere to absorb the individual energies and enthusiasm. Over time, most participants have been women and many are mothers. After the pandemic put in motion the required adjustment to virtual trainings, we were encouraged by the unexpectedly smooth transition and our successful efforts to remodel this topic of holding into a remote teaching opportunity. Whether in-person or virtual, the training class soon develops into a small group gathering of like-minded, well-trained therapists who collectively transform their ambition and passion for this work into something else. Something more vulnerable. Something exceptional.

The Shifting Tide

Roughly three decades ago, when a handful of pioneers in the field started handing out brochures and promoting the notion that some mothers did not feel good after the birth of their babies, reactions to this view were mixed. Most healthcare providers responded with a perfunctory, "Thank you, we'll get back to you," whereas mom-led groups and peer-support forums were relieved that finally there were words to what they were feeling but could not articulate. In 1994, the publication of *This Isn't What I*

DOI: 10.4324/9781003402145-12

Expected lent credibility to this campaign and broke ground in the uncharted territory of maternal mental health. I dare say that the predominance of male physicians were more impressed with my book, published by a fancy highfalutin New York publishing house, than they were with my individual plea for their consideration of this important matter. Either way, it got their attention. This was when my determined door knocking and offers of free lunch in exchange for an hour of their time eventually paid off. This is when the momentum shifted from obligatory support to a more legitimate endorsement of the appeal to take postpartum depression seriously. Some do take it seriously. Others continue to believe that postpartum depression is another name for baby blues no matter how clearly the distinction is made. Today, dedicated professionals and laypeople continue this crusade on behalf of postpartum women and their families who, by virtue of their symptoms, are not always in position to express what they need.

Is a Desire to Do This Work Enough?

There are many reasons why therapists decide to specialize in the treatment of perinatal mood and anxiety disorders. The following is a sample of some of the variables that motivate individuals to address the unique therapeutic needs of perinatal women in distress.

There Are Evidence-Based Statistics That Are Startling

1 An estimate that one out of seven women will develop depression in the year after they give birth has become a widely accepted statistic (Wisner et al., 2013). In lower socioeconomic areas, new mothers are twice as likely to develop depressive symptoms (Goyal et al., 2010).
2 Only 50% of women who screen positive for postpartum depression accepted follow-up treatment (Sim et al., 2023).
3 In the first few weeks after delivery, a woman's chance of requiring a psychiatric admission is seven times higher than at any other time in her life (Barker et al., 2016; Spinelli, 2009).
4 It has been reported that postpartum women find counseling to be a trustworthy source of support, but barriers and constraints make follow-up difficult (Negron et al., 2013).
5 Suicide accounts for up to 20% of postpartum deaths (Chin et al., 2022; Lindahl et al., 2005).
6 Self-harm ideation is as high as 19.3% when screening with the Edinburgh Postnatal Depression Scale (EPDS) according to one study (Wisner et al., 2013).
7 Women with a previous postpartum depression are at an increased risk for postpartum depression after a subsequent pregnancy.

8 It is estimated that 30% of women who show signs of depression after delivery had a history of depression prior to pregnancy (Wisner et al., 2013).

9 In the women studied, 40.1% of the depressive episodes began during the postpartum period, followed by 33.4% that began during pregnancy and 26.5% that began before pregnancy (Wisner et al., 2013).

10 More than two-thirds of the women also had signs of an anxiety disorder (Wisner et al., 2013).

11 Of the women who screened positive for depression, 22% had bipolar disorder (Wisner et al., 2013).

12 The postpartum period is a high risk time for the first lifetime onset of anxiety disorders such as panic and OCD (Sichel et al., 1993; Viswasam et al., 2021; Wisner et al., 1996).

13 Women with a history of bipolar disorder have a high risk of recurrence in the postpartum period (Conejo-Galindo et al., 2022).

14 A survey of Ob-Gyns found that 44% often or always screen for depression, 41% sometimes screen for depression, and 15% never screen for depression (Farr et al., 2011; LaRocco-Cockburn et al., 2003).

15 At the time of this writing, The American Academy of Pediatrics recommends that pediatricians screen mothers for postpartum depression (at 1, 2, 4, and 6 month visits). However, less than 50% of mothers are screened nationally (Lamere & Golova, 2022).

There Are Clinical Reasons That Are Compelling

1 Postpartum depression is a potentially life-threatening condition with a substantial impact on the quality of life of all family members.

2 Untreated postpartum depression places the mother and infant at risk and is associated with significant long-term effects on child development (Peindl et al., 2004; Slomian et al., 2019; Weissman et al., 2006).

3 Research indicates that a variety of effective psychological treatments exist to address and treat postpartum depression and anxiety, including supportive, cognitive behavioral, and interpersonal therapy (Dennis & Dowswell, 2013).

4 Identifying women at risk can facilitate appropriate action, including preventative and therapeutic interventions.

5 Proper screening is vital for maternal and infant well-being and can improve outcomes.

6 Interventions targeting at-risk mothers may be more beneficial and feasible than those including a general maternal population (Dennis & Dowswell, 2013).

7 Early intervention will augment treatment and recovery.

There Are Compassionate Reasons That Are Gut-Wrenching

1 Postpartum depression is the most common complication of childbirth.
2 Too many women are suffering after the birth of their baby.
3 The entire family suffers.
4 Despite the fact that the health risks and complications associated with maternal depression are well documented, pregnant and postpartum women who are depressed often do not get treatment due to their fear of disclosing how they feel with their providers (Declerq et al., 2002; Manso-Córdoba et al., 2020).
5 Women and their caregivers frequently overlook postpartum depression. Cultural norms that promote the expectation of happy moms continue to be pervasive.
6 Stigma silences women.
7 Women in the throes of a severe postpartum depression who state that their child would be better off without them believe this to be true.
8 Failure to disclose exacerbates guilt and suffering.
9 A shockingly high number of healthcare professionals continue to be misinformed.
10 Misinformation causes women to needlessly fear they are "insane," "losing their minds," or "going crazy."

There Are Personal Reasons That Are Hard to Articulate

1 Some therapists state they feel their own postpartum experience inspires them to change the focus of their existing clinical practice.
2 Some therapists state they are on a mission or feel they have a calling to be a part of this specialized work.
3 The work is both challenging and extraordinarily rewarding.
4 There is indescribable intimacy within the walls of a postpartum specialist's office, which propels the work forward even when words are not spoken.
5 Recent advocacy and persuasive awareness campaigns sanction any emotional impetus to do this work.

Consistent with the premise that therapists should examine their own motivation for doing this work and bearing in mind all areas of vulnerabilities, let's consider some variables that affect your commitment to this work. In reviewing these questions, you may discover strengths of yours that are in position for this work, as well as vulnerabilities that require attention as you proceed.

Are You a Good Therapist?

This is a question asked of each prospective therapist at The Postpartum Stress Center. I wait until she or he is comfortable with me, after some mutual pleasantries and a dutiful exchange of expectations, and so forth. Toward the end of the interview (which, by now, has mutated into casual chitchat because that's what happens to my grown-up self once I feel at ease), I ask them if they are a good therapist. This practice of mine has been criticized by one or two members of my team who feel it is a trick question because applicants might be afraid they would appear arrogant or conceited if they said they were a good therapist right off the bat like that. I disagree.

Surely, there are extenuating circumstances and disclaimers that would be appropriate to raise, such as, "I'm good with adults, but not with children." Or, "Yes, but I would not be comfortable dealing with clients with substance abuse." Or any of many stipulations that might qualify their response. I get it. Still, if I was interviewing for a new job today and was asked if I was a good therapist, I would reply, "Yes."

That is the answer I look for, too.

We can iron out the details and provisions of their strengths and challenges later. Notice that my question is not, "Do you think you are a good therapist?" Rather, it is "*Are* you are good therapist?" The distinction between *do you think you are* and *are you* potentially leads to a more objective perspective of your work, rather than a personal or esteem-based assessment. Similar to the question *how do you know if holding is working*, we explore *how do you know if you are a good therapist?* You just know. You know because you can feel it. You know because your clients tell you. You know because your clients connect well with you, they find meaning from their sessions, they learn, they grow, they feel better, they function better, they find successes or joy in their lives, they return for further sessions. You know because your work feels rewarding as you respond to the exchanges and outcomes that unfold before you. You know because you can feel the difference between clients you work well with and clients with whom you are not working well, for one reason or another, and that frustrates you, or bores you, and challenges you to seek supervision and guidance.

The answer to the question of whether or not you are a good therapist within the context of postpartum healing is directly related to your ability to hold. Not your desire to do it, nor your commitment to this population. Your ability, defined here as a combination of your skill set, your proficiency, and your confidence with specific regard to holding techniques, will determine whether or not holding is effective.

Is Holding Enough?

It should be. That being said, it cannot be disputed that what drives much of the energy behind the good work of therapists in this field is passion. Grounded enthusiasm and dedication toward making a difference, disseminating good, accurate information, and helping women reclaim their sense of self and well-being override almost everything else. Or so it seems. What may be too obvious to mention is that passion is not enough to sustain the intricacies of holding skills and excellent postpartum therapy. It is a good and an important start but requires the endorsement from advanced training and serious skill-building efforts. Remember, even dedicated therapists can continue to miss the mark and mistakenly believe that their devotion to their clients will earn them the success they desire. Holding is enough as long as the practitioner does not misinterpret holding as synonymous with compassion and kindness. Holding is skill-based, not to be confused with the sentiments that drive our passion for this work.

When considering each holding point, sincere passion needs to be bolstered by competency; for example: a) Grounding requires supportive interventions such as psycho-education, pertinent research references, and stabilizing exercises; b) Current state requires assessment tools, mental health/status evaluation inquiries; c) Expert requires belief in self, expertise, authority, the ability to exude confidence, and the ability to influence without intimidating or marginalizing; d) Design requires access to resources and referrals, knowledge of effective interventions, and execution of appropriate treatment plan options; e) Presence requires self-control management skills, emotional regulation skills, and mindful participation in proactive dialogue; and f) Safeguarding requires ongoing or emergency safety assessment and intervention as well as the use of language, tone, words, awareness, and actions to promote security, hope, and well-being.

After all is said and done regarding holding points, passion for this work is a close second in terms of prerequisites for exceptional work. On balance, without passion, holding techniques are not entirely genuine – they are only gestures. Without passion, this would just be a job.

Is Who You Are Enough?

Who you are. This is deep, existential, and way too complicated to tackle within the confines of this book. Although it is tempting. I can hear my mother telling me to leave this section out of this book because she is my best editor. *Too much hubris. Too much self-importance,* her cautionary words resound. There is, to be sure, a difference between confidence in who you are and an overinflated sense of self. Clearly, if your work is ego-driven, you have stepped out of the bounds of healthy holding and into the dangerous territory of is-this-more-about-you-than-your-client? Therefore, the reference to *who you are* speaks to your character and an honest awareness of your connection with your core self.

Consider these questions carefully. Sit with each one for a couple of minutes and run through the answer aloud in your head. If you are not truthful with yourself, you are not in a strong position to ask for this level of honesty from your clients.

- Do you know what you are good at?
- Do you know what you are not good at?
- Do you know why people like you?
- Do you know why people do not like you?
- Is your self-awareness an asset, or does your self-awareness intrude on your self-esteem and interfere with your ability to live wholeheartedly?
- Are you able to ask for help? Are you able to accept help?
- Are you proud of the choices you have made and continue to make?
- Do you believe you are a good role model for your clients, and if so do you think that's important for your work?
- Do you have secrets, pains, losses, shame, and disgraces that you need to come to terms with before you can sit with a vulnerable woman in distress?
- Are you living the life you want to be living?
- Are your primary relationships strong and satisfying?
- Do you have unfinished psychological work that needs attention?
- Are you making changes that need to be made?
- Are you accepting what needs to be accepted?
- Are you forgiving what/who needs to be forgiven?
- Do you like who you are? Why? Why not?

Remember this as you move forward with this work:

> Within the context of postpartum healing, wisdom is the balance between the knowledge you have and who you are.

There is no better way to say that who you are *does* matter in this work. It matters because it is conveyed through your presence in each session and through your use of holding points.

Symptoms of postpartum depression and anxiety can have a negative impact on a woman's self-esteem and your positive self-esteem can be contagious under these conditions. One of the best ways to model a strong sense of self to a woman who feels helpless is to embody it. Not with conceit, but with gentle and total knowingness. Knowing who you are is not projected with intent to influence. It is an energy that emits from a pure sense of being at one with yourself. Of course, this comes with tons of self-scrutiny and constant monitoring. Most importantly, it comes with authenticity.

Do You (Really) Believe in Yourself as an Expert?

This is an area that causes considerable anxiety in clinicians. If carrying yourself with the confidence of an expert sounds good to you but you are not sure how to gain this confidence, invest in any process that helps you understand what makes you feel uneasy. Some areas of vulnerability that may interfere with the development of this confidence include:

• Low self-esteem
• Limited experience
• Limited exposure to information and resources
• Uncertainty regarding the use of power/control
• Negative thinking
• Shyness
• Anxiety
• Fear of imposter syndrome
• Fear of rejection or failure

If these traits resonate for you, protect yourself and forge forward with tools to augment these areas. Try focused meditation, cognitive reframing, or grounding exercises. Belief in yourself and your ability to do this work underscores every step you take. Along with, of course, excellent supervision, mentoring, or professional consultation.

What Does Being Your Best Self Really Mean?

Throughout these chapters, references to your best self are used to remind you that whatever affects you on a personal or emotional level must be contained; you must refocus and defer to your work with your client. From a supervisor's perspective, I often find myself reminding a therapist to be their best self when they experience a strong emotional response – either positive or negative, usually negative – to something being said or occurring in a session. When a therapist experiences a highly charged emotion in a session, it is likely to obscure objectivity and potentially interfere with the process. If, when discussing the case, the therapist and I ascertain that they are indeed too angry, too frustrated, too overwhelmed, too upset, even in our discussion, we process this in order to determine the next best course of action when they revisit their client.

In our office, Marcie reminds our group to take a slow deep breath in, in conjunction with a hand motion. She demonstrates by taking one hand

and starting at the forehead, pulling her five fingers together with a rapid downward gesture (as if symbolically pulling and capturing the contents of your mind with the closed claw hand), and simultaneously pulling this hand down along an imaginary line from the head to the body's center. The gesture reminds us, as we breathe in deeply, that all controlled emotions involve both our head and our core self, and the motion made with our hand is actually quite centering. It can put a halt to emotions that are starting to run amok. Try it. As you pull from your forehead down to your belly button, breathe in slowly and deeply while thinking "be my best self."

Apply whatever words are meaningful to you, whatever words signify hard and honest work. Summoning your best self brings forth your integrity. As you hold a postpartum woman in distress, you will be tested time and time again. To endure, to tolerate, to absorb, to reassure, to guide, to calm, to educate, to encourage, to evaluate, to question, and, of course, to ground, assess, be an expert, make a plan, be present, and safeguard. That's a lot to do all at the same time! The only way you can do that efficiently is to bring your best and most centered self, into that moment. Without question, that is precisely who each postpartum woman in distress hopes to find on the other side of that office door she is about to enter.

What About Self-Disclosure?

Think about this: Did your own experience with postpartum depression affect your decision to go into this work? If so, is that helpful or not?

Unnecessary or careless self-disclosure is a clinical calamity. Every temptation to self-disclose demands meticulous consideration at the very least, leaving room for the possibility of postponement or rejection of the notion under consideration. The incentive to self-disclose within the postpartum context seems disproportionally high, often naively misconstrued as a means to establish a connection. As pointed out previously, there appears to be a high percentage of maternal mental health therapists who have experienced postpartum depression or anxiety themselves. Many of the therapists I meet reveal that their decision to concentrate on the treatment of pregnant and postpartum women is a direct result of their personal experience. Self-disclosure between a therapist and a perinatal client requires scrupulous boundaries, however, as your own experience may influence your perception of who will benefit from your disclosure – you, or your client.

The dangers of overidentifying with a client and allowing one's subjective experience to hinder impartiality are well known to therapists. Even so, a therapist's own experience with childbirth unites her to her client in a way that is hard to ignore. Identifying areas of common life experience may in fact provide an early connection for the postpartum woman trying to make sense out of coming to therapy, especially for those who are not familiar with therapy or who are hesitant to engage. Therapists who are eager to connect in a meaningful way may view their private experience as the ticket in. Earnestness to connect with a client by acknowledging your personal experiences can expose you in a way that contaminates the therapeutic process. Your client may believe she wants to know this about you, but your revelation can rapidly alter her perception of your ability to help her. Suddenly she believes you were as sick as she is. Or you were sicker. Or you were not nearly as sick. For some women, relating to you might be comforting, to see that you were ill and have recovered so well. For some you may sound fraudulent. For others, you may always cause them to wonder whether you are truly healthy enough to help.

The disclosure of personal information is generally frowned upon according to psychotherapy standards, although modern thinkers tend to support the belief that when pieces of personal information are germane to the work at hand, they may, when appropriately related, be useful to the client. Worth repeating is the statement that *all self-disclosure must benefit the client.*

Some rules of thumb regarding specific reference to your own personal postpartum symptoms and treatment are:

- If it has been *less than a year* since your own recovery from depression or an anxiety disorder, it is too soon to do this work.
- When in doubt, do not disclose.
- Even if you believe it will benefit the client, you may not be right about that.
- Boundaries, boundaries, boundaries. This session is for her. Not you.
- Your own treatment and your course of recovery will not necessarily work for her, nor will it necessarily be helpful for her to know.
- Be prepared for this work to be a constant trigger. Do not presume that your full recovery protects you from feeling entangled in her suffering.
- Supervision is obligatory.

If you do decide (be cautious about this decision) to disclose any portion of your own experience, heed these words of caution:

- Premature self-disclosure is a potential deal breaker for the relationship. Make sure you know who your client is and what is motivating their curiosity or your urge to disclose.
- Specifics are never a good idea, keep your self-disclosure brief.
- If you experience or express *any* emotion along with your disclosure, that is too much.

- Her engagement with your self-disclosure is likely to be distracting from and counterproductive for the therapeutic process.
- If at *any* point you begin to question your decision to disclose anything, stop and redirect.

As noted in *Therapy and the Postpartum Woman* (Kleiman, 2009), there are occasions when self-disclosure within this context may be helpful. When used appropriately, revealing personal information may be beneficial. Deliberate and appropriate self-disclosure can potentially:

1 Enhance the alliance
2 Promote trust
3 Facilitate engagement
4 Increase compliance

That said, self-disclosure must always be filtered through the lens of the bigger picture. For example, revealing that you have children is not the same thing as telling her you were hospitalized. Or revealing that you know how bad anxiety can feel in the context of being a mother is not the same thing as telling her that when you tried to wean from your anxiety medication, you suffered from prolonged panic attacks.

Therefore, you should ask yourself:

- What information am I sharing?
- Is it too much information?
- Why do I want to share it?
- Would it be better if I decide not to share it?
- Could there be a downside to sharing this?
- How do I think this will affect her?
- Is this information that the client is capable of dealing with?
- Do I know that for sure?
- Is this the right timing?
- Is there any other way to reach the result I am hoping to achieve via self-disclosing?

The decision to disclose should be based on two things: a) your active decision to do so, and b) ethically deciding that the disclosure is in the best interest of your client. Remember that no client ever needs to know you experienced postpartum distress. You can, might want to, or ethically may need to, decide it is not at all relevant to her treatment.

Therapists who have recovered from postpartum depression and anxiety report that they feel the force of two opposing perspectives. They feel their personal experience unites them with their client and facilitates trust in the relationship. Concurrently, they feel conspicuously raw and vulnerable. Once confidence has cracked, threads of doubt find their way into this work. Any hesitation of spirit, although uncomfortable and unnerving, should be managed with good clinical supervision. Without good supervision, a therapist with a history of depression and anxiety can feel overexposed in this work, which can weaken effectiveness in the following ways.

• You are at risk of overidentifying with your client and her experience.
• You are at risk of expressing inappropriate opinions about what works and what doesn't work that may or may not be relevant or helpful to your client.
• You are at risk of compromising your objectivity.
• You are at risk of feeling overwhelmed by your emotions.
• You are at risk of inadvertently influencing the course of your work together by allowing the impact of your own experience to invade the process.
• You are at risk of becoming symptomatic.

There may be general ways that your own experience with postpartum depression or anxiety can augment your clinical work and specific ways it could affect a particular client. Still, it is imperative that you put her needs first and remember that *words cannot be unheard.* Once you disclose something, it cannot be undone. Generally I believe that therapists should be discouraged from revealing specific information that relates to personal history of symptoms or treatment. The best way to bring that information into the session is to relate it as a story about someone else, an invented client, or a friend of yours.

Your relationship with your client is an intimate one, which might unexpectedly set the stage for self-disclosure, but it is also a business relationship, further bound by professional ethics. The more information you bring into the session that she perceives as even slightly irrelevant, the more likely you are to injure the relationship.

Motherself: How Does Your Own Experience with Your Mother and Your Child Influence Your Work?

You have seen how competent holding can echo a maternal relationship, whether you are examining it through the lens of psychoanalytic references or simply responding to the way it feels when you sit with a postpartum woman who is suffering. It is hard not to make the comparison between the holding connection and a maternal response to distress.

If there is merit to the analogy, it obliges you to be wary of your own issues with your mother and/or your children in order to prevent them from seeping into your work. Only you know how your relationship with your own mother and yourself as a mother, if that applies, affects the way you feel about yourself and your work. *Motherself*, first presented in *Therapy and the Postpartum Woman* (Kleiman, 2009), is a term used to describe the sense you have of yourself as a mother after you integrate who you expected yourself to be, including all the good and the bad that comes with that. In order to achieve the purest state of motherself, there must be sufficient separation from your perceived or real expectations of who you think you are and who you think you should be. That is not easy for any of us and surely it takes a lifetime. I am still working on my motherself, even after becoming a grandmother.

This term has been used to describe the process of helping a client sculpt a unique vision of and expectation for motherhood that is reasonable, attainable, and considerate of your client's sense of self. In the context of holding perinatal distress, this construct applies to you, as her therapist. You must discover your path to your motherself in order to guide your clients to theirs.

The work involved in the construction of your motherself identity requires close inspection and reconciliation with your own fantasies, expectations, and losses. Indefinite variables will find their way into your work when you least expect them, often when your client states something that raises a red flag for you. Grab that moment, set it aside, and be sure to return to it on your own time. Only then can you expect to see clearly enough to support her through the expectations and losses that belong only to her.

Therapists as Wounded Worriers

Even the most experienced therapists will agree that intrinsic to this work are panic-inducing flashes of imposter syndrome. If you tell your clients that they can be competent and symptomatic at the same time, likewise, you can be a competent therapist and still question your capability. Even the most skilled maternal mental health therapist needs to be alert and on guard for signs of trouble and, given the very high stakes inherent to the perinatal period, feeling unsure at times is expected. After all, you are aware of the difficulty your client might have disclosing her pain and level of distress, even to you. Your client might tell you she's fine, though she's having thoughts of harming herself. She might tell you she's eating, though she has an eating disorder; she might tell you her mother smacked her senseless when she was little, but she's "over it now." Thus, we listen, we notice, we try not to judge. Still we ask ourselves, *Is this okay? Is that okay? Is that too much? Am I right, or is she right?* And, of course, there are the absolute, definite concerns, such as, *Is she telling me the truth? Is she safe? Is the baby safe?*

Common Worries

Therapists in training state that this work makes them nervous. They report that they are both energized and terrified to dive into clinical practice. Many continue to report this juxtaposition of emotions after several years of clinical practice. I think that is good – it keeps you on your toes. It discourages apathy. It compels you to sharpen your skills. I feel it, too. It's an energy that strengthens my attention and forces me to make every postpartum woman I see believe she is the only one I work with.

The worries I hear most often from maternal mental health therapists are:

- I worry I might miss something and something catastrophic could happen.
- I worry she could become psychotic or suicidal and I won't know what to do.
- I worry about my own ability to intervene appropriately.
- I worry I might respond emotionally to some of her painful symptoms.
- I worry I won't be able to handle the stress of working with this fragile population.
- I wonder if I will really be able to help her.
- I worry that I might fail.
- I worry if I have what it takes to sustain a clinical practice.

By far, the list topper in bold is the worry that therapists express most often. *I worry I might miss something and something catastrophic could happen.* When polled through an informal survey, this worry beat out a long list of additional worries shared by therapists who specialize in this field. This predominant worry, as troubling as it might feel at times, is what keeps us on top of our game. These common worries are understandable and will, as previously mentioned, keep you attentive to details that you cannot afford to miss. The adaptive function of worry applies here, too. It keeps you alert to potential danger, much like the worry that characterizes postpartum women. It follows, then, that you, too, can learn to surrender some of the worry the way we teach our clients to let go of troubling thoughts.

Here are some thoughts to guide you through this:

• You are worried. Good. Be alert. Be smart. Be aware.
• Try to let go of over-worrying. Despite the dominant theme of this book, that your confidence is paramount, you do not have as much influence as you think you have (or wish you had).
• If something unforeseen and critical is going to happen, it will happen whether you are a good therapist or not. Any misstep you might make along the way will have less of an impact on her well-being than you think. You are in a perfect position to watch her and your work together. That alone puts her in a safer place than she would be without you. Trust yourself.
• I cannot emphasize this enough: If the unthinkable occurs, if tragedy descends upon you, if you are left reeling from the pangs of professional loss and grief, I implore you: do not think you allowed or caused this to happen. Bad things do happen. Hopefully they will not happen on your watch. If a suicide does occur, or if a baby dies as a result of a psychotic episode, it is most often the case that there was little you could have done to prevent either of those tragedies. These are brutal mental illnesses associated with radically impulsive behaviors. There should, and will, be sadness. There should not be guilt.
• Make sure you have excellent supervision. Collegial support from associates and others in this field is indispensable.

"I Have To"

Shortly after introducing herself for the first time and gathering the paperwork, Cindy, mother of an 8-month-old, sauntered into my office as if she a) had been there before, b) had not a care in the world, c) wanted me to see that she was totally in control, d) did not want her symptoms to show, e) was going to a business meeting or meeting me for coffee, f) had a script and was eager to start speaking lest she forget what she was going to say, g) wanted me to see how healthy she was, h) needed control of the session, or i) all of the above.

She took me by surprise when she sat down on the couch, leaned forward, and started our session with a congenial flair:

"So why do you do this work?"

"Well that's a fine how-do-you-do, as we say in St. Louis." I smiled in response to her inquisitive opening. "Why do you ask?"

"I dunno. I just wondered how you can sit and listen to so many people complain, I guess. I can't imagine listening to this all day long. It must be boring."

"I think that's an interesting question to start off with. Would you mind if we first talk about why you are here, and I'll answer that when we are done, because I do think it's an important question. Okay? And by the way, I do not hear any of this as complaining. I believe you must feel bad or you wouldn't be here."

Her introductory question was possibly a representation of her anxiety and ability to deflect focus; still, I found it an interesting, if not off-putting, introduction. She fell into line, however, and eased right into a 45-minute chronicle of unfulfilling and disturbing relationships that led up to this point. I heard stories of impaired relationships, dysfunctional family dynamics, early parentification, and saw evidence of her compensatory veneer of good mental health. It seemed that any postpartum issues were eclipsed by lifelong pangs of inadequacy that compelled her into a constant quest for control in her life. It also seemed she had never really been listened to, never felt heard, never felt as if her opinion mattered. Which was interesting to me because she was so assertive and articulate.

When our session had come to its conclusion, she reached for her purse. I broke the silence with, "Would you like me to answer the question you came in here with now?"

"Yes. I would love that."

"I think it's a good question because even though it sounds like you are asking about me, by asking that question you are, in a way, screening me, interviewing me, questioning who I am and wondering if I will be a good fit for you."

She nods.

"That is a valid concern and an interesting way for you to learn more about me, to see if this feels like a good place for you."

She smiles, listening to my explanation.

"You said it seems 'boring.' It makes more sense to me, now, that you might think this, doesn't it? When you think about the messages you received growing up? And how irrelevant you believed your feelings and thoughts were? How unappreciated you felt when you tried to express yourself? It makes sense that you would consider this kind of exchange as a burden, or something of little value to me, or question my motivation. But you know why I do this work? I have to. I actually feel like I have to. It's hard to explain, but it's a feeling I have deep inside me which draws me to it and I love the way it makes me feel. So, honestly, I have to."

"I love that answer. That is so perfect."

"Why is that, Cindy? It sounds a bit self-important to me," I grin with confidence and transparency.

"It's perfect. It's just what I need. I didn't even realize it's what I needed until you said that. It feels good to be heard, I guess. Especially from someone who wants to listen."

A rare, exquisitely timed moment of mutual awareness and fulfillment.

Isn't this really why we do this work?

Chapter 13

Holding Diverse Parents

Longing to feel heard, validated, supported, and cared for are natural human needs and are integral goals for every therapy environment. The holding therapist recognizes that while the clinical interventions learned in graduate school and other professional development avenues are critical components of treatment planning, establishing a space that meets these needs is the priority. When these essential needs go unmet, those clients who may still be willing to accept our invitation into the holding environment likely will not stay.

Everyone Needs to Feel Held

As a holding therapist, recognizing how my white, cisgender, female, birthing-mother experience influences my holding stance is critical to recognizing my strengths and challenges as a holder. In order to establish a holding space that feels truly safe for clients with different lived experiences, we must learn about how other cultural and environmental experiences influence what clients need from their holding environment. In a study by R.H. Keefe et al. (2016), African American and Latina mothers were asked to provide recommendations for mental healthcare providers caring for mothers with postpartum depression. Their recommendations to providers wishing to establish a strong therapeutic alliance with members of their communities included:

> (1) conveying knowledge and understanding of postpartum depression; (2) listening carefully to the mothers' concerns and empathizing with them; (3) offering validation and reassurance that the mothers' symptoms would improve; (4) providing emotional support; (5) building trusting relationships; and (6) establishing more services that are accessible, have flexible appointment times, and are parent- and child-friendly.
> (p. 9)

DOI: 10.4324/9781003402145-13

What is striking about their feedback in the context of holding is how well these recommendations align with the basic principles of the holding points:

1 Conveying knowledge and understanding (Expert)
2 Listening carefully and offering empathy (Grounding, Current state, Presence)
3 Offering validation and reassurance about symptom improvement (Design)
4 Building trust (Safeguarding)
5 Establishing accessible services (Expert, Design)

All human beings at some time in life benefit from and need to feel the unique comfort and power of a holding environment. The holding points are evergreen. Our challenge as providers is to identify the ways in which our own lived experiences inform our assumptions about what others need in and from the holding environment. When we develop this insight, we can practice compartmentalizing our assumptions to make space for learning about what others need by listening and attending.

Maya and her Six Children

Maya presented for therapy at seven months postpartum after giving birth to her sixth child, a daughter, Rachel. Maya reported experiencing symptoms of anxiety and depression, including many ego dystonic intrusive thoughts about her baby. She was having a very difficult time sleeping at night and talked about feeling guilty about her impatience. "My five older children and their dad have been such a help to me and they love Rachel. They ask me for so little and they don't deserve to have a mom who is irritable and snapping at them. I am just so tired, and I am stressed all the time."

Maya shared that she arrived at The Postpartum Stress Center for therapy after seeing two other therapists who also specialized in treating postpartum depression. She emphasized that these therapists were helpful but that they both focused on the size of her large family as a probable factor in her depression. Maya said "I liked both of the therapists I saw but felt like they really did not understand what I was trying to say. I know that I have a lot of children and of course that is stressful, but this is normal in my community, and I know in my heart that the size of my family is not the problem."

In response, Maya's therapist explored her cultural context and inquired with curiosity about Maya's community. Maya shared that she is part of a traditional Jewish community in which having many children is normative. She talked about support that exists within the community for each of her children, her husband, and herself and acknowledged ways she finds deep meaning and fulfillment in having a large family. While dealing with parenting stress was certainly a part of Maya's treatment design, her therapist was mindful of Maya's expectations, perspective, and needs. As Maya healed from her depression she reconnected with her sense of agency, confidence, and joyfulness and her family system, and their extensive support system, were essential to her recovery.

The Downside of Intuition

Chapter 11 explored the mechanics of holding, including the role of intuition. Many therapists consider themselves gifted with keen intuition and recognize that intuition can serve as a useful tool in the therapy space (Arnd-Caddigan & Stickle, 2017; Shapiro & Marks-Tarlow, 2021). Within the holding environment the first indication that our client is feeling held may be noticed intuitively. Many therapists who receive mentoring at The Postpartum Stress Center describe "just knowing" when holding takes place and express a feeling of confidence that the therapeutic alliance is growing stronger. This is intuition at work.

However, even the most experienced, attuned, attentive, well-intentioned, and intuitive therapist is vulnerable to cognitive and affective biases that developed in response to the therapist's own lived experience. When we are not mindful of these biases our personal belief systems and judgments may lead us down the wrong clinical path (Yager et al., 2021). While we can certainly change our biases by welcoming opportunities to practice within settings that may cause us discomfort, gaining additional training, and seeking out professional supervision, we must first become aware of our biases and be willing to confront them.

There are many courses, resources, and guides for you to explore that cover the topics of cultural humility, implicit bias, racism, and discrimination within healthcare (and all other domains of society) in greater detail than we will in this chapter. You are urged to consider seeking out these resources, as they are essential to your work as a therapist, and particularly as a holding therapist. The goal for the pages ahead is simply to increase your sensitivity to your own responses when confronted with someone who might be different from you. What thoughts come to mind? What are you feeling? What happens in your body? Why might you feel these ways? It is important to practice noticing these cues, especially the subtle cues, so that you can quickly recognize and deal with them when they arise in sessions.

The Holding Therapist and Implicit Bias

Throughout the book you have learned the history and basic tenets of holding, as well as ways to troubleshoot complexities of the holding environment. You have learned how the holding relationship honors your clients' experiences of loss and reflects their strengths. You have learned how the six holding points efficiently develop a therapeutic relationship that lends itself to a vulnerable and fearful postpartum woman's disclosure of terrifying symptoms. You have also learned that when a client does not feel held, they may resist or terminate treatment which can lead to persistent, pervasive, and severe symptoms that can be impactful for a lifetime.

Chapter 10 explored the concept of hard-to-hold and discussed how the needs of clients with certain symptoms or personality traits can impede upon the holding relationship. In this chapter we explore how the therapist's biases can hinder this relationship and interfere with holding well. Of course, every therapist arrives to their therapy space with lived experience, personal success and failure, trauma, and unique cultural contexts. We all arrive with bias. For example, all therapists have their own reproductive experience. Some have been pregnant, some have not. Some have given birth, some have not. Some have experienced loss, fertility treatments, and medical trauma, others have become pregnant easily and experienced their births as fulfilling and empowering. Some have experienced postpartum depression; others find bliss in perinatal parenting. Some have a uterus, many do not. Therapists who seek mentorship or supervision with the goal of holding better realize that processing their reproductive experiences is essential to ensuring that the focus of therapy remains on the client.

Like our clients, we may want or need to process our reproductive journeys, but we recognize that this work should happen in our own therapy, supervision, and peer support spaces. We become conscious of how our reproductive experiences impact us, our work, and our perspectives and learn how to set our experiences aside so they do not burden our client's holding environment. When we lose sight of our biases, whether related to reproduction or to race, ethnicity, religion, or gender, we risk the integrity of the therapeutic relationship and the holding environment. We risk harming our clients. It is therefore imperative that we identify and address any biases that we bring to the therapeutic relationship that may interfere with the holding relationship. Not only within this chapter, but as an ongoing practice for the duration of our careers.

Unquestionably readers of this book will arrive at this chapter with a wide range of experience in diverse communities. Some may be well-versed in the pursuit of equity and practice of cultural humility and others may just be recognizing that they too hold implicit bias. Some may identify with one or multiple marginalized groups and others may be newly awakened to their privilege. Again, this chapter and the exercises ahead are not intended to offer comprehensive training, perspective, or instruction on cultural diversity, inclusion, or eliminating your implicit biases. You are asked to consider the following vignettes and reflective questions to gain awareness of how reactivity to diverse parents may present in your body and mind. Keep in mind that the cases discussed represent only a very few examples of the countless diverse and unique parents whom we as healthcare providers will encounter. You may notice a blind spot in these pages, but if you do not, continue to explore diversity within your local and broader community and try to notice how it feels to engage with someone who is different from you.

Noticing Your Internal Responses

In the pages that follow you will read about the experience of a BIPOC mom, a Jewish mom, an Asian mom, a transgender dad, and a cisgender couple in which the father is experiencing postnatal depression. Following each example is a series of questions for your reflection. Consider taking notes on your answers and discussing them with a supervisor, mentor, therapist, and/or professional peers.

Marianismo and the Superwoman

As explored extensively in this book, care for postpartum clients can only be as effective as the client's willingness to disclose and participate in the therapy process. Some cultural perspectives on motherhood can limit a woman's inclination to engage in therapy or to seek support at all. For example, the concept of *marianismo*, which highlights values traditionally associated with feminine ideals such as self-sacrifice, passivity, and silence, can leave Latina mothers feeling ashamed, isolated, and unsure about whether or how to seek help (Sampson et al., 2021). Similarly, many African American women are expected to uphold values assigned to the superwoman schema, a paradigm of behavior that requires emotional suppression, acts of strength, and refusal to display vulnerability (Nelson et al., 2023). Both cultural constructs can interfere with help seeking among members of these communities due to fears associated with failing at motherhood and failing to meet expectations (Nelson et al., 2023; Sampson et al., 2021).

These constructs do not exist within a vacuum, however; rather they are a product of a rich and complex heritage that has sustained great periods of joy and the agony of trauma. When we, the therapist, are an outsider to the complexity of these dynamics, we lack context and empathy. Nelson et al. point out in their 2023 discussion of the superwoman schema that new research shows that while this paradigm is problematic for many women, some African American women find empowerment and resilience in this schema. Therapists entering their relationships with African American mothers risk offending, alienating, or negatively reinforcing inappropriate or harmful stereotypes when they make assumptions about how an individual mother may feel about what is culturally expected or normative.

Two years after the birth of her second child Lena, an African American mom, presented for her first therapy session. Lena reported that she liked being a mother and felt bonded to her children – she described her children as "my everything." She reported feeling supported by her husband and a wide network of friends and family members. Lena was especially close to her sisters whom she felt were always willing to help with her kids when she needed some extra hands. Still, since the birth of her second baby, Lena experienced symptoms of postpartum depression and anxiety and passive suicidal thoughts. Lena shared her emotions with her husband and some of her close friends and sisters, all of whom encouraged Lena to seek help. However, Lena resisted seeking help for two years, a choice she made due to feeling "weak and like a disappointment."

Lena explained that she shares a very close relationship with her mother. Her mother had a difficult childhood and worked extremely hard to raise her five daughters in a stable environment. She considered her mom a role model and hoped to emulate her mom in her own parenting. Lena never viewed her mother as anything but resilient, strong, and unwavering and took to heart the memories she had of her grandmother who presented the same way. Lena stated "I want so badly to be strong like my mother and her mother, and I am sure my great grandmother too. I am raising a daughter and I want her to learn resilience and strength from me. But here I am, so weak, I am a burden and a failure. And if my mother ever found out I was here, I just don't know how I could live with that."

Holding Questions for Reflection:

1 What are expectations for women and/or mothers in your cultural context? What is your opinion of these expectations?
2 How do these expectations impact your individual expectations of women and/or mothers in your life? How do these expectations impact your expectations of yourself?
3 What feelings, emotionally and in your body, do you notice having in response to the paradigm of the marianismo and the superwoman schema?
4 What might you feel emotionally and somatically in response to a client expressing a strong desire to uphold these values in their own family system?
5 How might your feelings impact your ability to support this client in reaching their goal?

Brit Milah

In the Jewish tradition babies traditionally assigned male at birth are welcomed into the Jewish community with a *brit milah*. A *brit milah*, or a *bris*, is a ritual circumcision ceremony held on the eighth day of life. The bris may be held in a synagogue, the parents' home, or in any other setting the family chooses. In addition to the circumcision process itself, the ceremony includes readings, blessings, and often a first announcement of the baby's name. A *mohel* is a professional trained in the ritual of *brit milah* as well as best practices in modern medicine's approach to circumcision. This person may be a medical professional, a member of the clergy, or a full-time mohel. Despite receiving reassurance from family members their baby does not feel pain, that ritual circumcisions are safe, and that this event is a beautiful and meaningful part of the sacred Jewish lifecycle, some Jewish mothers report feeling nervous, scared, guilty, or obliged to participate in this ritual. Further complicating the experience for modern mothers is a growing interest in the ethics of circumcision, including within the Jewish community itself (Moss, 2023). There is no equivalent procedure to circumcision for babies assigned female at birth, though in modern times Jewish ceremonies (without this surgical component) have been developed to celebrate all births and welcome all Jewish children into the community, regardless of gender assignment.

Annie contacted The Postpartum Stress Center for therapy when her son was 3 months old. Joey was her first child, and she was overjoyed to be a mother. Annie's journey to motherhood was complicated, involving a series of early pregnancy losses and two rounds of IVF. She experienced symptoms of depression and anxiety during this time but found comfort in her Jewish community. She participated in support groups for Jewish mothers navigating infertility, was the recipient of weekly prayers at her synagogue, and discovered that participating in a Jewish meditation class brought both comfort and hope. When Annie arrived for her intake session she reported, "I really don't have any symptoms of postpartum depression or anything like that. I feel like a good mom, I am happy, and I'm excited about Joey and our family. But I think every day about his bris and how horrible I felt on that day. I chose the mohel and he walked me step by step through the entire ceremony. I thought I was prepared and I thought I wanted this for our family. But when I watched my baby being held down, naked and crying, I did not feel the spiritual fulfillment I thought I would. I was excited about the bris; I wanted my baby to share the experience of his dad and his ancestors. I knew it might be emotional for me, I've been to a thousand other ceremonies for friends' babies, cousins, nephews. But when it was Joey's turn, I felt in that moment like a bad mom, an abusive mom. So now I'm struggling with all this guilt, guilt about what I put Joey through, guilt about feeling betrayed by this ritual, and guilt about regretting that we chose this for our son."

Holding Questions for Reflection:

1 What did you feel emotionally and in your body when you read Annie's story? What words did Annie use that were most impactful?
2 What are your opinions on circumcision, ritual circumcision, or Jewish tradition?
3 What have you been taught by your own community about these practices?
4 Have you needed to make similar choices for your own body or for your children?
5 How might your feelings about this ritual impact your ability to support a client like Annie? How might your feelings or opinions impact your choice of intervention or treatment goals?

La Cuarentena and Sitting the Month

Many cultures around the world expect postpartum mothers to participate in rest and healing focused practices that involve prescribed amounts of rest, dietary restrictions, and socialization habits. In Hispanic and Latino communities this practice is often called *la cuarentena*. Cuarentena occurs over a 40-day period during which new mothers abstain from eating certain foods and participating in certain activities. New mothers are instructed to rest, focus on their baby, and practice breastfeeding. Their bodies are viewed as "open" and la cuarentena provides the body an opportunity to close (Waugh, 2011). In some Asian cultures postpartum women are expected to participate in "sitting the month" or "doing the month." Like women participating in cuarentena, mothers who are sitting the month spend an extended period, in this case 30 days, eating specific foods, abstaining from certain activities, and participating in traditional Asian practices for self and infant care. Support for new mothers in both cultures is typically provided by other females in the community. This may include the new mother's own mother, sisters, female cousins, and elders. This may also include the women of the new mother's in-law family and other female members of the community. On one hand, mothers who experience a period of prescribed rest articulate the value of taking this time to engage in self-care and to experience feeling cared for by loved ones. On the other hand, the high expectations for the new mothers' compliance as well as conflict between the new mother and those caring for her can be a cause of distress and increase likelihood of developing risk factors for postpartum depression and anxiety (Zheng et al., 2019).

Kathy presented for therapy while pregnant with her second child. Her eldest child, a four-year-old daughter, Emme, was born in New York City. Kathy's parents immigrated from China when she was a young child. They maintain many of their traditions and Kathy enjoys participating and sharing them with her Caucasian American husband and their daughter. When Kathy gave birth to Emme her mother came to care for them both during the period of "sitting the month." Kathy described her relationship with her mother as close and reported that they often bonded over their shared love of their Chinese traditions and sharing these traditions with Kathy's growing family. For this reason, it was especially hard for Kathy to admit to her mother that sitting the month was not enjoyable or fulfilling for her. She felt cooped up in her home, longed to take a shower, and desperately wanted to eat take out from her favorite restaurants. She felt envious of her friends and especially of her sister-in-law who had a baby at a similar time. She watched as her sister-in-law took her newborn for walks, drank milkshakes, and enjoyed friends coming to visit. Kathy sought out therapy while pregnant a second time with the goal of working through her feelings about sitting the month a second time and her ambivalence about whether she wished to have this experience again.

Holding Questions for Reflection:

1 What did you feel emotionally and in your body when you read Kathy's story? What parts of Kathy's story were most impactful for you?
2 What are your opinions on rest, diet, and socialization during the postpartum period?
3 What have you been taught by your own community about rest during the postpartum period?
4 Have you experienced feeling in need of support from your community? Have you received this support for yourself? If so, what was that like for you? If not, how did that feel?
5 How might your experience of needing or wanting support impact your ability to support a client like Kathy? How might your feelings or opinions impact your choice of intervention or treatment goals?

Gender Expansive Parents

Many transgender and gender non-conforming people wish to maintain the option to give birth to their own children if they are physically able, regardless of their gender identities and expression. As an increasing number of gender expansive birthing parents present in the delivery room, the need for reproductive healthcare providers to develop sensitive, equitable, and non-discriminatory practices is increasingly urgent. In addition to experiencing the same perinatal challenges as cisgender parents, gender expansive parents are confronted with a variety of additional nuanced challenges. The trans and nonbinary community is incredibly diverse within itself, with birthing parents presenting at different stages of their gender transition processes, both biologically and emotionally. Gender dysphoria, or distress related to incongruent gender identity and sex assigned at birth, may be exacerbated or complicated by pregnancy, even when the pregnant person desired to become pregnant and give birth (Besse et al., 2020). Pezaro et al. (2023) describe transphobia among birthing professionals, trepidation due to fear of offending a patient by using incorrect terminology, and concern about birthing training and care that is cis-heteronormative. Furthermore, not all providers caring for trans parents are educated in the needs of chestfeeding parents (MacDonald et al., 2016). At the most basic level, each of these studies mention the importance of developing trust, which is understandably difficult to establish with members of a community so frequently facing misapprehension and discrimination, including in healthcare settings.

Prior to his appointment Bryan asked if our offices were baby friendly. Of course, we told him, babies are welcome to bottle, breast, and chest feed and you are welcome to bring a pump. Whatever meets your needs. Bryan expressed his gratitude and arrived for his session the next day. Our practice intake paperwork has been amended to ensure that gender expansive parents can share any information they wish about their gender identity prior to their session and to convey our acceptance of gender expansive parents. Bryan disclosed on his intake paperwork that he is a trans male, uses he/him pronouns, and will be called "dad" by his partner and their baby. Despite working hard to offer a safe environment for all parents, it remains unusual for a chestfeeding dad to arrive in our waiting room. His therapist greeted him and met his 4-month-old baby, Riley, and invited them back into the therapy space. Like so many new parents Bryan asked again in the therapy room whether it would be okay to feed Riley and, again, his therapist answered, "yes, of course." Bryan settled in, latched Riley, glanced up at the therapist and asked, "how many breastfeeding dads have sat here in this chair?"

Holding Questions for Reflection:

1 What did you feel emotionally and in your body when you read Bryan's story? What did you feel in response to Bryan's question?
2 How might you have answered Bryan's question? What feelings do you notice having emotionally and somatically when you consider responding?
3 What are your opinions on chestfeeding and gender expansive birthing parents?

4 What have you been taught by your own community about gender expansive birth?
5 How might your experience, or lack thereof, with gender expansive individuals impact your ability to support a client like Bryan? How might your feelings or opinions impact your choice of intervention or treatment goals?

Non-Gestational Parents

Historically postpartum depression and anxiety were attributed to the hormonal impact of giving birth. We now recognize that this is only one of many factors that influence a new parent's mental health during the early days, weeks, and months of parenthood. Non-gestational parents, or parents who do not carry and give birth themselves, include fathers, adoptive parents, parents who bring a child into the world via a surrogate or gestational carrier, and non-birthing partners. Many non-gestational parents experience mood and anxiety disorders after the birth of a child and increasingly non-gestational parents are seeking help and support for these symptoms. One feature of depression and anxiety symptoms experienced by non-gestational parents is a feeling of surprise that despite not having given birth and experiencing the related hormonal shifts, they too can experience postpartum emotional symptoms. Parents and members of their support systems may overlook the significance of the psychosocial adjustment to parenthood and may devalue the biological relevance of factors that impact all new parents, not only those who have given birth, such as sleep deprivation. Like birthing parents, non-gestational parents are still confronted with the emotional and practical challenges of becoming a parent including learning how to care for an infant, coping with new stressors within the family system, confronting a never-ending list of new anxieties, isolation, identity loss, and role confusion. Moreover, non-gestational parents, such as adoptive parents, may need to reconcile feelings about having depressive symptoms after finally bringing home a badly longed for baby (Foli et al., 2016). They too need the support and rallying of their community.

Lisa and Evan requested couples counseling at The Postpartum Stress Center. Lisa gave birth to their son Henry 8 months earlier. During her first few postpartum months Lisa received therapy for symptoms of postpartum anxiety. She had a difficult physical recovery from a very difficult and prolonged birth and said that by this point she is finally feeling more like herself. Lisa talked about the hardships she endured and expressed her gratitude for Evan's support during her physical and emotional recovery. Evan talked about the awe he felt when Henry was born and described Lisa as "the strongest person I have ever known." Evan admitted that over the past few months, however, he has been feeling angry, resentful, and depressed much of the time. Evan reported that he loves both Lisa and Henry but often feels like he is in the way. He describes Lisa's life as "full" and envies her growing circle of mom friends and awareness of activities Henry loves. Evan acknowledges that he is experiencing symptoms of depression and describes feelings of guilt and shame associated with failing to be a better partner to Lisa during this time. Lisa expresses empathy and compassion for Evan, but also acknowledges her own resentment at his bad moods, impatience, and low tolerance for some of Henry's normal behaviors. Lisa stated, "I spent all of this time recovering from such a horrible birth and terrible and scary postpartum anxiety. Evan was so supportive, and I want to support him now, but I feel so angry that he seems miserable all the time. I understand that he is depressed, and I know he loves us, but I am sick of feeling like I am doing everything for our life and everything for Henry because Evan just has no patience for him."

Holding Questions for Reflection:

1 What did you feel emotionally and in your body when you read Evan's story? What did you feel in response to Lisa's description of her feelings?
2 How do you feel about parents who have not given birth experiencing symptoms of depression or anxiety after welcoming a baby?
3 What is your comfort level witnessing and holding space for emotionally expressive men and fathers?
4 What have you been taught by your own community about the needs of new parents? What have you been taught about gender norms and emotional expression?
5 How might your experience as a birthing or non-birthing person impact your ability to support a couple like Lisa and Evan? How might your feelings or opinions impact your choice of intervention or treatment goals?

Holding While Addressing Personal Bias

Take some time to review your reflections. Take note of the feelings, sensations in your body, and beliefs you noticed while reading the last few pages. Were you honest with yourself? Did you allow yourself to admit to any discomfort you might have felt? Maybe you noticed feelings that were not resistant or negative; did you recognize an exciting pull to help or a fascination in response to one of these patients? If that happened to you, did you ask yourself whether you are feeling inappropriately captivated by something or someone you perceive as exotic? Was your excitement in some way self-interested? These are a few of the many questions we need to ask ourselves as part of our self-awareness practice, a key component of becoming a competent holding therapist.

Our work needs to be culturally informed, so we can be sensitive to ways in which cultural norms and values influence each client's story and script. Cultural context cannot be ignored in the practice of psychotherapy, and we must each be responsible for expanding our awareness and knowledge. Ask your clients about their identities and cultural backgrounds and seek additional training and supervision in the areas that are unfamiliar to you. While we cannot possibly know each nuance intrinsic to each diverse group, we can rely on the expert point, carry ourselves with confidence, and ask questions like:

- Can you describe how some of your behaviors or symptoms are perceived and understood by members of your family and community?
- What do you think I need to know to better understand your background or cultural context?
- Have you experienced frustration expressing what you need, either in here with me or with others?
- Are there differences that you notice between the two of us that make it hard for you to feel comfortable here with me?

If appropriate, follow up with a statement of gratitude for what your client has shared and reassurance that you will seek out more information to learn more about the issues they raised before their next session. Apprehension about being politically correct or carelessly offending your client may make you hesitate, but it behooves you to ask direct questions when you need clarification. While use of the holding points and consideration of the holding fundamentals can still work to invite diverse patients into your holding space, it is the work presented in this chapter that will help keep this space safe and free from judgment.

Chapter 14

Clinical Challenges and FAQs

Patricia hung up the phone in our office and looked at me, raising her eyebrows and pursing her lips. I couldn't help but notice her dissatisfaction with the outcome of the phone call. Patricia had worked at The Postpartum Stress Center for a while and discovered that it doesn't get easier when you feel that your attempts to engage a new caller are disregarded or misunderstood.

"Hard-to-hold?" I asked her.
"Yep. Really hard."
"What happened?"
"I don't know, actually. I was explaining how things work here in response to her many questions, you know, can I bring my baby, should my husband come, what if I need medication, how long do you think I will feel this bad, you know, like that. She seemed to want all that information. She kept asking me questions and I kept answering. She was anxious and I thought the information would help her feel more at ease with our first appointment. Then she sort of drifted off, like she wasn't interested or what I was saying wasn't helpful. I shifted my focus and asked her if this was too much information, and she said, no, I'm just not sure about making an appointment right now. I'll call you back."

Patricia grimaced again, revealing her frustration. It is hard when you extend yourself in the direction you think the caller wants or is asking for and then either you were mistaken about that perception or she pivots in another direction. Knowing what we know about the ambivalence, shame, and tentativeness surrounding this difficult first phone call, we try hard to zero in on those fine distinctions between desperately wanting our help and not.

DOI: 10.4324/9781003402145-14

"So what do you think? Was this about her? Was this about you? What happened here?"

I have high expectations of the therapists who work with me. It can be an occupational asset and hazard, which keeps me in tune, in touch, and acutely critical. Sometimes that's a good thing. Other times, not so much.

"Good question. It was probably a little of both of us," Patricia responded.

"How so?"

"Well, I mean, she wanted answers, so I offered them. Right?"

"Maybe."

This is when some therapists start to take on the burden and responsibility of a phone call or session gone astray. When pressed to scrutinize the trajectory of the exchange, anything less than an optimal outcome might generate feelings of inadequacy in the therapist.

But it shouldn't.

There are always other choices you can make and other pathways you can take; even so, it may not be the one that particular woman wants, needs, expects, or can handle. You might be off course for her, but that doesn't make it wrong. Sometimes, in fact, you may be very right, and it doesn't feel right to her, for any number of reasons.

"Do you think I should not have answered all of her questions?"

"I'm not sure, Patricia. It's true that sometimes information can ease anxiety. It is also true that too many questions with too many answers can agitate a restless brain. So, we cannot be sure. The only way to assess that is to feel how it is going and to monitor her response and stay attuned and if in doubt, pause."

Anytime you discount the usefulness of an exchange or intervention, you introduce an object of inspection that needs to be followed up with before moving forward. Most likely, you are responding to a signal the client has put out there, but it could just as easily originate from you. Either way, the doubt factor is a call to attention and recalibration is in order. Doubt in this context is not a negative reference. Your awareness of even the slightest disconnect will initiate a hesitation that can make the difference between successful holding or not. This split-second pause will enable you to process a critical instant in this early contact.

"I think it was fine," Patricia continued to assess. "As soon as I noticed I was losing her attention, I asked if this was too many questions and I told her we could address all of her concerns when she came in. I think that made her nervous, if you know what I mean. Just when I thought I was saying something to help her feel better, I made it worse?"

"No, I don't think you made it worse. She might have responded the same way no matter what you said. It's hard to know exactly how our words will be heard by any single caller, especially if we have no prior relationship with her. Often it's a crap shoot, no matter how carefully we pick our words and how gently we try to guide her."

That notion can be both reassuring and exasperating to the postpartum therapist who is focused on holding a new postpartum caller.

Protect Her Wisely

This scenario shows how tenuous this work can be and illustrates another distinguishing feature of the postpartum population. You need to be forever mindful of the possible ways your words, your actions, or your feelings may affect her. What you say or do may immediately calm her. Or it may impinge upon her fragile emotional state. Again, you are obliged to make sure she is grounded, check her current state, maintain the expert stance, consider your plan, stay present with her, and keep her feeling safe at all times.

Any postpartum intake, assessment, first contact, or subsequent session can entail an explosive combination of her palpable discomfort, her inner turmoil, and your high-priority attempt to hold. As a compassionate person, you might wonder how to respond therapeutically to the surges of emotion that may occur at any point in time. Balancing the feelings you have toward what you are hearing with what is best for her is a challenge that you must tend to at any given moment. One of your most crucial tasks is to assess with rapid and spot-on discernment.

Because, what if you are wrong?

What if your immediate interpretation of her narrative is off course or spun in a direction that is poised to better meet your needs than hers? If suffering is subjective, how do you appraise whether it is too much? What if you reach a conclusion that is not accurate or reflects your level of arousal rather than her experience?

Self-awareness is key. It is your ultimate professional tool. It does not come without a price, and the burden associated with heightened self-awareness can emerge as anxiety, self-doubt, compassion fatigue, and burnout, which will be discussed subsequently. For now, regard your self-awareness as your compass. You should trust the signals you receive but proceed with careful consideration of all unknown possibilities.

There is a classic mindfulness exercise, courtesy of Jimmy Harmon (although I confess that an exhaustive search failed to find a reputable citation). A psychology teacher was presenting stress management strategies to her students. She raised a glass of water and asked, "How heavy is this glass of water?"

Answers called out ranged from 8 oz to 20 oz.

She replied, "The absolute weight doesn't matter. It depends on how long I hold it. If I hold it for a minute, it's not a problem. If I hold it for an hour, I'll have an ache in my arm. If I hold it for a day, my arm will feel numb and paralyzed. In each case, the weight of the glass doesn't change, but the longer I hold it, the heavier it becomes."

She continues, "The stresses and worries in life are like that glass of water. Think about them for a while and nothing happens. Think about them a bit longer and they begin to hurt. And if you think about them all day long, you will feel paralyzed – incapable of doing anything."

Remember to put the glass down, we are reminded by this story.

At first glance, this analogy works well for many of our clients who are walking around carrying too many worries, too many obligations, too many tasks. Giving them permission to prioritize, let some things go, and take better care of their own needs is a prerogative of our therapeutic authority. It is a premiere holding task.

Let's spin this story from the perspective of the holding therapist. Imagine each of your postpartum clients holding this metaphorical glass of water. Now imagine that this glass of water contains the sustenance your client needs. If you hold it in the palm of your hand reaching out toward your thirsty client with intent to offer it, you can only do that for so long. It appears like a giving gesture, but soon, if she doesn't accept it, you will tire. As your arm becomes heavy, you will lose concentration and either the contents will spill or you will become more focused on what you are doing than on how she is experiencing it.

The mistake many new perinatal therapists make is offering the glass of water too soon, too abruptly, too insistently, or too vehemently. The postpartum client feels too parched to realize that water will even help. Dehydration feels like a permanent state of being. The holding power does not only refer to how to best meet her needs. It also refers to knowing how to hold your magic, how to hold the power of the therapeutic relationship, how to hold the water. Imagine this: take the glass into both hands to secure it; rest it on your lap. Got that image? Hold it gently in place. It will not spill. It will not weigh you down. It will rest comfortably until she is ready. In the meantime, you do your work. And you just hold the glass. You don't need to show her. You do not need to offer it. You know it is there (*I have what you need*). She will know, too.

Frequently Asked Questions: Clinical Challenges

The following pages address =common questions asked during trainings, mentoring, team meetings, and supervision sessions. Although each question deserves considerably more attention than this book allows, each brief review should guide you in the right direction if you are faced with any of these clinical challenges:

- Is holding different with male clients who are depressed?
- Is it possible to hold virtually via telehealth?
- How do you hold a mom who endured an unimaginable loss?
- How do you hold when she has limited resources?
- How do you hold when her emotions run high and push your buttons?
- Do male therapists hold differently?
- How do you hold if conflicting feelings are aroused?
- How do you hold when her partner may be sabotaging?

1 Is Holding Different with Male Clients Who Are Depressed?

Up to one in ten fathers fit diagnostic criteria for major depression during the first year of fatherhood (Scarff, 2019). Interestingly, but perhaps unsurprisingly, having a wife who has been diagnosed with postpartum depression is a risk factor for the development of postnatal depression in fathers (Eddy et al., 2019). Despite the high prevalence of paternal depression and recognition that, like maternal depression, depression in fathers can significantly impact both the individual and the entire family system, paternal postnatal depression remains highly stigmatized, often misunderstood, and poorly recognized (Guillemette et al., 2023). However, men are four times more likely than women to die by suicide (CDC Vital Statistics, 2023) and also more likely to engage in substance abuse (NIDA, 2022). The need for intervention and treatment is urgent.

Hesitation, or even unwillingness, among men to seek mental healthcare is well known and researched. Traditional gender roles and beliefs about masculinity and male behavior in particular are often factors inhibiting help seeking in men with depressive disorders (Eggenberger et al., 2023). Research shows that facilitating peer support between men, increasing male exposure to positive, gender sensitive messaging about mental healthcare, and highlighting ways help seeking builds upon strengths can improve male openness to engaging in therapy (McKenzie et al., 2022). The development of gender informed treatment approaches for the treatment of depression in men also shows promising results (Eggenberger et al., 2023). Still, best practices for treatment of depression in men, particularly those with a strong attachment to conventional masculine expectations, remain underdeveloped and non-existent in the specific niche of postnatal male depression.

The therapeutic alliance is paramount in therapy, regardless of patient gender. The process for developing a therapeutic relationship, however, is unique and varies based on each individual's needs, lived experiences, and world views. Holding a male client in distress is therefore fundamentally the same. We use our holding points to gain access to his specific needs and to learn how best to help him remain engaged and present.

At this time in our society, fathers are increasingly encouraged to become more involved than ever in childcare, childrearing, and in experiencing new parenthood. It is unsurprising that many therapists share that they are seeing more and more fathers in their practices who are struggling with identity and adjustment.

For example, Jason said he and his wife agreed that he would stay home because her business was self-owned and quite successful. Jason felt "ready to work less" in the office since becoming a father and could freelance out of their home. All went smoothly until Jason noticed he was feeling more irritable and short of patience on a regular basis. He said he expected it "to be hard" but didn't feel prepared for how "empty" it would feel "just being a dad." He stated he felt unproductive and unimportant. The longer he went dismissing his emotions, the more entrenched the feelings became. Symptoms of depression brought him to The Postpartum Stress Center.

Jason's therapist responded to his distress through the lens of a holding framework:

- Initially, it was important to **ground** Jason by acknowledging the importance of his presence in the therapy space. His therapist affirmed that his decision to come to therapy is the best thing he can do right now for himself and for his partner and new baby, and shared that he is one of many fathers who have found relief from symptoms at the center. This way, Jason's therapist validated any discomfort he was experiencing and reassured him that he is not alone in this experience. He stated this was encouraging to hear and he proceeded to tell his story by recounting the life events that have led to this point of distress.
- Like all therapists, Jason's therapist attended to his current state and presenting symptoms. Jason's therapist however listened carefully to how Jason's distress may be related to his experience of becoming a new father. When asked about the quality of his sleep and separately about how his baby's sleep and his wife's sleep were impacting his, Jason responded "you're right, my sleep is so affected by theirs, I never really thought of that until now."
- As an **expert**, it is important to convey your confidence in holding his emotional vulnerability by tolerating his distress with unconditional acceptance. Many therapists remark that the male expression of emotions can be particularly provocative and strangely captivating. This may be the result of our culture's constraint on male expressiveness or any particular therapist's limited exposure to or bias around it. Regardless, holding dictates that we become comfortable with and

unaffected by sitting with strong emotions experienced and expressed by a male client. In supervision after Jason's intake, his therapist noted feeling overwhelmed by his exposure of emotions at first, but quickly was able to recognize this personal distress and take a few breaths to remain centered. Jason expressed feeling slightly self-conscious. In response, his therapist normalized this feeling and shared some psycho-education to increase his comfort. Jason was surprised to hear that 10% of new dads experience depression after the birth of their baby and that expressing emotions and vulnerability is extremely helpful toward recovery. This feedback helped Jason feel that he was in the right place.

- The **design** for Jason's treatment was clear, practical, and sincere, accounting for Jason's preferences. Jason stated he preferred a goal-oriented, time-limited program of intervention which would enable him to follow up and achieve his desired result. Jason, like many, admitted he avoids asking for help and tends to depend on self-reliance. These factors should be considered in working with Jason.
- Remaining **present** helped Jason connect to the therapeutic process. Take extraordinary care to examine any biases you carry related to males' participation in therapy. If you over sympathize or stereotype, he may feel patronized. If you miss the intensity of his pain because he is minimizing it and you fail to recognize this mask, he may mistrust your expertise. If you prematurely validate his suffering without connecting with him personally, he may retreat. Jason's therapist conveyed responsivity, authenticity, and neutrality from the start which helped Jason feel comfortable.
- The best way to **safeguard** a dad who is depressed is to confidently state how important, albeit difficult, this decision to seek support is and that his doing so will help him get symptom relief sooner rather than later. Jason's therapist spent some time in each session exploring what Jason found helpful and what might not be working. This enabled his therapist to engage him in the process and to track his progress. Jason later shared that this was encouraging for him and motivated him to attend sessions even when he felt reluctant or like his sessions might not be helping.

Fathers are often underappreciated and underrecognized during the post-partum period, whether they are depressed or not. The majority of consideration is given to mothers during this time, although we have seen that this is lacking, also. Given that social support is well established as a protective factor against perinatal distress (Biaggi et al., 2016), our attention needs to be placed on how the couple has been affected, regardless of the object of our therapeutic focus at the moment.

Thus, our objective in supporting fathers is two-fold. First and foremost, we want to identify and sufficiently treat any mental health vulnerability or symptom in order to provide relief. Secondly, our goal is to help them return to their previous level of functioning to position them as a reliable source of support for mom and to fortify the well-being of the entire family. Supporting fathers, whether they are the client or the partner of a client, is essential, and fosters a more inclusive and empathetic environment for fathers to feel encouraged and included during this challenging time.

It is noteworthy that there is a push toward a couple-focused treatment approach, recognizing the impact of both maternal and paternal depression (Pilkington et al., 2016). Even if couple-focused treatment is not desired, it is always prudent to check in on the mental health of a partner in order to have a comprehensive understanding of the total picture and all variables impacting the family.

2 Is It Possible to Hold Virtually?

With exploding technology, this question is increasingly relevant as psychological support services become more digitalized and clients express a desire for remote therapy options. After COVID-19 accelerated the shift toward telehealth, virtual psychotherapy came into view as the next best thing in therapeutic support. Or better, some would say.

It probably won't surprise readers that I am not a great fan of virtual therapy. Like any alternative treatment option, if it works, then it's wonderful. I support that. It is not something I am completely comfortable with for my own work because, as noted previously, I rely heavily on in-person, real-time energy. That being said, as we all continue to adapt to the seismic demands on our professional flexibility and commitment to this work, many of us have found virtual therapy to be surprisingly successful. My early resistance morphed into compliance, and eventually acceptance of a process that began to take on a life of its own.

Since even before the pandemic, telehealth has been shown to be effective and increases access to care and can improve service delivery (Hilty et al., 2013; Smith et al., 2011). Some therapists also use additional electronic means, such as phone calls, text messages, and/or emails to provide therapeutic interventions. It has been shown that during COVID-19, people in psychological distress increasingly used these forms of support when seeking help. It has been suggested that some of the support for this increase includes the improved accessibility, affordability, and the general acceptance of psychotherapy being offered by way of online formats (Joshi, 2020).

The Upside

On the plus side, there are good reasons to engage with technology for perinatal support:

- Perhaps the most notable benefit to virtual therapy is the increase in access for people in rural areas, people who are geographically isolated, or anyone who has difficulty attending in person. This advantage is huge and enormously relevant when considering our ongoing effort to support as many perinatal women in distress as possible.
- Scheduling and logistical steps are more convenient and may be accompanied by less anxiety or stigma.
- People with anxiety, particularly social anxiety, may be more likely to reach out to an online therapist.
- Lack of a physical waiting room can feel more private and less stigmatizing.
- Less need for childcare arrangements.

The Downside

There are some pitfalls to virtual sessions, particularly through a holding lens:

- Technological constraints and internet connection failures are unpredictable, creating session flow interruptions, sometimes at very vulnerable moments.
- Virtual therapy may not be ideal for certain diagnoses such as suicidal intent or psychosis. While not impossible, it does warrant meticulous attention and care.
- Connecting online can feel awkward to some people and takes getting used to. Be straightforward in your effort to check out your client's comfort level as part of the process. After a while, you and your client find a flow that works for both of you.
- Lack of ability to perceive body language or micro-expressions can hinder assessment. Eye contact is tricky, distractions are abundant, and concentration can be fickle, depending on the environment and focus of the client and the provider.
- Perceptions may be distorted. Poor lighting and other environmental conditions may misrepresent the surroundings that could lead to misinterpretations, such as, *Is she pale and not feeling well?*
- Distractions could interfere with boundaries, concentration, and efficacy.
- Ever changing technologies raise potential ethical issues related to privacy and confidentiality.
- Crisis intervention is more challenging when working online.

Regardless of whether therapy is provided through telehealth or in person, given the value attributed to the therapeutic relationship as a predictor of treatment responses (Tryon et al., 2018), it is prudent to evaluate whether or not the client is comfortable with the mode of therapy. This seems like a prerequisite for proceeding with therapy.

3 How Do You Hold a Mom Who Has Endured an Unimaginable Loss?

When immersed in this work, you quickly learn how important it is to accommodate the high levels of grief and pain inherent within this population. Intense suffering is intimidating for the unskilled, including for therapists unfamiliar with, or perhaps too personally familiar with, bereavement. For many therapists, holding a woman who has lost a pregnancy or infant is especially painful. This is partly due to the immeasurable sorrow, partly because it is so hard to heal, and partly because it represents a level of bereavement that one cannot fathom. Unless you have experienced a similar loss, and then your job is appreciably more complicated.

When a woman suffers a reproductive loss, her excruciating grief is normal and going to therapy does not always make sense to her. A therapist cannot bring back her baby. As we have discussed, the tenets of holding apply regardless of diagnosis, complexity, and circumstance. When holding a client with a clinical diagnosis, however, our design will feature the integration of tools to encourage symptom relief. In contrast, new mothers experiencing grief following a reproductive loss often express frustration with pressure they feel to heal. Many grieving mothers will describe the well-meaning attempts of others to help them "feel better," "move on," or "find joy." What is the same about holding grieving mothers is that your holding environment may be the one place where she can express her emotions fully. What is different about holding grieving mothers is that you must take care not to convey any feelings of your own urgency for her to feel better.

It can help if you collect some information about reproductive loss in general as well as her specific loss prior to your meeting. Are you familiar with the causes and consequences of various reproductive crises, such as ectopic pregnancy, neonatal death, termination of a wanted baby, miscarriage, stillbirth, and abortion? Do you have a basic knowledge about sudden infant death syndrome and sudden unexplained death in childhood? Are you informed of some of the genetic anomalies that may be relevant to her loss or the resources she may benefit from such as specific diagnosis-related support groups? Be informed. Do your homework. Review the nature of her loss so you are familiar with some of the terms she may use. It is fine to let her know you are not an expert in this or perhaps this is the first time you have learned of this particular genetic disorder, for example. Still, you may decide to read up on it so you can discuss some of the details with her, especially if she has some difficult decisions to make.

The following is a review of the holding points as they relate to a perinatal loss:

- **Ground** her by validating her grief. Let her feel what she needs to feel. Each and every bit of it.
- Identify her **current state** as a normal bereavement condition, along with any difficult emotions that accompany it. Differentiate this from any present or developing pathology.
- Secure your position as **expert** by demonstrating your ability to hold her level of suffering. There is a very fine line between showing her how much you care and showing her how much it hurts. Be mindful of this. When suffering is acute and hard for you to sit with, there may be times when you may experience strong urgency for the pain to resolve. It can be tempting to move toward use of misattuned reassurance ("good things will come again"), platitudes ("everything happens for a reason"), and well intentioned directives ("let's talk about the good times"). Remember that it is vital for you as a holding therapist to have the courage to sit with and hold space for immense pain. Resisting the urge to console her by offering surface-level sympathy is key to holding in this circumstance. Most of the time, *I'm sorry* is a powerful and poignant compassionate statement, while you fortify your holding response. It may be difficult when you are distracted by the strong emotions you are feeling. So breathe, stay focused on her, and rely on your own supervisors or therapists to hold your distress outside of your client's session.
- Augment the **design** for treatment by gathering any information you need to accompany her through this intricate journey from despair to acceptance. Evaluate your own ability to proceed as you carry the weight of this much pain.
- Stay **present** with the grief by attending to her story with compassion and awareness of how this is affecting her. Make sure she feels safe enough to say what she needs to say. Specifics of her experience may or may not be pertinent to her healing at any given moment, but she will likely feel less burdened if she feels safe to disclose her darkest thoughts and fears as well as the most incidental details. Details have a subtle way of haunting the healing process so encouraging her to verbalize them may ease any guilt or shame.
- **Safeguard** her by assessing her current level of support. Lack of perceived social support is a known risk factor for prolonged grief disorder (Mason et al., 2020). Reactions to loss are deeply personal and vary from woman to woman. Often, we see temporary impairment of

day-to-day functioning, withdrawal from social activities, intrusive thoughts, and numbness, all of which can persist for varying lengths of time. These are natural and normal responses to loss. Therapists who are in a position to support bereaved parents should be on the lookout for prolonged, pervasive symptoms that significantly disturb functioning. If those symptoms set in, the client should be evaluated for prolonged grief disorder, which can have a substantial psychological impact on the family.

If you are seeing a grieving couple together, you may find yourself face to face with two people who grieve differently and may each require an individualized method of holding concurrently. The best way to tackle this disparity is to put words to it and share your observation with the couple. They will be relieved to learn that neither of them is more right or more wrong than the other, and your identification and support of this will provide a small amount of comfort for their aching hearts.

There is no template for grief. At times grieving parents surrender instinctively to their own unchecked, unrestrained impulse to withdraw from the world and at other times they may scream with outrage to the universe. The best way to support them is to sit there and let them feel what they feel and say what they need to say. That enables you to hold them, together and independently, as a couple. Do not underestimate your ability to do that and do that well. Most friends and family cannot, understandably, endure that level of sorrowfulness for extended periods. It can take your breath away. Listen to each of them. Support each of them equally. Unless their grief response is detrimental to the family dynamics or the well-being of the relationship, each should be honored and allowed to run its course. Accompanying them through the pounding pain of life's most cruel loss can be the most heartbreaking hold you are asked to perform.

The weight of profound physical and psychological loss and trauma can produce an ache that saturates the space between you and your client no matter how hard we try to maintain our professional presence. This rouses the most poignant irony: we must be sensitive souls to master our craft and we must be able to remain objective and detached. Regardless, we are destined to be forever touched and changed.

It is worthwhile here to mention that despite the enormous differences between working with parents experiencing uncomplicated bereavement and those with symptoms of PTSD, working with parents who have been diagnosed with PTSD can be similarly difficult for a therapist to hold. The stories of clients who have survived reproductive trauma can be highly distressing for therapists to hear. This is especially true for therapists who have experienced a perinatally related trauma themselves. Therapists supporting parents who have experienced trauma must convey unwavering presence and tolerate extraordinary levels of suffering. In addition to applying principles of holding to hold yourself (a concept further explored in the Epilogue), all therapists are encouraged to seek strong support for themselves personally and professionally.

4 How Do You Hold When She Has Limited Resources?

I am reminded of a woman who had given birth to her fifth child, the father of her baby worked the night shift for minimum wage, and she was estranged from her extended family. She struggled to access transportation and childcare that would enable her to come to her sessions (at this time telehealth was unavailable). She had a history of significant mental illness in her family, had no medical insurance, her phone had been disconnected due to a delinquent account, and she often wasn't sure how she would get through the next day. Her new baby had some gastrointestinal issues that forced them back and forth to the pediatrician. It was recommended that she see a specialist but she knew that was not going to happen due to extraordinary cost. Her only close friend was in rehab for long-term substance abuse.

In cases when resources are inadequate, sometimes severely so, that level of overwhelm can infiltrate your holding environment, instantly making you feel beset by more questions than answers. *How do I fix this? What can I possibly do to help? What resources are out there? Who can I consult with to get more information on what's available for her? Am I the best person to help her when my own knowledge of resources is so incomplete?* These initial restless queries that rush into your head are likely followed by others: *Is she depressed or is this an appropriate response to the situation? Can we even consider therapy if she is currently deprived of fundamental support and any assets that could assist her? Should we be offering crisis or practical intervention options and postpone further assessment at this time?* She needs money, childcare, help with her house, transportation. She is isolated and exhausted. *Does she need a case manager instead of a therapist? Should I be the one providing the case managing?*

Each therapist will respond to this heightened request for urgent support from her own set of experiences and information. And it goes without saying that each individual case will provoke different responses for different reasons. The bottom line is that it would behoove you to familiarize yourself with local free or low-cost resources so they are at your fingertips. Keep handy a list of options such as church, synagogue, or community groups that have programs focusing on maternal support. Seek out websites that offer subsidized childcare or babysitting swapping. Google financial assistance programs. How much of this work should *you* be doing on her behalf? As much as you are comfortable doing to launch her into a more stable state. You can, when feasible, do some of this together. Asking her to do one more thing may feel impossible for her. Doing it together can empower her and hold her at the same time. It is perfectly okay to make some phone calls on her behalf if that is what you are inclined to do. Ask her first, join her, and explore resources together.

You might have to think outside the box while searching what is available. One of my clients told me about her local yoga studio, which offered free babysitting one night a week for moms of new babies. Or, if telehealth is not an option, you might agree to her other three children accompanying her to the office and set them up in a spot where they can be safely supervised or otherwise engaged while you and mom talk.

In cases where access to resources is severely restricted, most therapists will be reminded of what attracted them to this work in the first place: the desire to help others work through life's challenges. In these most challenging cases, we might compress all holding points into one action taken or a decision to make a phone call together. For example: How *do* you get her to the office when she cannot get herself there? Explore options with her: public transportation, friends, virtual sessions, referral to a closer facility. These rapid actions that feel more like case-management coordination than therapy should be limited to the early assessment time frame and should focus on helping her get on track toward recovery. If too much is needed from you regarding concrete tasks, she would benefit more from a referral to a case worker who can help her access more resources that can provide longer term and wider spectrum relief.

5 How Do You Hold When Her Emotions Run High and Push Your Buttons?

What happens when she is enraged or when you don't like the way she is making you feel? What do you do if you do not like her or her words and emotional expression make you uncomfortable? What if she is making choices that are inconsistent with how you would do things? Or how you think she should do it?

Your inner monologue can be the key to how you respond to the challenge of provocative moments in session. It is hard to empathize when you feel threatened in some way. It is also hard to be compassionate and perform competently when working with someone who is prone to outbursts or becomes insulting or someone who is non-compliant or argumentative. There is no end to the number of circumstances that may, at any moment, feel confrontational, intimidating, or demanding in some way. These are moments that often generate flashes of a loud, critical inner voice: *What should I do? This feels terrible. Why is she so upset? I'm not sure how to proceed.*

Ethan Kross, a Professor of Psychology at the University of Michigan, set out to address the following question: Does the language people use to refer to the self during introspection influence how they think, feel, and behave under social stress? (Kross et al., 2014). Although his research can apply to your role as therapist and the self-reflective work that entails, it is also an effective tool for you to utilize in your direct work with postpartum women, particularly women who experience relentless negative thoughts.

Essentially, Kross determined that how we conduct our inner talk can boost our confidence and self-control by creating what he refers to as psychological distance. He found that when individuals under stress use the pronoun "I," they are more likely to become agitated and perform poorly. When they addressed themselves by their own name, performance soared. Have you ever found yourself doing this? When appropriate, I will coach a client with this practice and demonstrate that if she can gain distance by referring to herself in the third person, she might be surprised to notice that ruminations decrease and objectivity is within reach. This is referred to as "harnessing language to promote self-regulation" (Kross et al., 2014, p. 304).

Psychological distance backs us away from our innate egocentric viewpoint, thereby increasing our capacity to gain self-control in stressful situations. It appears to make it easier to observe and accept our feelings. You can encourage this by asking your client to step back from herself and imagine herself becoming an observer in a stressful moment, so she can watch and gain perspective on her own thoughts, emotions, and behaviors. We all know that it feels less complicated to help someone else than it does to help ourselves. It seems that Kross's research supports this by teaching us how to talk to ourselves more productively so we feel better and think more clearly.

For example: Can you imagine sitting with a client who is actively stirring things up for you, arousing a cascade of worry and idle introspection? The moment feels heavy with the pressure to respond appropriately while your head is screaming, *This feels awful, I have no idea what to do, I wish she would leave, why am I so upset*? Needless to say, these feelings are incompatible with holding techniques and require immediate regulation. Remember that the small shift in the language from *I* to the use of your own name can significantly influence your ability to regulate your own thoughts, feelings, and behavior under stress. Check out an example of my inner talk during a stressful moment in session.

Kristin was angry. At her family, at her husband, at her treatment-resistant illness. She was not thinking clearly, nor was she responding to medication the way we had hoped. She was compliant in terms of our treatment plan, but she was tired of feeling "bullied" by everyone who seemed to be telling her what to do, how to think, and talking behind her back about what's best for her.

Her soliloquy seemed to take on a life of its own as she sank into a state of agitated despair. I had known Kristin for several years, and she chose to be primarily mad at me. She felt betrayed when I agreed with her psychiatrist that she take an antipsychotic medication for her severe thought disorder. She said she knew her thinking wasn't right and yes, she can be tangential and irrational, but she feels better that way and wishes people would just leave her alone. She especially wished I would leave her alone.

When I asked why she was still coming for therapy if it feels so bad, she told me she is a good girl, she is doing what she is told; she is compliant. But her words stung and her eyes were dark with contempt. She was tired. We were all tired. Her team of clinical and medical support, along with her family, had watched Kristin descend into vortex of non-responsive symptoms and an impressive lack of insight.

She snarled at me and I contemplated my best, neutral response. She did not want to be held. Any attempt of mine to appease her, educate her, clarify for her led straight to a contrary response, usually ending up in a murmur of exasperation, "you don't understand." And of course, I didn't. She had delusional symptoms that encased her with illogical presumptions. Nothing I said made complete sense to her. Still, I knew she was there because she trusted me, because she knew I had safely helped her through a previous bipolar episode. I knew she resorted to anger because she was out of control and unable to access her repertoire of coping skills. Even so, it felt laborious and painstakingly unproductive. My chest tightened and my breathing became shallow.

It started with this unsupportive inner monologue:

Why are you snapping at me? Why aren't you listening to a word I am saying? The others in adjoining offices will hear your voice. Shhhhhhhhhhh. You are making yourself feel worse, see how agitated you are getting? We have worked so hard to help you feel better and now you are ungrateful? Enraged? Unappreciative?

That is when I knew I had to shift my thinking. I was blaming her for how bad I was starting to feel. Not good. Quickly, it progressed to this:

Karen, okay, slow down. This is fine. You know exactly what is going on here. Breathe. This is about her, not you. These are her symptoms talking. You know what to do. You are good at this. Help her contain her rant. Sit with it. Stay focused. Help her see what is happening here and keep her safe.

Ah, the internal roadmap to mastery. No one has to know the secret to your composure. Try this:

- **Distance** yourself by referring to yourself in the third person *by name*. Observe what is happening. Refrain from attaching the words *I* or *me*.
- **Self-direction.** Tell yourself what you need to do in order to achieve the desired result.
- **Affirmations** are useful ways to gain perspective and not be sucked into the same vortex that your client is swirling around.

Here, we regulate our emotional response and, by doing so, hold her, paradoxically, by *not* reacting. By tolerating. By remaining attentive to her misguided thoughts, addressing her strengths, and ensuring that she receives the treatment necessary to maintain her safety. But first and foremost, in any moment that inflames our sensibilities, we must hold ourselves.

6 Do Male Therapists Hold Differently?

The brief answer is no. The gender identity of the therapist has little bearing on the ability to apply holding practices to pregnant and postpartum women. At The Postpartum Stress Center, we feel it is important for male therapists to work on our team. It is helpful to have a male perspective and it is helpful to have a male therapist available to support dads who wish to see a male provider, whether they are partners of a depressed spouse or whether they are suffering from depression themselves. However, the question of whether or not a postpartum woman in distress feels as comfortable with a male as a female therapist raises additional questions. The majority of pregnant and postpartum women queried through an informal poll at The Postpartum Stress Center prefer a female therapist. This will not be true across the board, but it is an issue that comes up now and then, and repeatedly there is partiality toward female therapists.

This may be a function of common life experiences and perhaps a bias that female therapists are more empathic. Moreover, a postpartum woman, reeling from pregnancy, childbirth, and demands of the postpartum period, is excruciatingly vulnerable. Depending on her recent experience, she may have very strong positive or negative feelings about the medical community or perceived persons of authority or her feeling vulnerable in general. Vulnerability is not new for a postpartum woman. She has most likely already begun to open her heart and open her mind to her new baby. She has opened her legs to various levels of invasive inspection; she has learned how to bleed, discharge, poop, and lactate in front of strangers with little regard to judgment or consequences. It is not easy to do, but she does it. It often goes with the territory of giving birth. However, the vulnerability that comes with admitting you have thoughts of harm coming to your baby, or when you feel like your baby would be better off with another mother, or perhaps you made a mistake getting pregnant in the first place, or feeling that your body betrayed you, well, these are states of nakedness that may feel too hard to bear. And too hard to share. For some women, it is easier to talk about vaginal discharge and nipple soreness with another woman. In this way, female therapists have a leg up on male therapists in this field.

Research shows female graduate students significantly and consistently outnumber male graduate students in both master's level and doctoral level psychology programs (Fowler et al., 2018). Within a field dominated by female practitioners and within a subspecialty that so often involves a uniquely female experience, I suspect the men who are drawn to this work are wildly compassionate, wouldn't you think? The men I have encountered in this field certainly are. What perinatal women in distress need is a good therapist: one who can hold, one who can empathize, and one who can help her find her way back to her *self*. The gender of that therapist is not as important as it might feel to her at the moment if she is given a choice. Who that therapist *is* matters most. There are superb male perinatal therapists as well as not-so-fabulous female perinatal therapists. Whenever possible, you should honor the gender preference of anyone who seeks professional support if he or she expresses one. There may be a myriad of reasons behind a preference for one gender over the other.

7 How Do You Hold When Conflicting Feelings Are Aroused?

Many therapists have confessed that one major frustration is when the client isn't responding as anticipated. Perhaps she doesn't like the intervention, or she responds passive aggressively, or isn't choosing the path we believe would be in her best interest. One therapist reported she was annoyed that her client wasn't complying or doing things the way she thought she should. Things seemed pretty straightforward, but her client was making choices that contradicted what the therapist was asking her to do and she wasn't feeling better. "I asked her to fill out a CBT worksheet, but she didn't have time. I suggested she take a short walk each day, but she couldn't fit that in. We practiced breathing exercises together, but she reported she 'forgot' to do it on her own. She seems motivated enough to keep coming, but she is continuously late for sessions and I honestly don't feel like I'm helping her."

Intermittent or partial compliance can leave a therapist disappointed in themselves or reflecting on what they must surely be doing wrong. It is tempting to take it personally when the course of treatment goes awry. The single best technique to rescue a client who might be off track is to process what you observe by bringing it to her attention and discussing it. Remember that presence and safeguarding entail good-mother wisdom, keeping the larger picture in mind while leading her to the path that is tolerable to her. Surely you must honor and balance what she wants with what you think might be best. All the while keeping in mind that you could be mistaken about what you believe is best for her. She is the author of her story. It is her voice, her beliefs, that matter. Your interpretation of the various twists and turns gently guide her. Inevitably, she will dictate which way she wants this to go.

There will be times when holding feels impossible. There will be mamas who are difficult or situations that feel untenable. There will be times when you are sure you are not the right therapist for her and times when her reaction to her situation is the antithesis of how you would approach things. There will be women you do not like working with and women who do not like working with you. There will be sessions that seem to last an eternity. There will be partners that sabotage. There will be gut-wrenching decisions that violate your moral code and pierce your heart.

When things feel complicated, let her feel, and do your best to stay present with her and sit with her suffering. When cases provoke strong emotions in you, identify and externalize your uncertainty, focus on remaining present and make sure you take the time to sort out your emotions after the session with a professional who can help you put meaning and perspective behind your responses and feelings.

8 How Do You Hold Her When Her Partner May Be Unintentionally Sabotaging?

I met Stephanie with her 1-month-old baby and her husband, Marc, who made it clear in the first 15 minutes that he was a super fan of her continuing to breastfeed (Stephanie was currently nursing her newborn and her 2-year-old. Her 5-year-old stopped nursing when she became pregnant with this new baby). Marc was also an enthusiastic supporter of co-sleeping (all three children end up in bed with them by midnight each night), and they were adamant about not taking any medications, "We don't even take aspirin" (euphemism for we-would-never-put-anything-chemical-in-our-natural-bodies-even-if-it-means-we-might-suffer-longer). He said she was "tough" and "smart" and "strong."

She *was* tough and smart and strong. She was also drowning in her own high expectations of perfection. She denied suicidal thoughts but stated she wanted to sleep forever. She was shrouded with guilt and did not make eye contact with her husband when she spoke. She was ashamed of disappointing him. She had been such a good mother. Now she felt broken.

I liked both of them right from the start. Liking a client typically suggests connectability and high holding potential. Stephanie was bent over on the couch, swaying back and forth in rhythm with her nervous breath.

"How long will I have to feel this way?" A question often asked, with no good answer. "It depends" is never a suitable answer, but, of course, it does depend. It depends on how sick she is; how severe and pervasive her symptoms are; how significant her history of depression is; how long she's been sick; how much support she has; how supportive she perceives her support to be; how anxious she is about how she is feeling; how good her coping skills are; how strong her marriage is; how resourceful and resilient she is; how much sleep she is getting; how many external stressors she has in her life right now; how open to help she is; how intrusive her thoughts are; how she has responded to symptoms and treatment in the past. And, of course, when symptoms are moderate to severe, there is the dreaded: *How open is she to the possibility of taking medication?*

Marc was clear. No medication. Stephanie was not so clear. "I don't want to take medication. Really. But I don't know what to do. I don't want to feel this way for too long. I just can't." The three of us did the medication cha-cha for a while, back and forth and around again, the advantages, disadvantages, why she might benefit, why she might be okay without meds, how depression is a brain disorder that sometimes requires medical intervention, and so on. He didn't buy it, because, well, *she's so strong.*

My first impulse is to join with both partners, reiterating their desires and validating each. Next, I asked mom to come by herself to the next session. This way, I might better determine her position regarding treatment options without the loving interference from a man who is scared and may not have all the information he needs to come to the best decision. In this particular case, when I met with Stephanie alone, her opposition to medication weakened as her symptoms persisted. She remained reticent and sought repeated reassurance. We discussed the options she had; we also talked about her marriage, which was good, and soon thereafter, we brought Marc back into the session so the three of us could move onto the same page. It became clear that Stephanie had failed to express to Marc the extent to which she was suffering. It was equally clear that he did not want her to suffer. Not for a minute. That's all it took to get him on board.

In this chapter we have reviewed a sample of the issues that therapists may be confronted by in their clinical practices and how these issues may influence holding. As you look closely at these and all clinical challenges, you will gain a deeper understanding of how holding points are not the treatment, as such. They are the gateway to treatment options; the essential and foremost intervention.

Chapter 15

Holding and Letting Go

When preparing the final pages of the first edition of this book, it seemed appropriate to conclude with a chapter on recovery. The recovery process is as individualized as the woman herself, thus, holding inevitably evolves and recalibrates as recovery progresses. If your client continues in therapy through and beyond recovery for ongoing support, you continue to hold her. The urgency may subside, but her need for continual grounding, assessment, expertise, presence, treatment plans, and safeguarding will continue throughout her sessions with you. As I thought about the changing needs of the postpartum woman in recovery and how best to address them in the concluding chapter, I found my thoughts shifting in a different direction. A direction that took me back to you, to the role and well-being of the holding therapist. Although the emphasis of this book has been to highlight the therapeutic care of postpartum women, you have learned that this is best achieved by holding on tightly, philosophically, psychologically, spiritually, respectfully, self-assuredly, and fundamentally to *who you are*. Armed with that wisdom, it is my fervent hope that readers of this book are better prepared to pursue this work with renewed enthusiasm and greater confidence.

The psychological experience of motherhood has gained attention in the public and academic spheres and as an area of professional specialty appealing to therapists on both a professional and personal level. As discussed, many therapists choose to specialize in this area as a result of their personal experience. Intermingled with their strong desire to help postpartum women is their own history of positive and negative experiences and expectations related to their own reproductive journeys. The complexity of each individual's private inner journey is a driving force behind the desire to do this work and the capacity to hold. You have learned that therapy with perinatal women involves far more than use of tools, techniques, and strategies of intervention. It is also about your own self-discovery and the intricate process of synthesizing who you are with what your client needs.

DOI: 10.4324/9781003402145-15

For these reasons, discussion of holding points and techniques is most aptly concluded with an overall view of best practices when it comes to holding postpartum women from the perspective of the therapist. This provides a closing effort to *hold you* as you advance through your professional path. In supervision, I find it unsatisfactory to discuss holding a postpartum woman without ensuring that the therapist feels sufficiently held in her dealings with this particular client. These two experiences are inextricably intertwined.

Principles of Excellent Clinical Practice

During my time in graduate school, it wasn't popular to engage in open discussions about how one's personal experience or emotions weave into the practice of psychotherapy. At that time, it was perceived as something one should discuss in private with one's supervisor. We didn't have dialogues in class about how countertransference felt or, heaven forbid, how our delicate vulnerabilities were affecting our work. Countertransference was strictly a theoretical phenomenon that was conspicuously left out of intimate group discussions. Although it was a serious consideration since early in 1910 when Freud first explored the concept of countertransference (Freud, 1910), our studies were focused more on the academics and processes. Concentrating on how our work made us feel, in or out of session, felt rather indulgent, if not superfluous. Today, the psychological community is more forgiving, and therapists are encouraged to take notice of their own emotional responses and make use of them on behalf of their clients.

I tell trainees at our program to "work well." Best practices include keeping up with current research, advocating and implementing programs to enhance public awareness, expanding screening protocols, improving access to healthcare and treatment options, and, of course, keeping your finger on the pulse of the postpartum woman herself, who remains your best source of information. Working well incorporates the following principles as they guide your actions and help you synchronize the delicate balance between loving your work and doing it well. The following principles sum up much of what we have discussed in earlier chapters. Live by these principles as you hold your postpartum clients and move through your clinical practice. If it isn't already clear, you will eventually see how your work with your postpartum client and your work on yourself are interrelated. Ultimately, successful holding is really about you.

Principle 1: Believe in Yourself

Cliché or not, belief in yourself is first and foremost the groundwork from which successful holding evolves. Whether you are a beginning therapist or a wise experienced practitioner, believing in your ability to make a difference will propel you forward in this work. You are at the helm. Although that level of control is both invigorating and daunting, it is precisely this paradoxical energy that sparks your passion and keeps us invested.

It still surprises me when accomplished clinicians confess how nervous this work makes them at times. Or how concerned they are about the details of assessment and treatment with postpartum women when they have been practicing in the mental health field for years. There is a tenderness to this population that supersedes any previous acknowledgement or appreciation of one's skill set and expertise. After all, there is a baby involved. That's part of it. It is also because a postpartum woman is so incredibly raw, physiologically and emotionally. The fiber of her being, her innermost nerves and guts, are exposed, leaving even master clinicians to question whether they have what it takes to compete with these forces of nature. As if depression isn't bad enough, this is depression with the cruelest twist of all. It is an illness that takes everything a woman believes she loves the most and makes it all unreachable. There is an incomprehensible numbness: an inner horror that, when clashing with the outside world, is shocked into total motionlessness. She cannot move. She cannot breathe. When she comes to you for air, you either convince her that you can help or she will never come back. There is little in between.

Principle 2: Choose Your Words Carefully

Your words are indispensable tools of intervention. They can also lead to serious negative repercussions. Small modifications can turn your words of empathy into words of judgment. Do not underestimate how easily she can misinterpret and obsess with her distorted analysis of what you did not mean to say. Unless you know her extremely well, be cautious when relying on humor or sarcasm, which can quickly sabotage your best efforts if she misreads your intentions. In the early sessions, when you focus on grounding and assessment, you may find you need to be more reserved and mindful of your words so as not to veer off course, even slightly. After she begins to feel some degree of relief, you may notice you are more comfortable expressing yourself with less apprehension about potential misunderstandings.

Remember she is being inundated by intolerance from social media, critics of political correctness, images of phony perfection, and constant critiques of what she is doing or not doing. She is trying her best to operate under her own set of objectives and reasons that make the most sense to her. She may privately wonder if her choices and decisions are good ones, but she clings to them, nonetheless. When choices are easy, everything makes sense. Things feel nice and balanced. When choices are complicated, desperation can pierce a previously sanctioned belief. She is plagued by random judgments and family and cultural pressures, as well as her own distrustful thoughts. Sensitivities and preferences become intractable.

When uncertainty takes precedence, your impartiality and purposeful guidance become indispensable. Remember that her proclivity to think obsessively during this time means that *anything you say cannot be unsaid.* Or unheard by her. Choose your words wisely. Do your best to help her reach her own conclusions. Hold her while you support her priorities and beliefs without necessarily letting her know how you feel about the choices she is making, unless, of course, she chooses something that is not in her best interest.

Principle 3: Beware of Assumptions

Take an honest account of your biases. Your work is loaded with emotionally laden material. Complicated issues such as childbirth and delivery choices, psychopharmacologic options, terminations, assisted reproduction, unplanned pregnancies, adoption, infertility, genetic testing and screening procedures, selective termination, and multiple pregnancies are just a few of the life-altering circumstances with which your clients may be grappling.

- Is your client adequately informed?
- Does she have access to appropriate resources?
- Do you have a strong opinion of what you need to be watchful?
- Are you able to support her unconditionally even if you do not personally agree with the choices she is making?
- Do you need to research this further so you are adequately informed?
- Other issues that may be less of a crisis can be just as emotionally loaded, especially when she is highly symptomatic. Making assumptions is tempting yet misleading. There will be times when it is hard to not make assumptions.

Examples of Some Assumptions You Might Make Are:

If she is breastfeeding, you might assume she likes it.
  Ask her.

If she looks healthy, you might assume she is not suicidal or that she does not have access to a gun in her house.
  Check it out. Ask the hard questions.

If she tells you her husband is perfect, you might assume her relationship is as good as she says it is.
  It might be. It might not be. He could be contributing to her distress in some way. Explore this.

When she answers your questions, you might assume she is telling you everything you need to know.

Perhaps she is. Perhaps she is not. Be mindful. Ask more questions.

Clients may withhold the truth, confabulate, or neglect to mention pieces of their history or current stressors, either intentionally or inadvertently. Typically, it is a therapist's nature to lean toward accepting what the client reports as her truth to be true. Keep an eye and ear open to the possibility that her truth may be shrouded, either by her symptoms or her shame.

Principle 4: Know Your Areas of Vulnerability

Take a good hard look at yourself. In this context, "knowing" your area of vulnerability means identify it, acknowledge it, understand it, accept it, and work with and around it. Being vulnerable is a good thing. It makes you bravely human, and it opens your heart to the changes that are possible within your sessions and in your own life. Without vulnerability, you will be the very therapist she is trying to avoid.

One of the clinicians in our training class revealed her struggle with this: "My greatest strength is my greatest weakness. I know that my empathy makes me a good therapist. It is also what drains me and makes me worry way too much about my clients." Many therapists confess similar sentiments; what makes them feel most vulnerable is their tendency to become overly involved. Not surprising, most also report their capacity for empathy and compassion to be their most indispensable asset.

Various responses to the question of personal vulnerability from The Postpartum Stress Center trainees are listed below. Take a minute to reflect on these statements, and if any resonates for you pay attention to its meaning and give some thought to how you might tackle this in order to reinforce your resilience.

- I question my own competence.
- I wonder about my inability to separate emotionally.
- I have been told I can work harder than my clients at times.
- I have trouble setting limits.
- I have difficulty focusing on self-care.
- Self-disclosure. I tend to feel my story will help my client relate to me and feel better.
- Self-confidence in my abilities. I feel I never have enough knowledge.
- If a client is overwhelmingly stuck, I can feel that way too.
- I absorb a great deal of the stress in this work but try not to let it interfere with my personal life.

- Self-doubt. I tend to think I am not doing a good enough job.
- I have a tendency to overextend and overcommit myself.
- I hesitate to ask for help.
- I am hard on myself and a perfectionist.

Trust and protect your tenderness. Fortify your work with a genuine scrutiny of all that is meaningful and difficult for you. Maturity in this field requires acceptance of these vulnerabilities and the attributes that make you feel insecure in this work. Keep an eye on how you feel and use it to nourish this process.

Principle 5: Know Your Limits

Most of the time, you learn what your limits are when you reach beyond them. That's because most individuals who go into this work are propelled by an incredible work ethic and lofty personal expectations. If you insist on waiting until you are burned out, or exhausted, or angry, or overwhelmed, use that moment in your career to make certain you stop and pay attention. Ideally, you will learn in retrospect that you waited too long and you can intervene earlier next time before you are negatively impacted.

Knowing your limits in terms of a) *logistics* (hours, commitments, energy spent, projects taken on); b) *clients* (boundaries, contact availability, expectations, responsibilities); and c) *personal space* (say no, self-care, overextended desires, or behaviors) will enable you to break free from the excruciating model of perfectionism.

On a more global level, knowing your limits also refers to coming to terms with just how much of a difference you really can make. We may want to obliterate all sources of distress and pain, but alas, we cannot. We may want to advance the knowledge of all providers who come in contact with each and every perinatal woman, but we cannot. We may hope that our efforts, our teachings, our perfect holding responses will have long-lasting and wide-reaching influence on women near and far, but how could they possibly? When we consider how long we have been trying to get the message out that postpartum depression and anxiety are real and are worthy of legitimate and vigilant responsiveness, it can be disheartening. Just when we think our local or more widespread endeavors are making a difference, we notice highly educated individuals oftentimes ignore warnings or misread cues. Still, each of us knows how good it feels to connect with a woman who has listened to our words, applied the interventions, and was restored to good health as a direct result of our skills and goodwill. That is our preeminent professional accomplishment.

I am reminded of this familiar tale:

A young man is walking along the ocean and sees a beach on which thousands and thousands of starfish have washed ashore. Farther along he sees an old man, walking slowly and stooping often, picking up one starfish after another and tossing each one gently into the ocean.
"Why are you throwing starfish into the ocean?" he asks.
"Because the sun is up and the tide is going out and if I don't throw them farther in they will die."
"But, old man, don't you realize there are miles and miles of beach and starfish all along it! You can't possibly save them all; you can't even save one-tenth of them. In fact, even if you work all day, your efforts won't make any difference at all."
The old man listened calmly and then bent down to pick up another starfish and threw it into the sea.
"It made a difference to that one."[1]

Principle 6: Turn Weakness into Strength

As with most constructs in therapy, we will be the best teachers of tools and skills if we are good at them ourselves, in our own lives, and if we can successfully model them for our clients. One of my great joys is to point out to a perfectionistic client who professes to vacuum before she leaves the house every day how comfortable she is in my not-so-organized office. I ask her how it feels to sit in this room, with papers strewn across my desk, and books out of whack on the shelf, and oh yes, the magic wand hanging precariously out of place. She looks around. "It feels good," I often hear.

"You see," I explain, mocking my authority in messy offices, "see how good it can feel to just be? To not worry if things are in place around you? Perhaps the best thing I can teach you is how to live with your mess. See how well I do it?"

We both laugh. We both know that someone else's mess is never as bad as your own. That's for sure. More importantly, the metaphor of letting go, loosening the grip, relinquishing control is easier for her to see when it is presented outside of herself. Holding her within the confines of this "mess" demonstrates that I can be in control of my work and my life even though I have not taken steps to tidy up the busyness around me. Most postpartum women tell me they want to learn how to do that, how to be okay with things out of place. After all, that is basically the quintessential task and the most pressing paradox of becoming a new parent:

How do I maintain control while learning how little control I really have?

Learning how to reframe someone's perceived weakness into a strength is a skill that can transcend almost any other therapeutic intervention. It may not be easy for her to hear or believe, but you can help her accept her anxiety, help her live with her disappointments, help her rethink her negative appraisals with the flick of a cognitive switch – she can begin to believe that she has control over the way she thinks and feels. After we repeat what we believe she said (*Let me make sure I understand you correctly*), we might explore: *What if there were other ways to view this? Are there alternative ways for you to think about this? What if this were a good attribute and not something you needed to feel bad about? Let's look at it that way together for a moment.* But first, you have to learn how to do that for yourself.

Principle 7: Know Your Own Underlying Triggers

Of course, we always remind ourselves that therapists are human and can experience strong emotional reactions. The indisputable responsibility of the therapist is to manage these emotions professionally at all times. Still, we have mentioned throughout this book that working with the perinatal population can be especially triggering for therapists, especially for those who have personally encountered similar circumstances. Understanding what may trigger you is an essential part of your professional preparation for this work. This cannot be stressed enough, and it is different from knowing your vulnerabilities. Your triggers can emerge from your family of origin, your personal battleground, your history of mood and anxiety disorders. Triggers can touch old wounds and entirely derail a session. Lack of awareness around your triggers can cause you to react impulsively. This breach of boundaries is never good from a professional perspective. If you find yourself in a moment of unchecked reactiveness, breathe through it and resume focus on your client instantly.

Be aware. Be in touch. Be in supervision.

If you watch for it, you may notice that sometimes you can pick up a mood or a posture that your clients exhibit. Before you know it, you find yourself sliding into the emotional whirlpool. Sit up. Refocus. Protect yourself from feeling provoked by the moods of your client. The therapeutic space can only stay clear and clean if you are aware of and responsible for your own emotional reactions. Your objective is to keep your issues separate from hers and minimize any impact.

Principle 8: Break Some Rules

Rules and boundaries are fluid, at times.

This statement only works in the therapeutic setting when therapists have a comprehensive, well-developed and steadfast understanding of what appropriate therapeutic boundaries mean. And they mean different things for each client.

As I've purported, ad infinitum, I am a living, breathing, behind-the-times contradiction. Ask any one of my clients: my list of No's is extensive. Please do not call my cell phone. I will not answer. Please do not text me. I am busy. If I text you because I choose to check in, please do not interpret that as permission to text me later. No, I cannot see you on Saturday. No, I will not see you at my home since we are virtual now. No, I will not call you when I am home writing, but I will have someone call you and make sure your need is addressed...

However:

- If I am worried about her, I may go see her in the hospital after her baby is born.
- If I don't like the way she sounds, I will call her at night to check in and maybe every day after that until I see her again.
- If she is incapacitated by symptoms, I will make endless phones calls on her behalf, with her and for her, so we can facilitate a path to treatment together.
- If she cannot find the words, I will sit in the silence and fill in some of the spaces with comforting reassurance and suggestions to help her feel better.
- If she would prefer not to tell me something, I will honor that whole-heartedly and will also do my best to convince her that she will feel better if she shares it with me.
- If I do not like the way she clinically sounds or looks, I will let her know this and contact her partner and family members, with her permission, to enlist their help and support.
- If I am worried about her and she does not call me back, I will call her. And then, I will call again, and maybe once more, to make sure she is okay.

Here again, knowing who you are, knowing your limits and vulnerabilities and understanding your strengths, will enable to you to continue holding while you pursue the best treatment options. Sometimes this involves breaking your own rules or those you were taught in graduate school, because, as we've said over and over in this book, the needs of postpartum women are fragile, they are urgent, and there is a baby in the picture.

Principle 9: Engage in Self-Care

I have previously emphasized the value of self-care and self-compassion and can only reiterate the life-altering impact that some small regular routines can have on your well-being. It doesn't have to be transcendental;

it can be adding a teaspoon of fiber to your diet. As long as you take action on behalf of your mind, your body, your emotions, and your relationships, you are investing in your *self* and will have far more to give your clients.

At the time of this writing, therapists are enduring difficult times personally and professionally. This present reality imposes tremendous constraints on our time, our energy, our motivation, and our mental health. Taking care of ourselves is no longer just about comfort and indulgence. It is crucial to our well-being. It is also very subjective. What works for you will not be what works for someone else. Listen to your body and your heart. Find ways to rest, soothe, and reset. Your work-life balance is key. The time-honored standards, e.g. exercise, mediation, play, music, sleep, etc., will work, and many are sanctioned by research (Posluns & Gall, 2020), but self-care efforts will benefit you most if they are accompanied by self-compassion and intention.

Finally, if taking care of yourself doesn't agree with you as a primary objective, remember that it is one of the most constant ways to protect you and your clients from negative clinical outcomes. Burnout or any compromised resilience will put you and your work at an increased risk for poor quality of life and professional impairment (Butler et al., 2017).

Try framing self-care as self-compassion, and as part of your responsible caring for your client. Your greatest worth to your clients emerges from a belief in your own worthiness.

Principle 10: Be Informed

The principles we apply to ourselves as the facilitator of postpartum healing also apply to ourselves as experts in the treatment of postpartum depression. There exists an ever-growing body of knowledge that underpins our work, and our awareness of the literature and relevant research will enhance our clinical practice. Information is changing all the time. Stay connected with communities and resources that serve as conduits for this information if you do not have direct access. In addition to the implications this information will have for your clients' well-being, you may feel inclined to promote the cause at large. We need to make every effort to reduce patient- and provider-based barriers to effective diagnosis and treatment.

Practicing and committing to the ten principles described above will help sharpen your skills as a holding therapist and keep you focused on being your best (professional) and authentic (personal) self. As we've seen, this work is both incredibly gratifying and emotionally demanding. It is important not to lose sight of the ongoing necessity to reflect on and assess our purpose, our well-being, and our holding skills.

Holding Hope

Andrew Solomon, author of *The Noonday Demon*, has a wonderful way of articulating complicated concepts in a straightforward manner. In an interview on NPR with *Fresh Air*'s Terry Gross, Solomon said, "I go and see a psychotherapist every week, not so much because what happens in any individual session is transformative, but because I feel it's important that there be someone, a trained professional, who is watching what is going on" (Solomon, 2015). Many postpartum women express similar sentiments. Many say it feels good to know someone else is on board, someone objective, someone with no agenda, keeping an eye on things.

Defining and understanding depression is tricky. As much as we learn about it through rigorous research and as much as we claim to know what helps and what doesn't, the experience of depression remains elusive and subjective. I have seen women with irrepressible suicidal thoughts function at work every day. I have also seen women incapacitated and homebound resulting from a single unimaginable intrusive thought. Although we have a reliable, validated measure of postpartum depression in the EPDS, there is much this scale does not tell us. And although we profess to understand some of the biological, genetic, psychological, emotional, and social influences, depression remains a very personal and shattering hell, with few definitive markers. Surely, we have clusters of symptoms that we can identify and treat successfully. And we have evidence-based therapies that can mitigate symptoms and provide relief. Still, the shock of misaligned expectations, disorganized thinking, and extraordinary levels of distress occurring at a time when a woman expected to feel magnificently joyful makes maternal depression fundamentally different from other clinical depressions. Resounding ambivalence, utter frustration, and unthinkable resentment toward her own beloved baby provokes an earth-shattering sense of failure and despair.

It follows, then, that treatment options would follow a similar imprecise trajectory. Some women prefer to take a pill. Others prefer to talk it out. Despite the many declarations of medical breakthroughs and psychopharmacologic concoctions, when we sit in the office with a postpartum mother aching from a decaying sense of self, treatment options can feel hard to pin down, if not slightly irrelevant, at those moments. Sometimes, the best we can do, in the beginning, is contain her pain.

There is no real consensus on the best treatment for postpartum depression, so those of us who bear witness to successful treatments must have an answer when asked how we do it. When asked, "How do you treat postpartum depression?" by journalists determined to support our plea for a public conversation, we invariably feel pressure to subscribe to a tried and true set of psychological interventions to be recited with authority. Those of us on the front line understand that treating postpartum depression and anxiety is complicated by all kinds of factors, many mentioned throughout these chapters. Resistance gets in the way. Babies take precedence. Families misunderstand. Personal histories dictate. Medical communities are unacceptably misinformed. Stigma sidetracks recovery before it even begins. Shame silences mothers.

When we talk about containing her pain, we talk about holding. If we hold correctly and contain her pain, we enable the suffering to shrink, ever so slightly. In this complicated realm of depression, it may feel impossible for her to feel better, but it actually takes very little to let her know and help her feel that she can have hope that her symptoms will subside, and recovery is within reach.

One hard truth in this work is that relationships, marriages, mental health, and well-being all flourish in direct proportion to the attention placed upon them. We learn to appreciate something by devoting our time and energy to it. This is true for you and for your clients. Although therapy during the postpartum period may present an oxymoron at first, it may actually be a first step a new mother takes to sit with herself and determine what she needs during a time when she is so intently focused on others. Your earnest request that she stay present with this process can set in motion her mission for true peacefulness as a mother.

Shortly after we moved into our home, almost 40 years ago, my husband and I went across the street with our new neighbors to see the hand-crafted bookshelves they had installed. Eager to share the excitement of owning a new home, we followed them on a tour of their house, room after room. We couldn't help but notice the freshly painted walls up against the striking crown molding, bedrooms that looked like they had just been prepared for a magazine photo shoot, kitchen counters that were bare other than one lonely coffee maker. Beds were tidy, decorative pillows were in position, faucets were sparkling. Noticeably missing were random pieces of mail, paper piles, dog hair, stray socks on the floor, keys out of place, crumbs on the floor. *Where was all their stuff?* I thought for sure we had entered a model display home. Suddenly I found myself feeling 12 years old. *Maybe one day, when I grow up, I can have a house like this. Wait. I am grown up. I do have a house like this. Why doesn't mine look like this? Why will mine never look like this?* For an instant, I was overcome with envy. I don't have the skills, the propensity, the desire, or the wherewithal to make my home look like this. Or, did I?

My husband and I said our gracious goodbyes and walked across the street. We entered our house, the same exact house, constructed by the same builder in our development of sweet cookie-cutter homes. Few distinguishing features from the outside. But from the inside…

We walked in. I started with my flair for whimpering. "Do you think our house will ever look like a grown-up house?"

My husband chuckled. He is amused by my overanalytical preoccupations. "Our house is perfect," he reassures. "It's us. It's cozy."

"That's sweet. And true. But still, our house looks like we are still in college."

"It does. That's who we are. That's why people like coming over here. It feels comfortable, lived in. It makes people want to be here. It makes us want to be here. It's our home."

I can't say I entirely stopped comparing myself to others at that moment in time, but I can say it's when I began to consolidate a more developed sense of self along with greater comfort with who I was and where my life had taken me. Your comfort with yourself, who you are and what you have to offer will translate through your holding skills as confidence in your ability to help her. She is looking to you for that.

Becoming comfortable with who you are is a task that all therapists must take seriously in their own lives before expecting to accompany your client down that path. That's because perinatal illness is not all about biology and hormones. It is also about becoming a mother and transitioning into a new dimension of oneself. Just when you start to believe that you understand the impact perinatal illnesses can have on a woman and her family, you find yourself confronting a new symptom, a new manifestation, a new life circumstance or challenge that demonstrates the extraordinary nuances of these illnesses. This premise of remaining open to the overarching emotions and conflicts is crucial to your work and to her well-being. She comes to you, hoping you will understand this, hoping you will understand how she battles the inequities she endures at home, at her workplace, online, on the playground, in the mirror, with her family, and in her heart. Her simultaneous wish to be the best mother she can be with her desire to vanish into thin air can feel impossible to reconcile. It also illuminates her primary request of you. Can you embrace her ambivalence? Will you be able to tolerate her emotional deprivation juxtaposed with the neediness of her baby? Are you able to help her make sense out of her longing to disappear? This is the language of a mother losing hope. Her world at this moment is equally fed by her desire to take care of and be cared for.

Thus, you hold her.

As you hold, you heal, enabling her to hold her illness, her symptoms, her suffering with greater acceptance and less despair. When she is able to oppose them less and reinterpret her suffering as a call to listen and take care of herself, perhaps she can rest more easily within this transitional space. This is when you see her sheer exhaustion transmute into the hope of retrieving her lost self.

Hope is a legitimate and necessary intervention.

When you hold a postpartum woman, you hold her symptoms and her illness. When she alone holds her symptoms, she is panicked by the flailing, the fight-or-flight response, *the slimy deer*. There is nothing to hold on to, to secure her grip. She locks herself into her system of suffering and cannot find her way out. She wrangles through the labyrinth, often worsening her symptoms. When you hold, you create the opportunity for her to pay attention to her symptoms, embrace them, listen to them, as you escort her back home to herself. Her time with you calls this into perfect view. She yearns for you to know *who she was* before depression robbed her of her being. She desperately seeks to reclaim her previous healthy self, the life she knew and owned with the simplicity of what was.

With the increase in attention to perinatal depression and anxiety disorders, more healthcare providers are becoming aware of the high stakes involved. Consequently, providers are beginning to understand how these illnesses affect their clinical practices, and some are recognizing the seriousness of maternal mental health and referring women at risk for treatment.

Whether or not you incorporate advocacy into your clinical practice, whether or not you are driven to immerse yourself in the legislative, political, social, or medical implications inherent in this work, you cannot escape the repercussions of these influences that inform your work. A postpartum woman is inundated by mandates, directives, and obligations that complicate her already challenging experience of having a baby. By the time she reaches your office, she is counting on you to absorb the assault.

Holding her and holding yourself are two sides of the same work. Do not do one at the expense of the other. There is no greater reward in this work than the privilege of accompanying a postpartum woman through the trials and triumphs of this awesome life transition. As she begins to find relief, so, too, will you reap the benefits of working hard on her behalf. That synergy is magical.

So, does a postpartum woman in distress need to see a postpartum specialist?

I believe so. This is where you bring your humanness and your healing energy into the space between her and you. This is how the therapeutic alliance transforms into something else. Something distinctly personal. Although it is all about her, it is also about you. With your training, passion, skills, magic, expertise, and your best self, *you* are precisely what she needs right now.

She will get better if you believe in your ability to help her.

Note

1 Adapted from Loren Eiseley's essay "The Starfish Story.".

Epilogue
Therapist, Hold Thyself

The COVID-19 pandemic, along with various global crises, continue to impact families with unprecedented stress. As a result, it has become more commonplace for parents to seek professional support as stressors mount and challenges multiply. What makes this preponderance of stress particularly complicated is that it presents itself equally across the board leaving both clients and therapists grappling with similar issues. This unusual occurrence of parallel stressors creates new challenges for therapists who must make taking care of themselves a top priority as they tackle the urgent needs of their clients. Never before have we been asked to place so much attention on how we are doing, how we are coping, and how we are feeling, in order to ensure we are there for our clients, unequivocally.

For this reason, we decided to add this epilogue, to provide tools for you to take care of yourselves as you continue to monitor the well-being of your clients. While we touched on this in Chapter 15, we now urge you to take this seriously and make sure you leave time in your day to stretch, take a walk, sit in the sunshine, listen to music, and move your body, in order to preserve your energy, increase your resilience, and enable you to focus on your work. Practice some of the exercises we present below so you can establish healthy boundaries and avoid overextending yourself. Remember that the very sensitivity that makes you good at this work can also put you at risk for over caring and burning out. It is not how much you care; it's how you care, for your client, and for yourself.

It is not easy to sit with and absorb the suffering of others. Emotions and behaviors such as raging, blaming, self-annihilating, sarcasm, criticizing, panicking, hyperventilating, denying, weeping, obsessing, despairing, lamenting, self-loathing, and mourning can defy every attempt to hold a postpartum woman in distress. Brutal emotions can sabotage an unsuspecting new mother. They can also sway her into self-sacrificing or hyper controlling demeanors that are hard to break and equally difficult to live with. Some of these emotional manifestations may be personality driven and some may be symptomatic of a particular diagnosis. Regardless of

DOI: 10.4324/9781003402145-16

their origin or the myriad of factors contributing to them, when they are expressed in tandem with the demand for immediate resolution, we are tempted to respond with our own compelling need to fulfill this request. Our anxiety to subdue her panic is a natural response to seeing another person in acute discomfort. Even so, this unmistakably sympathetic response must remain our secret as we intuitively search for tools of intervention.

It is not exactly news that therapists are better at taking care of others than they are of themselves. Why is that? Are we too busy? Too devoted to our work? Too undeserving? Too empathetic, leaving little left for ourselves at the end of a day? Do we not endorse the merit of our own words? Do we not have the proper skills? Does our hypocrisy negate the value of our work?

Or, at the end of the day, are we immobilized by the work and simply too tired?

Empathy is at once your greatest asset and liability. If you are good it, it can exhaust you. It can deplete your emotional reservoir. It can make you vulnerable to burnout. The accumulation of stress can knock the healthiest therapist off balance.

In her book, *Help for the Helper*, Babette Rothschild (2006) refers to the mechanism of mirror neurons, a small circuit of cells in the premotor cortex and inferior parietal cortex. To oversimplify a complicated series of scientific explanations of brain functioning, research explains that we are hardwired and primed to experience each other's joy and pain. The most fascinating part of the literature on mirror neurons is that there is a physical process to the pathway to our emotional response. For example, when we see someone smile, our own mirror neurons for smiling fire up too, initiating a surge of neural activity that is associated with smiling. It enables us to experience (to a lesser degree) what the other is experiencing (Iacoboni, 2008).

However, emotions can be misperceived. One's own mix of experiences, combined with any number of factors that add to the interpretation and misinterpretation of another's emotional experience, can lead one off course. My daughter and I share a peculiar ache in our chests whenever we catch a glimpse of (either a photograph or in real life) a being (person or animal, usually extremely old or young) who we *perceive* is in some vulnerable state (lonely, frightened, sad, misunderstood). Mind you, we *attribute* these emotional states to them; we have no knowledge of the situation. We merely witness the image and instantly feel the pain. We observe an elderly man eating alone and feel a physical pang of loneliness. We see a newborn baby orangutan being cared for in a nursery, and we feel the pain of abandonment. We assume the aging man has no family and presume he is sad eating alone. Similarly, we deduce the baby orangutan has been separated from its mother.

Perhaps we are right, perhaps we are not. We experience pain, regardless.

Therapists can misconstrue emotions. Therapists tell me they are frustrated when clients don't respond the way the therapist feels they "should" or the way they themselves would. They say, *I would never let my husband talk to me that way.* Or, *I would feel so much better if I meditated. I don't know why she is resisting this.* Or, *I would love it if someone taught me how to relax; why isn't she relieved? Why isn't she practicing what we talked about?*

Neuroscience aside, even our experience of countertransference can lead us astray when it comes to reading the emotional responses of our clients. We must remain attuned to how easily this can happen in order to ensure that we empathize more strategically with our clients. If empathy is rooted in our bodies, you need to pay attention to your physical responses in order to harness your emotions and use them effectively in your work. Harnessing them means using your awareness and skills to decelerate an interfering emotion or cut short your brain's rush to overidentify with a particular moment that may not be in your client's best interest.

Burnout, Vicarious Trauma, Compassion Fatigue

It has been suggested that, on average, the productive life span of a psychotherapist is approximately ten years before burnout is likely to develop (Grosch & Olsen, 1994). That's sobering, isn't it? Burnout in our profession is understood in part as a process of declining interest, waning spirit, or disconnect from one's original passion in the helping profession. Christine Maslach (2003) defines burnout as a syndrome of emotional exhaustion, depersonalization, and reduced personal accomplishments that occurs in response to chronic emotional strain. It is so commonplace that burnout has been described as "the single most common personal consequence of practicing therapy" (Kottler, 2003, p. 158).

There are various concepts that overlap in meaning that refer to the emotional depletion that can result from working in the helping profession. Whether we refer to *burnout* (Skovholt, 2001) or *compassion fatigue* (Joinson, 1992) or *vicarious trauma* (Pearlman & Saakvitne, 1995), the emotional impact of our work with the perinatal population is exacting and demanding. These three terms are complementary yet different. *Burnout* is a term that has been used since the early 1980s to describe the physical and emotional exhaustion that professionals can experience as a result of low job satisfaction and feelings of overwhelm and powerlessness (Mathieu, 2011). *Compassion fatigue* refers to the intense emotional and physical depletion that occurs when therapists (or other helping professionals) are unable to refuel and regenerate. *Vicarious trauma* (also known as secondary traumatic stress) describes the penetrating shift in world view that occurs in helping professionals when working closely with trauma victims. Some professionals reveal that their fundamental beliefs about the world have been altered by repeated exposure to traumatic content.

The distinction between burnout, compassion fatigue, and vicarious trauma is less relevant for our purposes than the awareness that if you lose touch with your best self, it is a signal that you are in a danger zone that requires immediate attention and corrective action. If you are mindful that burnout, compassion fatigue, and vicarious trauma are to be expected in psychotherapeutic work – rather than experienced as a character flaw or indicators of inadequacy – you are in a better position to identify the warning signs and respond effectively when overly stressed.

Know When to Hold Yourself

Maslach (2003) emphasized that burnout might just be the price a therapist pays for overly empathizing with clients. To some extent, most good therapists believe this to be true. Additionally, there are many aspects of this work that put us at risk, such as large caseloads, lack of professional support or supervision, excessive idealism, or overidentifying with clients, for example. As mentioned earlier, in your work with the perinatal population, the risk is high that you will overidentify with your client. As a human being with a reproductive system and journey, you are at risk for overidentifying with your client. If you have a personal history of depression or anxiety, or a family history of depression or anxiety, or if you had prenatal or postpartum depression or anxiety – whether you had treatment or not – any or all of these variables increase the probability that you could experience a disproportionate empathetic response. The importance of checking in with yourself to assess and reassess your own level of burnout cannot be overstated. Consider reviewing your answers to these prompts periodically, maybe every three months, six months, or year.

To What Extent Do These Feelings Interfere with Your Satisfaction, Work, and/or Personal Functioning?

- **Overwhelmed?**
  All the time. Sometimes. Rarely. I don't feel this way right now.
- **Drained?**
  All the time. Sometimes. Rarely. I don't feel this way right now.
- **Exhausted?**
  All the time. Sometimes. Rarely. I don't feel this way right now.

- Overloaded?
  All the time. Sometimes. Rarely. I don't feel this way right now.
- Angry, enraged in response to your client?
  All the time. Sometimes. Rarely. I don't feel this way right now.
- Joyless?
  All the time. Sometimes. Rarely. I don't feel this way right now.
- Apathetic?
  All the time. Sometimes. Rarely. I don't feel this way right now.
- Fatigued?
  All the time. Sometimes. Rarely. I don't feel this way right now.
- Depressed?
  All the time. Sometimes. Rarely. I don't feel this way right now.
- Overly emotionally involved with your client (positive or negative emotions)?
  All the time. Sometimes. Rarely. I don't feel this way right now.
- Isolated and alienated in your work?
  All the time. Sometimes. Rarely. I don't feel this way right now.
- Numb or detached?
  All the time. Sometimes. Rarely. I don't feel this way right now.
- Preoccupied with thoughts of your clients outside of work?
  All the time. Sometimes. Rarely. I don't feel this way right now.
- A loss of hope, pessimistic, more cynical?
  All the time. Sometimes. Rarely. I don't feel this way right now.
- Insecure about your self-worth or capabilities?
  All the time. Sometimes. Rarely. I don't feel this way right now.
- Dissatisfied with your work?
  All the time. Sometimes. Rarely. I don't feel this way right now.
- A high overall distress level?
  All the time. Sometimes. Rarely. I don't feel this way right now.
  That you can help every client who enters your office?
  All the time. Sometimes. Rarely. I don't feel this way right now.
- Avoidant of traumatic stories that are difficult or triggering for you?
  All the time. Sometimes. Rarely. I don't feel this way right now.
- Urgency to distance yourself from your clients?
  All the time. Sometimes. Rarely. I don't feel this way right now.
- Distracted in session?
  All the time. Sometimes. Rarely. I don't feel this way right now.
- Maintaining boundaries with your clients is difficult or triggering?
  All the time. Sometimes. Rarely. I don't feel this way right now.
- Unfocused or sleepy in session?
  All the time. Sometimes. Rarely. I don't feel this way right now.
- Doubtful of your competence and ability to help your client?
  All the time. Sometimes. Rarely. I don't feel this way right now.

Worried that no matter what you do, it will **not be enough?**
All the time. Sometimes. Rarely. I don't feel this way right now.
- **Unsure about whether you have chosen the right line of work?**
All the time. Sometimes. Rarely. I don't feel this way right now.
- Take things **too personally**
All the time. Sometimes. Rarely. I don't feel this way right now.

Now notice your vulnerabilities and try to determine the level of intervention you need. Are you feeling many of these ways all the time? Perhaps you need to consider how to take a day or two off, reduce your caseload, seek additional supervision or therapeutic support for yourself. Are you feeling these ways sometimes or rarely? Maybe implementing increased self-care and self-help will be rejuvenating and prevent you from worsening symptoms. Feeling well right now? Keep taking good care of yourself and remember it is never a bad idea to increase self-care if you can, even when you feel good.

The Art of Holding Yourself

Taking good care of yourself is not easy but your success at holding is contingent upon your ability to treat yourself with the same respect and attention you impart on your clients. Start with small and achievable goals. Be realistic. Discover what works for you, what feels good, what feels right. Disregard what seems to work for others. Pay little attention to the memes that flash on the internet or the promises of well-being. What does work is for you to find and utilize simple and doable techniques that resonate for you personally.

I am well aware of what forms of self-care work best for me. It is difficult for me to invest myself in a mindfulness practice, anxiety provoking to take a yoga class, and I loathe gyms. I have a love-hate partnership with my treadmill. I am, however, good at working hard and equally good at doing nothing with zero guilt. I recognize that the practice of doing nothing sometimes is my self-regulation strategy, my self-care. I can binge-watch *a good show on Netflix* for hours with no guilt about the fact that my husband is folding laundry beside me. I can choose to take a long walk with the dogs when I should be writing for a deadline. People who know me well know that I am seriously good at spoiling myself, putting my needs first, and spending endless hours sharing cozy space with people I love, along with an occasional Dorito. Spending enough time taking care of myself allows me to start my days with plenty of space to hold. But that space fills quickly with the distress of my clients and their demands. We know that if we are mentally, physically, or emotionally depleted we will not be effective. Therefore, I rely on a few favorites for taking care of myself as well as in-the-moment self-regulation, as needed:

Dr. Andrew Weil's 4-7-8 Breathing

On his website and in his videos Dr. Andrew Weil (n.d.) teaches the *4–7–8 breathing exercise*:

Exhale completely
Close your mouth and inhale through your nose for the count of 4.
Hold your breath to the count of 7.
Exhale completely through your mouth to a count of 8.
This is one breath.
Repeat the cycle three more times for a total of four breaths.

Dr. Weil claims this diaphragmatic breathing can be calming and invigorating at the same time. With practice, this becomes second nature and no one can tell your breathing pattern has changed.

Kristin Neff's Self Compassion Break

Kristin Neff, PhD (2011), a pioneer in research on self-compassion, points out the irony that being good to yourself in fact will help you be good to others. Neff's body of research suggests increasing evidence to indicate that self-compassion helps us sustain compassionate actions, develop coping skills, decrease negative emotions and fear of failure, and increase accepting thoughts, capacity for forgiveness, resiliency, and motivation, Furthermore, studies suggest that a capacity for self-compassion may help protect against anxiety and depression (Neff, 2003; Neff et al., 2007) and is associated with psychological strengths such as happiness, optimism, wisdom, curiosity and exploration, personal initiative, and emotional intelligence (Heffernan et al., 2010; Hollis-Walker & Colosimo, 2011; Neff et al., 2007).

I often recommend that clients and therapists I mentor learn Neff's self-compassion break. As an antidote on behalf of your clients' broken spirit and propensity for putting the needs of others ahead of their own, self-compassion offers the courage to soothe the aching soul by momentarily letting go of negative emotions. It is believed that the negative feelings will continue to fade over time as long as one doesn't intensify them by resisting or perseverating on them. Self-compassion is a way of actually *being with* the pain, learning to tolerate it, and eventually move through it. This is a priceless lesson for you and for your clients.

In moments of distress, say to yourself:

(Neff suggests putting your hands gently upon your chest)

1 *This is a moment of suffering* (mindfulness).
2 *Suffering is a part of life* (humanity).
3 *May I be kind to myself in this moment* (kindness).

Dr. Sandra Bond Chapman's Brain Rest

Dr. Sandra Bond Chapman, author of *Make Your Brain Smarter: Increase Your Brain's Creativity, Energy, and Focus* (2014), suggests a resting principle for the brain where you take a break from whatever you are involved with, five times a day for at least five minutes, to reset the brain. She says that resting the brain is a more efficient way to use its power, increasing mental productivity and preventing what she calls "brain drain" (p. 12).

After the pandemic, Dr. Chapman said our world has been "turned upside down" which takes a toll on the brain. On an episode of "Brain Storm," Dr. Chapman offers strategies to help teach our brains how to cope with stress:

- Understand your individual stress, learn what makes it change from manageable to high levels of distress.
- Breathe in slowly, then breathe out. Repeat this a few times.
- Spend time in nature, look at flowers, touch the grass.
- Come up with two things you can do in 30 minutes to accomplish a small victory.
- Focus on one or two positive things that have happened during the day.
- Laughter is excellent medicine for the brain. Try to find things to laugh about every day.
- Reduce the amount of negative information (social media, news reports). Too much exposure builds negative neural networks that your brain locks onto.
- Take breaks, give yourself permission to step back from the burden of responsibility, for example, to experience the joy of being a family.
- Try to avoid worries over one to two months from now. Your brain can figure out a way through shorter time frames.

Although none of us can expect to remain immune from the slings and arrows of this delicate work, there are steps we can take to protect ourselves from the unavoidable emotional toll. Appropriate self-care demonstrates a healthy respect for yourself and your clients. Because our psychological well-being directly affects the therapeutic process and the well-being of your client, this is not a luxury. It is essential.

References

ACOG. (2018). ACOG Committee opinion no. 757: Screening for perinatal depression. *Obstetrics and Gynecology, 132*(5), e208–e212. doi:10.1097/AOG.0000000000002927

Adlington, K., Vasquez, C., Pearce, E., Wilson, C. A., Nowland, R., Taylor, B. L., Spring, S., & Johnson, S. (2023). "Just snap out of it" – the experience of loneliness in women with perinatal depression: A meta-synthesis of qualitative studies. *BMC Psychiatry, 23.* doi:10.1186/s12888-023-04532-2

Akik, B. K., & Batigun, A. D. (2020). Perinatal post-traumatic stress disorder questionnaire-II (ppq-11): Adaptation, validity, and reliability study. *The Journal of Psychiatry and Neurological Sciences, 33,* 340–350. doi:10.14744/DAJPNS.2020.00102

Akinci, E., Wieser, M. O., Vanscheidt, S., Diop, S., Flasbeck, V., Akinci, B., Stiller, C., Juckel, G., & Mavrogiorgou, P. (2022). Impairments of social interaction in depressive disorder. *Psychiatry Investigation, 19*(3), 178–189. doi:10.30773/pi.2021.0289

American Psychiatric Association. (2022). *Diagnostic and statistical manual of mental disorders* (5th ed., text revision). doi:10.1176/appi.books.9780890425787

Appelbaum, A. H. (2005). Supportive psychotherapy. *Focus, 3*(3), 438–439.

Aragón, O. R., Sharer, E. A., Bargh, J. A., & Pineda, J. A. (2014). Modulations of mirroring activity by desire for social connection and relevance of movement. *Social Cognitive and Affective Neuroscience, 9*(11), 1762–1769. doi:10.1093/scan/nst172

Arnd-Caddigan, M., & Stickle, M. (2017). A psychotherapist's exploration of clinical intuition: A review of the literature and discussion. *International Journal of Integrative Psychotherapy, 8,* 79–102.

Atwood, M. (1988). *Cat's eye.* Doubleday.

Baier, A. L., Kline, A. C., & Feeny, N. C. (2020). Therapeutic alliance as a mediator of change: A systematic review and evaluation of research. *Clinical Psychology Review, 82.* doi:10.1016/j.cpr.2020.101921

Bajaj, M. A., Salimgaraev, R., Zhaunova, L., & Payne, J. L. (2022). Rates of self-reported postpartum depressive symptoms in the United States before and after the start of the COVID-19 pandemic. *Journal of Psychiatric Research, 151,* 108–112. doi:10.1016/j.jpsychires.2022.04.011

Balaram, K., & Marwaha, R. (2022, June 7). *Postpartum Blues*. StatPearls. www.ncbi.nlm.nih.gov/books/NBK554546/

Barker, L. C., Kurdyak, P., Fung, K., Matheson, F. I., & Vigod, S. (2016). Postpartum psychiatric emergency visits: A nested case-control study. *Archives of Women's Mental Health, 19*, 1019–1027.

Battle, C. L., Salisbury, A. L., Schofield, C. A., & Ortiz-Hernandez, S. (2013). Perinatal anti-depressant use: Understanding women's preferences and concerns. *Journal of Psychiatric Practice, 19*, 443–453.

Beck, C. T. (2001). Predictors of postpartum depression. *Nursing Research, 50*(5), 275–285.

Beck, C. T. (2006). Postpartum depression: It isn't just the blues. *American Journal of Nursing, 106*(5), 40–50.

Besse, M., Lampe, N. M., & Mann, E. S. (2020). Experiences with achieving pregnancy and giving birth among transgender men: A narrative literature review. *Yale Journal of Biology and Medicine, 93*(4), 517–528.

Biaggi, A., Conroy, S., Pawlby, S., & Pariante, C. M. (2016). Identifying the women at risk of antenatal anxiety and depression: A systematic review. *Journal of Affective Disorders, 191*, 62–77. doi:10.1016/j.jad.2015.11.014

Boath, E., & Henshaw, C. (2001). The treatment of postnatal depression: A comprehensive literature review. *Journal of Reproductive and Infant Psychology, 19*(3), 215–248.

Bradshaw, H., Riddle, J. D., Salimgaraev, R., Zhaunova, L., & Payne, J. L. (2021). Risk factors associated with postpartum depressive symptoms: A multinational study. *Journal of Affective Disorders, 301*, 345–351.

Bright, K. S., Charrois, E. M., Mughal, M. K., Wajid, A., McNeil, D., Stuart, S., Hayden, K. A., & Kingston, D. (2020). Interpersonal psychotherapy to reduce psychological distress in perinatal women: A systematic review. *International Journal of Environmental Research and Public Health, 17*(22), 8421. doi:10.3390/ijerph17228421

Buchholz, J. L., & Abramowitz, J. S. (2020). The therapeutic alliance in exposure therapy for anxiety-related disorders: A critical review. *Journal of Anxiety Disorders, 70*. doi:10.1016/j.janxdis.2020.102194

Butler, L. D., Carello, J., & Maguin, E. (2017). Trauma, stress, and self-care in clinical training: Predictors of burnout, decline in health status, secondary traumatic stress symptoms, and compassion satisfaction. *Psychological Trauma: Theory, Research, Practice, and Policy, 9*(4), 416–424. doi:10.1037/tra0000187

Canty, H. R., Sauter, A., Zuckerman, K., Cobian, M., & Grigsby, T. (2019). Mothers' perspectives on follow-up for postpartum depression screening in primary care. *Journal of Developmental and Behavioral Pediatrics: JDBP, 40*(2), 139–143. doi:10.1097/DBP.0000000000000628

Carney, D., Cuddy, A. J., & Yap, A. (2010). Power posing: Brief nonverbal displays affect neuroendocrine levels and risk tolerance. *Psychological Science, 21*(10), 1363–1368.

CDC Vital Statistics. (2023, November 29). *Suicide data and statistics*. Centers for Disease Control and Prevention. www.cdc.gov/suicide/suicide-data-statistics.html

Chapman, S. (2014). *Make your brain smarter: Increase your brain's creativity, energy, and focus*. Simon & Schuster.

Chew-Graham, C. A., Sharp, D., Chamberlain, E., Folkes, L., & Turner, K. M. (2009). Disclosure of symptoms of postnatal depression, the perspectives of health professionals and women: A qualitative study. *Biomed Central Family Practice, 10*(1), 7–9.

Chin, K., Wendt, A., Bennett, I. M., & Bhat, A. (2022). Suicide and maternal mortality. *Current Psychiatry Reports, 24,* 239–275. doi:10.1007/s11920-022-01334-3

Collardeau, F., Corbyn, B., Abramowitz, J., Jansen. P., Woody. S., & Fairbrother, N. (2019). Maternal unwanted and intrusive thoughts of infant-related harm, obsessive-compulsive disorder and depression in the perinatal period: Study protocol. *BMC Psychiatry, 19,* 94. https://doi.org/10.1186/s12888-019-2067-x

Conejo-Galindo, J., Sanz-Giancola, A., Álvarez-Mon, M. Á., Ortega, M. Á., Gutiérrez-Rojas, L., & Lahera, G. (2022). Postpartum relapse in patients with bipolar disorder. *Journal of Clinical Medicine, 11*(14), 3979. doi:10.3390/jcm11143979

Connelly, D. M. (1993). *All sickness is home sickness*. Wisdom Well Press.

Corrigan, C. P., Kwasky, A. N., & Groh, C. J. (2015). Social support, postpartum depression, and professional assistance: A survey of mothers in the midwestern United States. *The Journal of Perinatal Education, 2*(1), 48–60. doi:10.1891/1058-1243.24.1.48

Corwin, H. (2012). A secure attachment base is ideal to be a great learner. *Journal of Prenatal and Perinatal Psychology and Health. 27,* 38–46.

Cox, J. L., Holden, J. M., & Sagovsky, R. (1987). Detection of postnatal depression: Development of the 10-item Edinburgh Postnatal Depression Scale. *British Journal of Psychiatry, 150,* 782–786.

Cuddy, A. J., Wilmuth, C. A.,Yap, A. J., & Carney, D. (2015). Preparatory power posing affects nonverbal presence and job interview outcomes. *Journal of Applied Psychology, 100*(4), 1286–1295.

Daehn, D., Rudolf, S., Pawils, S., & Renneberg, B. (2022). Perinatal mental health literacy: Knowledge, attitudes, and help-seeking among perinatal women and the public – a systematic review. *BMC Pregnancy Childbirth, 22.* doi:10.1186/s12884-022-04865-y

Declerq, E. R., Sakala, C., Corry, M. P., Applebaum, S., & Risher, P. (2002, October). *Listening to mothers: Report of the first national US survey of women's childbearing experiences*. Maternity Center Association by Harris Interactive. https://nationalpartnership.org/wp-content/uploads/2023/02/listening-to-mothers-i_2002.pdf

DeFife, J., & Hilsenroth, M. (2011). Starting off on the right foot: Common factor elements in early psychotherapy process. *Journal of Psychotherapy Integration, 21*(2), 172–191.

DeMarneffe, D. (2004). *Maternal desire*. Little Brown & Co.

Dennis, C. L., & Dowswell, T. (2013). Psychosocial and psychological interventions for preventing postpartum depression. *Cochrane Database of Systematic Reviews, 2.* doi:10.1002/14651858.CD001134.pub3

Eddy, B., Poll, V., Whiting, J., & Clevesy, M. (2019). Forgotten fathers: Postpartum depression in men. *Journal of Family Issues, 40*(8), 1001–1017.

Eggenberger, L., Ehlert, U., & Walther, A. (2023). New directions in male-tailored psychotherapy for depression. *Frontiers in Psychology, 14.* doi:10.3389/fpsyg.2023.1146078

Elkjær, E., Mikkelsen, M. B., Michalak, J., Mennin, D. S., & O'Toole, M. S. (2022). Expansive and contractive postures and movement: A systematic review and meta-analysis of the effect of motor displays on affective and behavioral responses. *Perspectives on Psychological Science, 17*(1), 276–304. doi:10.1177/1745691620919358

Epp, R., Malcolm, J., Jolin-Dahel, K., Clermont, M., & Keely, E. (2021). Postpartum thyroiditis. *BMJ (Clinical research ed.), 372,* (n495). doi:10.1136/bmj.n495

Fairbrother, N., & Abramowitz, J. (2007). New parenthood as a risk factor for the development of obsessional problems. *Behaviour Research and Therapy, 45,* 2155–2163.

Farr, S. L., Dietz, P. M., Williams, J. R., Gibbs, F. A., & Tregear, S. (2011). Depression screening and treatment among nonpregnant women of reproductive age in the United States, 1990–2010. *Preventing Chronic Disease, 8*(6), A122.

Feinberg, E., Declercq, E., Lee, A., & Belanoff, C. (2022). The relationship between social support and postnatal anxiety and depression: Results from the listening to mothers in California survey. *Women's Health Issues, 32*(3), 251–260.

Field, T. (2014). Integrating left-brain and right-brain: The neuroscience of effective counseling. *The Professional Counselor, 4,* 19–27. doi:10.15241/taf.4.1.19

Foli, K. J., South, S. C., Lim, E., & Jarnecke, A. M. (2016). Post-adoption depression: Parental classes of depressive symptoms across time. *Journal of Affective Disorders, 200,* 293–302. doi:10.1016/j.jad.2016.01.049

Forray, A., Focseneanu, M., Pittman, B., McDougle, C. J., & Epperson, C. N. (2010). Onset and exacerbation of obsessive-compulsive disorder in pregnancy and the postpartum period. *Journal of Clinical Psychiatry, 71*(8), 1061–1068. doi:10.4088/JCP.09m05381blu

Fowler, G., Cope, C., Michalski, D., Christidis, P., Lin, L., & Conroy, J. (2018). Women outnumber men in psychology graduate programs. *Monitor on Psychology, 49*(11), 21.

Freud, S. (1910). *The future prospect of psychoanalytic therapy* (Standard ed.). Hogarth Press.

Gaynes, B. N., Gavin, N., Meltzer-Brody, S., Lohr, K. N., Swinson, T., Gartlehner, G., Brody, S., & Miller, W. C. (2005). Perinatal depression: Prevalence, screening accuracy, and screening outcomes. *Evidence Report/Technology Assessment (Summary), 119,* 1–8. doi:10.1037/e439372005-001

Goldstein, E. (2015). *Uncovering happiness: Overcoming depression with mindfulness and self-compassion.* Atria Books.

Good, G., & Beitman, B. (2006). *Counseling and psychotherapy essentials: Integrating theory, skills, and practice.* W.W. Norton & Company.

Goodman, J. H., & Tyer-Viola, L. (2010). Detection, treatment, and referral of perinatal depression and anxiety by obstetrical providers. *Journal of Women's Health, 19*(3), 477–490.

Gorka, S. M., Young, C. B., Klumpp, H., Kennedy, A. E., Francis, J., Ajilore, O., Langenecker, S. A., Shankman, S. A., Craske, M. G., Stein, M. B., & Phan, K. L. (2019). Emotion-based brain mechanisms and predictors for SSRI and CBT treatment of anxiety and depression: A randomized trial. *Neuropsychopharmacology*, *44*(9), 1639–1648. doi:10.1038/s41386-019-0407-7

Goyal, D., Gay, C., & Lee, K. (2010). How much does low socioeconomic status increase the risk of prenatal and postpartum depressive symptoms in first time mothers? *Women's Health Issues*, *20*(2), 96–104.

Grosch, W. N., & Olsen, D. C. (1994). *When helping starts to hurt*. Norton.

Grover, S., Avasthi, A., & Jagiwala, M. (2020). Clinical practice guidelines for practice of supportive psychotherapy. *Indian Journal of Psychiatry*, *2*(Suppl 2), S173–S182. doi:10.4103/psychiatry.IndianJPsychiatry_768_19

Guillemette, T. N., Monn, J. L., & Chronister, M. (2023). An evidence-based project to improve paternal postpartum depression. *The Journal for Nurse Practitioners*, *19*(4). doi:10.1016/j.nurpra.2022.11.005

Guintivano, J., Manuck, T., & Meltzer-Brody, S. (2018). Predictors of postpartum depression: A comprehensive review of the last decade of evidence. *Clinical Obstetrics and Gynecology*, *61*(3), 591–603.

Gutheil, T. G., & Gabbard, G. O. (1998). Misuses and misunderstandings of boundary theory in clinical and regulatory settings. *American Journal of Psychiatry*, *155*(3), 409–414.

Heffernan, M., Quinn Griffin, M. T., McNulty, S. R., & Fitzpatrick, J. J. (2010). Self-compassion and emotional intelligence in nurses. *International Journal of Nursing Practice*, *16*, 366–373.

Held, L., & Rutherford, A. (2012). Can't a mother sing the blues? Postpartum depression and the construction of motherhood in late 20th-century America. *History of Psychology*, *15*, 107–123.

Henshaw, C. (2003). Mood disturbance in the early puerperium: A review. *Archives of Women's Mental Health*, *6*, Suppl 2, S33–S42.

Heyne, C. S., Kazmierczak, M., Souday, R., Horesh, D., Lambregtse-van den Berg, M., Weigl, T., Horsch, A., Oosterman, M., Dikmen-Yildiz, P., & Garthus-Niegel, S. (2022). Prevalence and risk factors of birth-related posttraumatic stress among parents: A comparative systematic review and meta-analysis. *Clinical Psychology Review*, *94*, 102157. doi:10.1016/j.cpr.2022.102157

Hills, P. J., & Lewis, M. B. (2011). Sad people avoid the eyes or happy people focus on the eyes? Mood induction affects facial feature discrimination. *British Journal of Psychology*, *102*(2), 260–274.

Hilty, D. M., Ferrer, D. C., Parish, M. B., Johnston, B., Callahan, E. J., & Yellowlees, P. M. (2013). The effectiveness of telemental health: A 2013 review. *Telemedicine Journal and E-Health: The Official Journal of the American Telemedicine Association*, *19*(6), 444–454. doi:10.1089/tmj.2013.0075

Hollis-Walker, L., & Colosimo, K. (2011). Mindfulness, self-compassion, and happiness in non-mediators: A theoretical and empirical examination. *Personality and Individual Differences*, *50*, 222–227.

Horvath, A. O., & Symonds, B. D. (1991). Relation between working alliance and outcome in psychotherapy: A meta-analysis. *Journal of Counseling Psychology*, *38*, 139–149.

Iacoboni, M. (2008). The mirror neuron revolution: Explaining what makes humans social. *Scientific American.* www.scientificamerican.com/article/the-mirror-neuron-revolut/

Inekwe, J. N., & Lee, E. (2022). Perceived social support on postpartum mental health: An instrumental variable analysis. *PloS one, 17*(5), e0265941. doi:10.1371/journal.pone.0265941

Jamshaid, S., Malik, N. I., Ullah, I., Saboor, S., Arain, F., & De Berardis, D. (2023). Postpartum depression and health: Role of perceived social support among women. *Preprints.* doi:10.20944/preprints202301.0018.v1

Joinson, C. (1992). Coping with compassion fatigue. *Nursing, 22,* 116–122.

Jones, A. (2022). Postpartum help-seeking: The role of stigma and mental health literacy. *Maternal and Child Health Journal, 26,* 1030–1037. doi:10.1007/s10995-022-03399-1

Joshi, S. (2020, June 25). Online health platforms see spike in mental health queries amidst COVID-19 pandemic. *Times of India.* https://timesofindia.indiatimes.com/home/sunday-times/online-health-platforms-see-spike-in-mental-health-queries-amidst-COVID-19-pandemic/articleshow/76630185.cms

Kaplan, V. (2023). Mental health states of housewives: An evaluation in terms of self-perception and codependency. *International Journal of Mental Health and Addiction, 21,* 666–683. doi:10.1007/s11469-022-00910-1

Keefe, R. H., Brownstein-Evans, C., & Rouland Polmanteer, R. S. (2016). Having our say: African American and Latina mothers provide recommendations to health and mental health providers working with new mothers living with postpartum depression. *Social Work in Mental Health, 14*(5), 497–508.

Kendall-Tackett, K. A. (2014). Birth trauma: The causes and consequences of childbirth-related trauma and PTSD. In D. L. Barnes (Ed.), *Women's reproductive mental health across the lifespan* (pp. 177–195). Springer.

Kirsch, I. (2019). Placebo effect in the treatment of depression and anxiety. *Frontiers in Psychiatry, 10.* doi:10.3389/fpsyt.2019.00407

Kleiman, K. (2009). *Therapy and the postpartum woman: Notes on healing postpartum depression for clinicians and the women who seek their help.* Routledge.

Kleiman, K. (2022). *Therapy and the postpartum woman.* Routledge Mental Health Classic Edition.

Kleiman, K., & Raskin, V. D. (1994). *This isn't what I expected: Overcoming postpartum depression.* Da Capo Press.

Kleiman, K., & Raskin, V. D. (2013). *This isn't what I expected: Overcoming postpartum depression* (2nd ed.). Da Capo Press.

Kleiman, K., & Waller, H. (2023). The art of holding perinatal women in distress. *Women's Health Reports, 4*(1), 111–117. doi:10.1089/whr.2022.0083

Kleiman, K., & Wenzel, A. (2017) Principles of supportive psychotherapy for perinatal distress. *Journal of Obstetric, Gynecologic & Neonatal Nursing, 46*(6), 895–903.

Kleiman, K., Wenzel, A., Waller, H., & Adler-Mandel, A. (2020). *Dropping the baby and other scary thoughts: Breaking the cycle of unwanted thoughts in motherhood* (2nd ed.). Routledge.

Klerman, G. L., Weissman, M. M., Rounsaville, B., & Chevron, E. (1984). *Interpersonal psychotherapy for depression.* Basic Books.

Kottler, J. A. (2003). *On being a therapist* (3rd ed.). Jossey-Bass.

Kross, E., Bruehlman-Senecal, E., Park, J., Burson, A., Dougherty, A., Shablack, H., Bremner, R., Moser, J., & Ayduk, O. (2014). Self-talk as a regulatory mechanism: How you do it matters. *Journal of Personality and Social Psychology, 106*(2), 304–324.

LaCour, N. (2009). *Hold still.* Dutton Books.

Lamere, K., & Golova, N. (2022). Screening for postpartum depression during infant well child visits: A retrospective chart review. *Clinical Pediatrics, 61*(10), 699–706. doi:10.1177/00099228221097272

LaRocco-Cockburn, A., Melville, J., Bell, M., & Katon, W. (2003). Depression screening attitudes and practices among obstetrician-gynecologists. *Obstetrics & Gynecology, 101*, 892–898.

Lazarus, R. S., & Folkman, S. (1984). *Stress, appraisal, and coping.* Springer.

Leichsenring, F., Sarrar, L., & Steinert, C. (2019). Drop-outs in psychotherapy: A change of perspective. *World Psychiatry, 18*(1), 32–33. doi:10.1002/wps.20588

Lewis, H. B. (1986). The role of shame in depression. In M. Rutter, C. E. Izard, & P. B. Read (Eds.), *Depression in young people: Developmental and clinical perspectives* (pp. 325–339). Guilford.

Li, X., Laplante, D. P., Paquin, V., Lafortune, S., Elgbeili, G., & King, S. (2022). Effectiveness of cognitive behavioral therapy for perinatal maternal depression, anxiety, and stress: A systematic review and meta-analysis of randomized controlled trials. *Clinical Psychology Review, 92.* doi:10.1016/j.cpr.2022.102129

Lindahl, V., Pearson, J. L., & Colpe, L. (2005). Prevalence of suicidality during pregnancy and the postpartum. *Archives of Women's Mental Health, 8*(2), 77–87.

Liu, R. T., Bettis, A. H., & Burke, T. A. (2020). Characterizing the phenomenology of passive suicidal ideation: A systematic review and meta-analysis of its prevalence, psychiatric comorbidity, correlates, and comparisons with active suicidal ideation. *Psychological Medicine, 50*(3), 367–383. doi:10.1017/S003329171900391X

MacDonald, T., Noel-Weiss, J., West, D., Walks, M., Biener, M., Kibbe, A., & Myler, E. (2016). Transmasculine individuals' experiences with lactation, chestfeeding, and gender identity: A qualitative study. *BMC Pregnancy Childbirth, 16.* doi:10.1186/s12884-016-0907-y

Malhotra, S., & Sahoo, S. (2017). Rebuilding the brain with psychotherapy. *Indian Journal of Psychiatry, 59*(4), 411–419. https://doi.org/10.4103/0019-5545.217299

Manso-Córdoba, S., Pickering, S., Ortega, M. A., Asúnsolo, Á., & Romero, D. (2020). Factors related to seeking help for postpartum depression: A secondary analysis of New York City PRAMS data. *International Journal of Environmental Research and Public Health, 17*(24), 9328. doi:10.3390/ijerph17249328

Marks-Tarlow, T. (2012). *Clinical intuition in psychotherapy: The neurobiology of embodied response.* W.W. Norton.

Maslach, C. (2003). *Burnout: The cost of caring.* Malor Books.

Mason, T. M., Tofthagen, C. S., & Buck, H. G. (2020). Complicated grief: Risk factors, protective factors, and interventions. *Journal of Social Work in End-of-Life & Palliative Care, 16*(2), 151–174. doi:10.1080/15524256.2020.1745726

Mathieu, F. (2011). *The compassion fatigue workbook: Creative tools for transforming compassion fatigue and vicarious traumatization* (Psychosocial Stress Series). Routledge.

Maushart, S. (2000). *The mask of motherhood: How becoming a mother changes our lives and we never talk about it*. Penguin Books.

Mauthner, N. S. (1999). Feeling low and feeling really bad about feeling low: Women's experiences of motherhood and postpartum depression. *Canadian Psychology, 40*(2), 143–161.

Mauthner, N. S. (2002). *The darkest days of my life: Stories of postpartum depression*. Harvard University Press.

Mayo Clinic Staff. (2023, February 11). *Fatigue*. Mayo Clinic. www.mayoclinic.org/symptoms/fatigue/basics/causes/sym-20050894

McGowan, F. J. (1957). The doctor talks about postnatal blues. *McCall's, 84*(4), 143.

McKee, K., Admon, L. K., Winkelman, T. N. A., Muzik, M., Hall, S., Dalton, V. K., & Zivin, K. (2020). Perinatal mood and anxiety disorders, serious mental illness, and delivery-related health outcomes, United States, 2006–2015. *BMC Women's Health, 20*, 150. doi:10.1186/s12905-020-00996-6

McKenzie, S. K., Oliffe, J. L., Black, A., & Collings, S. (2022). Men's experiences of mental illness stigma across the lifespan: A scoping review. *American Journal of Men's Health, 16*(1), 15579883221074789. doi:10.1177/15579883221074789

Milgrom, J., Gemmill, A. W., Bilszta, J. L., Hayes, B., Barnett, B., Brooks, J., Ericksen, J., Ellwood, D., & Buist, A. (2008). Antenatal risk factors for postnatal depression: A large prospective study. *Journal of Affective Disorders, 108*(1–2), 147–157.

Mills, R. S. (2005). Taking stock of the developmental literature on shame. *Developmental Review, 25*, 26–63.

Morgan, A. (2000). *What is narrative therapy? An easy-to-read introduction*. Dulwich Centre Publications.

Morgan, A. (2002). Beginning the use a narrative approach in therapy. *The International Journal of Narrative Therapy and Community Work, 1*, 85–90.

Moss, L. (2023). Proudly Jewish – and averse to circumcision. *Narrative Inquiry in Bioethics, 13*(2), 86–89.

Naji Rad, S., & Deluxe, L. (2023, June 12). *Postpartum Thyroiditis*. StatPearls. www.ncbi.nlm.nih.gov/books/NBK557646/

Neff, K. D. (2003). Self-compassion: An alternative conceptualization of a healthy attitude toward oneself. *Self and Identity, 2*, 85–101.

Neff, K. D. (2011). *Self-compassion*. William Morrow.

Neff, K. D., Rude, S. S., & Kirkpatrick, K. L. (2007). An examination of self-compassion in relation to positive psychological functioning and personality traits. *Journal of Research in Personality, 41*, 908–916.

Negron, R., Martin, A., Almog, M., Balbierz, A., & Howell, E. (2013). Social support during the postpartum: Mother's views on needs, expectations, and mobilization of support. *Maternal Child Health Journal, 17*, 616–623.

Nelson, T., Cardemil, E. V., Overstreet, N. M., Hunter, C. D., & Woods-Giscombé, C. L. (2024). Association between superwoman schema, depression, and resilience: The mediating role of social isolation and gendered racial centrality. *Cultural Diversity & Ethnic Minority Psychology, 30*(1), 95–106. doi:10.1037/cdp0000533

Nelson, T., Tomi, C. L., & Gebretensay, S. B. (2023). (Re)framing strength: How superwoman schema may impact perinatal anxiety and depression among African American women. *Women's Health Issues, 33*(6), 568–572.

Ngai, F-W., & Gao, L-L. (2022). Effect of couple-based interpersonal psychotherapy on postpartum depressive symptoms: A randomised controlled trial. *Asian Journal of Psychiatry, 78.* doi:10.1016/j.ajp.2022.103274

Nicolson, P. (2001). *Postnatal depression—facing the paradox of lost happiness & motherhood.* Wiley.

NIDA. (2022, May 4). *Sex and gender differences in substance use.* NIDA. https://nida.nih.gov/publications/research-reports/substance-use-in-women/sex-gender-differences-in-substance-use

O'Hara, M. W., & Swain, A. M. (1996). Rates and risk of postpartum depression – A meta-analysis. *International Review of Psychiatry, 8,* 37–54.

Orchard, E. R., Rutherford, H. J. V., Holmes, A. J., & Jamadar, S. D. (2023). Matrescence: Lifetime impact of motherhood on cognition and the brain. *Trends in Cognitive Sciences, 27*(3), 302–316. doi:10.1016/j.tics.2022.12.002

Orena, A. J., Mader, A. S., & Werker, J. F. (2022). Learning to recognize unfamiliar voices: An online study with 12- and 24-month-olds. *Frontiers in Psychology, 13.* doi:10.3389/fpsyg.2022.874411

Papousek, M. (2007). Communication in early infancy: An arena of intersubjective learning. *Infant Behavior & Development, 30,* 258–266.

Pearlman, L. A., & Saakvitne, K. W. (1995). *Trauma and the therapist: Countertransference and vicarious traumatization in psychotherapy with incest survivors.* W.W. Norton.

Peindl, K. S., Wisner, K. L., & Hanusa, B. H. (2004). Identifying depression in the first postpartum year: Guidelines for office-based screening and referral. *Journal of Affective Disorders, 80*(1), 37–44.

Pereira, A. T., Araújo, A., Azevedo, J., Marques, C. C., Soares, M. J., Cabaços, C., Marques, M., Pereira, D., Pato, M., & Macedo, A. (2022). The postpartum obsessive-compulsive scale: Psychometric, operative and epidemiologic study in a Portuguese sample. *International Journal of Environmental Research and Public Health, 19*(17), 10624. doi:10.3390/ijerph191710624

Peterson, Z. (2002). More than a mirror: The ethics of therapist self-disclosure. *Psychotherapy: Theory, Research, Practice, Training, 39*(1), 21–31.

Pezaro, S., Crowther, R., Pearce, G., Jowett, A., Godfrey-Isaacs, L., Samuels, I., & Valentine, V. (2023). Perinatal care for trans and nonbinary people birthing in heteronormative "maternity" services: Experiences and educational needs of professionals. *Gender & Society, 37*(1), 124–151. doi:10.1177/08912432221138086

Pilkington, P., Milne, L., Cairns, K., & Whelan, T. (2016). Enhancing reciprocal partner support to prevent perinatal depression and anxiety: A Delphi consensus study. *BioMed Central Psychiatry, 16*(1), 23.

Pitt, B. (1973). Maternity blues. *British Journal of Psychiatry, 122,* 431–433.

Posluns, K., & Gall, T. L. (2020). Dear mental health practitioners, take care of yourselves: A literature review on self-care. *International Journal for the Advancement of Counseling, 42*(1), 1–20. doi:10.1007/s10447-019-09382-w

Raphael, D. (1973). *The tender gift: Breastfeeding.* Prentice-Hall.

Reik, T. (1948). *Listening with the third ear: The inner experience of a psychoanalyst*. Grove Press.

Rogers, C. (1957). Training individuals to engage in the therapeutic process. In C. R. Strother (Ed.), *Psychology and mental health* (pp. 76–92). American Psychological Association.

Rogers, C. (1975). Empathic—an unappreciated way of being. *The Counseling Psychologist, 5*(2), 2–10.

Roseth, I., Binder, P., & Malt, U. F. (2011). Two ways of living through postpartum depression. *Journal of Phenomenological Psychology, 42*(2), 174–194.

Ross, E., Murphy, S., O'Hagan, D., Maguire, A., & O'Reilly, D. (2023). Emergency department presentations with suicide and self-harm ideation: A missed opportunity for intervention? *Epidemiology and Psychiatric Sciences, 32*, E24. doi:10.1017/S2045796023000203

Rothschild, B. (2006). *Help for the helper: The psychophysiology of compassion fatigue and vicarious trauma*. W.W. Norton & Company.

Sampson, M., Yu, M., Mauldin, R., Mayorga, A., & Gonzalez, L. G. (2021). "You withhold what you are feeling so you can have a family": Latinas' perceptions on community values and postpartum depression. *Family Medicine and Community Health, 9*(3), e000504. doi:10.1136/fmch-2020-000504

Scarff, J. R. (2019). Postpartum depression in men. *Innovations in Clinical Neuroscience, 16*(5–6), 11–14.

Shapiro, Y., & Marks-Tarlow, T. (2021). Varieties of clinical intuition: Explicit, implicit, and nonlocal neurodynamics. *Psychoanalytic Dialogues, 31*(3), 262–281.

Sichel, D. A., Cohen, L. S., Dimmock, J. A., & Rosenbaum, J. F. (1993). Postpartum obsessive-compulsive disorder: A case series. *Journal of Clinical Psychiatry, 54*, 156–159.

Sim, C. S. M., Chen, H., Chong, S. L., Xia, O. J., Chew, E., Guo, X., Ng, L. P., Ch'ng, Y. C., Ong, J. L. H., Tan, J., Ng, D. C. C., Tan, N. C., & Chan, Y. H. (2023). Primary health level screening for postpartum depression during well-child visits: Prevalence, associated risk factors, and breastfeeding. *Asian Journal of Psychiatry, 87*. doi:10.1016/j.ajp.2023.103701

Simhi, M., Sarid, O., & Cwikel, J. (2019). Preferences for mental health treatment for post-partum depression among new mothers. *Israel Journal of Health Policy Research, 8*(1), 84. doi:10.1186/s13584-019-0354-0

Skovholt, T. M. (2001). *The resilient practitioner: Burnout prevention and self-care strategies for counselors, therapists, teachers, and health professionals*. Allyn & Bacon.

Slomian, J., Honvo, G., Emonts, P., Reginster, J-Y., & Bruyère, O. (2019). Consequences of maternal postpartum depression: A systematic review of maternal and infant outcomes. *Women's Health, 15*. doi:10.1177/1745506519844044

Smith, R. E., Fagan, C., Wilson, N. L., Chen, J., Corona, M., Nguyen, H., Racz, S., & Shoda, Y. (2011). Internet-based approaches to collaborative therapeutic assessment: New opportunities for professional psychologists. *Professional Psychology: Research and Practice, 42*(6), 494–504.

Sockol, L. E. (2015). A systematic review of the efficacy of cognitive behavioral therapy for treating and preventing perinatal depression. *Journal of Affective Disorders, 177*, 7–21.

Solomon, A. (2015). *Pregnant women with depression face tough choices, no easy answers.* NPR. www.npr.org/sections/health-shots/2015/06/04/411978777/pregnant-women-with-depression-face-tough-choices-no-easy-answers

Spinelli, M. G. (2009). Postpartum psychosis: Detection of risk and management. *American Journal of Psychiatry, 166*(4), 405–408.

Tobin, E. J. (2020). Infant-directed speech of Australian English mothers and fathers: A high and variable pitch with a more breathy and less creaky voice quality. Macquarie University. Thesis. doi:10.25949/19444619.v1

Tolle, E. (2004). *The power of now.* Namaste Publishing.

Tosto, V., Ceccobelli, M., Lucarini, E., Tortorella, A., Gerli, S., Parazzini, F., & Favilli, A. (2023). Maternity Blues: A narrative review. *Journal of Personalized Medicine, 13*, 154. doi: 10.3390/jpm13010154

Tryon, G. S., Birch, S. E., & Verkuilen, J. (2018). Meta-analyses of the relation of goal consensus and collaboration to psychotherapy outcome. *Psychotherapy, 55*(4), 372–383. doi:10.1037/pst0000170

Usmani, S., Greca, E., Javed, S., Sharath, M., Sarfraz, Z., Sarfraz, A., Salari, S. W., Hussaini, S. S., Mohammadi, A., Chellapuram, N., Cabrera, E., & Ferrer, G. (2021). Risk factors for postpartum depression during COVID-19 pandemic: A systematic literature review. *Journal of Primary Care & Community Health, 12*, 21501327211059348. doi:10.1177/21501327211059348

Viswasam, K., Berle, D., Milicevic, D., & Starcevic, V. (2021). Prevalence and onset of anxiety and related disorders throughout pregnancy: A prospective study in an Australian sample. *Psychiatry Research, 297*, 113721. doi:10.1016/j.psychres.2021.113721

Walsh, T., Davis, R., & Garfield, C. (2020). A call to action: Screening fathers for perinatal depression. *Pediatrics, 145*(1), e20191193.

Waugh, L. J. (2011). Beliefs associated with Mexican immigrant families' practice of la cuarentena during postpartum recovery. *Journal of Obstetric, Gynecologic, & Neonatal Nursing: Clinical Scholarship for the Care of Women, Childbearing Families, & Newborns, 40*(6), 732–741. doi:10.1111/j.1552-6909.2011.01298.x

Weil, A. (n.d.). *Spirit & inspiration: Breathing: Three exercises.* Dr. Weil. www.drweil.com/drw/u/ART00521/three-breathing-exercises.html

Weissman, M. M., Wickramaratne, P., Nomura, Y., Warner, V., Pilowsky, D., & Verdeli, H. (2006). Offspring of depressed parents: 20 years later. *American Journal of Psychiatry, 163*(6), 1001–1008.

Wenzel, A., & Kleiman, K. (2014). *Cognitive behavioral therapy for perinatal distress.* Routledge.

White, M. (1997). *Narratives of therapists' lives.* Dulwich Centre Publications.

Whitton, A., Appleby, L., & Warner, R. (1996a). Maternal thinking and the treatment of postnatal depression. *International Journal of Psychiatry, 8*, 73–78.

Whitton, A., Warner, R., & Appleby, L. (1996b). The pathway to care in postnatal depression: Women's attitudes to postnatal depression and its treatment. *British Journal of General Practice, 46*, 427–428.

Winnicott, D. W. (1953). Transitional objects and transitional phenomena – a study of the first not-me possession. *International Journal of Psychoanalysis, 34*, 89–97.

Winnicott, D. W. (1956). Primary maternal preoccupation. In *Through paediatrics to psychoanalysis* (pp. 300–305). Basic Books.

Winnicott, D. W. (1960). The theory of the parent-infant relationship. In *The maturational processes and the facilitating environment: Studies in the theory of emotional development* (pp. 585–595). International Universities Press.

Winnicott, D. W. (1963) From dependence towards independence in the development of the individual. In *The maturational processes and the facilitating environment* (pp. 83–92). Karnac.

Winnicott, D. W. (1965). The maturational processes and the facilitating environment: Studies in the theory of emotional development. In *The international psycho-analytical library* (Vol. 64, pp. 1–276). The Hogarth Press and the Institute of Psychoanalysis.

Winnicott, D. W. (1967). Mirror-role of the mother and family in child development. In P. Lomas (Ed.), *The predicament of the family: A Psychoanalytical symposium* (pp. 26–33). Hogarth Press.

Winnicott, D. W. (1969). The use of an object. *International Journal of Psychoanalysis*, *50*, 711–716.

Winnicott, D. W. (1987a). *Babies and their mothers (A Merloyd Larence Book)*. Da Capo Press.

Winnicott, D. W. (1987b). *The child, the family, and the outside world*. Addison Wesley.

Winnicott, D. W. (1992). *Through paediatrics to psychoanalysis*. Basic Books.

Winnicott, D. W. (2002). *Winnicott on the child*. Da Capo Press.

Winnicott, D. W. (2005). *Playing and reality* (2nd ed.). Routledge.

Wisner, K. L., Peindl, K., & Hanusa, B. (1996). Effects of childbearing on the natural history of panic disorder with comorbid mood disorder. *Journal of Affective Disorders*, *41*, 173–180.

Wisner, K. L., Sit, D. Y., McShea, M. C., Rizzo, D., Zoretich, R., Hughes, C., Eng, H., Luther, J., Wisniewski, S., Costantino, M., Confer, A., Moses-Kolko, E., Famy, C., & Hanusa, B. (2013). Onset timing, thoughts of self-harm, and diagnoses in postpartum women with screen-positive depression findings. *Journal of American Medical Association Psychiatry*, *70*(5), 490–498.

Yager, J., Kay, J., & Kelsay, K. (2021). Clinicians' cognitive and affective biases and the practice of psychotherapy. *American Journal of Psychotherapy*, *74*(3), 101–138.

Yang, L., Long, Z., Cao, D., & Cao, F. (2017). Social support and depression across the perinatal period: A longitudinal study. *Journal of Clinical Nursing*, *26*(17–18), 2776–2783. doi:10.1111/jocn.13817

Zauderer, C. (2009). Postpartum depression: How childbirth educators can help break the silence. *The Journal of Perinatal Education*, *18*(2), 23–31.

Zheng, X., Watts, K., & Morrell, J. (2019). Chinese primiparous women's experience of the traditional postnatal practice of "doing the month": A descriptive method study. *Japan Journal of Nursing Science*, *16*(3), 253–262. doi:10.1111/jjns.12232

Zur, O. (2007). *Boundaries in psychotherapy: Ethical and clinical explorations*. APA Books.

Index

breaking the rules 79, 80–85,
  252–253
breathing, 4-7-8 265
brit milah (circumcision ceremonies)
  218–219
Broadbent, E. 1
burnout 261–262

careful choice of words 247–248
casual conversation, value of 82–83
Chapman, S.B. 266
cheated, feeling 62
checking in with client 179
children's books, reading to clients
  165–166
chitchat, value of 82–83
clinical challenges: conflicting feelings
  242–243; grieving mothers/fathers
  234–237; heightened emotions,
  holding and 238–241; limited
  resources, clients with 237–238;
  male clients, holding and 229–232;
  male therapists, holding by 241–
  242; sabotage by partners 243–244;
  virtual holding 232–234
cognitive behavioral therapy (CBT) 43,
  44–45
comfort with yourself 256–257
common experience 7–9
compassion fatigue 261–262
competency, passion and 200
confidence, therapist's 134–135,
  137–138
conflicting feelings 242–243
confusion | powerlessness domain
  124–125
connectedness, desire for 8
Connelly, D. 39–40, 51–52, 59
control: holding statements of
  127–128; and motherhood,
  incompatibility between 9–10
countertransference 246, 261
cries for help, not ignoring 188
crises, holding in 191–192
la cuarentena (sitting the month)
  219–220
Cuddy, A. 146
culture, motherhood and *see* diverse
  parents
current state point 89, 92–93, 96, 97,
  102, 230

de-centering the therapist 46
definitions, evolution of 3
DeMarneffe, D. 63
Dependency | shame domain 128–131
depression: as distraction 153–154; as
  elusive and subjective 255; fathers
  229; grounding techniques 154;
  stigma associated with 65; voice of
  depression 109–110; *see also*
  postpartum depression; voice of
  depression
design point 90, 96, 97, 103, 231, 235
devotion 73
diagnostic knowledge: baby blues 29;
  postpartum anxiety 30–31;
  postpartum bipolar disorder 33–34;
  postpartum depression 30;
  postpartum obsessive-compulsive
  disorder 31–32; postpartum panic
  disorder 33; postpartum
  posttraumatic stress disorder 32–33;
  postpartum psychosis 34;
  postpartum stress syndrome 29–30
disclosure of personal experiences by
  therapists 22, 81–82, 203–206
distorted thinking, technique for
  coping with 97
distraction, symptoms as 152–159
distress: holding and 63–64;
  normalization of 64–65
diverse parents: African-American
  mothers 212–213; biases and
  214–216; circumcision ceremonies
  218–219; *la cuarentena* (sitting the
  month) 219–220; cultural views on
  motherhood 10; fathers 17–18,
  222–223; gender expansive parents
  220–222; Hispanic parents 219–220;
  holding points and 212–213; holding
  questions 217, 219, 220, 221–222,
  223; internal responses to 216–224;
  Jewish traditions 218–219;
  knowledge of, expanding 224; large
  families as cultural norm 213–214;
  Latina mothers 212–213, 219–220;
  marianismo 216–217; non-
  gestational parents 17–18, 222–223;
  resources for therapists 214;
  superwoman schema 216–217; trans
  parents 220–222
doing the month 219–220

For Product Safety Concerns and Information please contact our EU
representative GPSR@taylorandfrancis.com Taylor & Francis Verlag GmbH,
Kaufingerstraße 24, 80331 München, Germany

Printed and bound by CPI Group (UK) Ltd, Croydon, CR0 4YY
08/06/2025
01897006-0004